Psychotrichology

Yuliya Ovcharenko • Anna Lyakhovitsky
Mohammad Jafferany
Editors

Psychotrichology

Psychiatric and Psychosocial Aspects of Hair Diseases

Springer

Editors
Yuliya Ovcharenko
V. N. Karazin Kharkiv National University, University Clinic "Trichology Institute"
Kharkiv, Ukraine

Mohammad Jafferany
Department of Psychiatry and Behavioral Sciences
Central Michigan University, College of Medicine
Saginaw, MI, USA

Anna Lyakhovitsky
Department of Dermatology
Sheba Medical Center, Tel Hashomer, Affiliated with the Faculty of Medicine and Health Sciences, Tel Aviv University
Tel Aviv, Israel

ISBN 978-3-031-64082-7 ISBN 978-3-031-64083-4 (eBook)
https://doi.org/10.1007/978-3-031-64083-4

This Springer imprint is published by the registered company Springer Nature Switzerland AG
The registered company address is: Gewerbestrasse 11, 6330 Cham, Switzerland

Dedication

I dedicate this book to my family with gratitude for their help in choosing a path, faith and support at every stage of my formation and development.

Yuliya Ovcharenko

I acknowledge this work to those who seek to understand the profound connection between the psyche and the hair—may this book serve as a bridge between science, compassion, and healing.

Mohammad Jafferany

Description

This is a fundamental work in the field of hair research based on the great clinical experience of the authors and launching the beginning of the development of an independent medical direction. For the first time in the world of science and practice, the authors of this collective monograph gathered, analyzed, and systematized unique data on the psychiatric and psychosocial aspects of hair diseases. The book shows modern views on the psychosocial significance of hair, the effect of stress on the hair follicle, proposes a classification of psychotrichological disorders, and gives a description of clinical and pathogenetic data and differential-diagnostic algorithms for conditions related to trichological and psychiatric pictures. The monograph presents the principles of therapy and features of medical management of psychotrichological patients, which involves interdisciplinary interaction of dermatotrichologists, psychiatrists, psychologists, and general practitioners.

Preface

The definition of health by the World Health Organization emphasizes the inseparable unity of mental, somatic, and social principles. This principle of unity is the basis of the biopsychosocial model of disorders, and an interdisciplinary strategy is suggested to be important when considering all issues related to health and illness. Psychotrichology from global perspective, implements a complex biopsychosocial concept based on the interaction and mutual influence of the mental and somatic principles in normal and pathological conditions. The study of the mental component associated with trichological manifestations reflects the modern personalized approach to the patient, which is characteristic of integrative medicine.

The emergence of psychotrichology was preceded by a range of factors and clinical observations, notably the broad spectrum of disorders exhibiting interconnected trichological and psychiatric symptoms. Along with primary psychiatric diseases, such as self-induced hair loss, somatoform disorders, dysmorphophobia, psychoimmunological disorders are highly spread, also there is a large spectrum of psychocomorbid pathology that occurs with hereditary, congenital, and acquired hair diseases, often leading to significant emotional stress against the background of a decrease in self-esteem and a deterioration in the quality of life of patients. In addition, psychosomatic pathology can complicate the process of psychophysiological adaptation to hair loss. The suffering of some patients can reach a level comparable to the consequences of life-threatening diseases. A similar response to previous hair loss may contribute to the maintenance or worsening of the disease and create a self-perpetuating vicious circle.

Due to recent achievements in the field of psychoneuroimmunology, scientists have opened up new opportunities for understanding the pathophysiology of hair diseases and developing new therapeutic concepts. In the context of these conditions, interrelationship of psychological factors and the potential consequences of their influence leading to a deterioration in the quality of life is insufficiently assessed. The lack of understanding of psychological factors and recognition of their influence, both on the part of doctors and patients, is one of the main obstacles in the treatment of psychotrichological disorders. The situation is further aggravated by the fact that most postgraduate programs still do not cover such topics as psychotrichology or psychodermatology.

Common practice shows that a trichologist is often the main specialist to whom a patient turns for help in the treatment of a primary disease, even if it is a psychiatric one, as he fears the stigmatization of treatment by a psychiatrist. Management of such patients is a real challenge for trichologists.

These factors served as the basis for the creation of this book, the purpose of which is to present an effective approach to the diagnosis and treatment of psychotrichological disorders. In the collective monograph created with the participation of the world's leading specialists in dermatology, psychiatry, and psychology, unique material on psychiatric and psychosocial aspects of hair and scalp diseases was collected, analyzed, and systematized for the first time. The book presents modern views on the psychosocial significance of hair, which goes far beyond the scope of diagnosis and treatment of trichopathology, the effect of stress on the hair follicle, a proposed classification of psychotrichological disorders, and clinical-pathogenetic data and differential-diagnostic algorithms are described, which have a link between trichological and psychiatric pictures. Rich illustrated material complements the description of pathologies. The monograph presents the principles of therapy and features of the medical management of psychotrichological patients, which involves the interdisciplinary interaction of dermatotrichologists, psychiatrists, psychologists, and general practitioners.

We hope that this first work on psychotrichology will be an incentive for further study of the psychological basis of hair diseases and approaches to their treatment and will allow specialists to expand their clinical competence and therapeutic arsenal in order to effectively manage psychodermatological cases in their practice.

We express our sincere gratitude to the team of author who supported our bold idea and made an invaluable contribution to the creation of this book.

Saginaw, MI, USA — Mohammad Jafferany
Tel Aviv, Israel — Anna Lyakhovitsky
Kharkiv, Ukraine — Yuliya Ovcharenko

Contents

Editors and Contributors

About the Editors

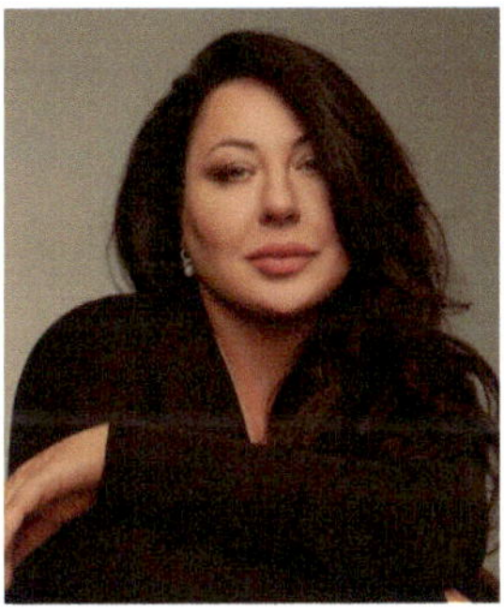

Yuliya Ovcharenko is Professor and Head of the Dermatovenereology Residency Program of the Karazin Kharkiv National University Medical School, Head of the University Clinic Trichology Institute and currently President of the Ukrainian Hair Research Society (UHRS), Treasurer of International Trichoscopy Society (ITS), Vice-President of the Eastern European and Asian Hair Research Society (EEAHRS), and a former Board Member of the European Hair Research Society (EHRS). Her main professional directions include trichoscopy, psychotrichology, alopecia areata, androgenetic alopecia, and hair and scalp conditions in children. Yuliya S. Ovcharenko is a pedagogue who trained a pleiad of talented dermatologists practicing in the field of trichology. She is author and co-author of over 100 scientific publications, 5 patents of Ukraine; co-author of national clinical guidelines, author and co-author of 8th books on hair.

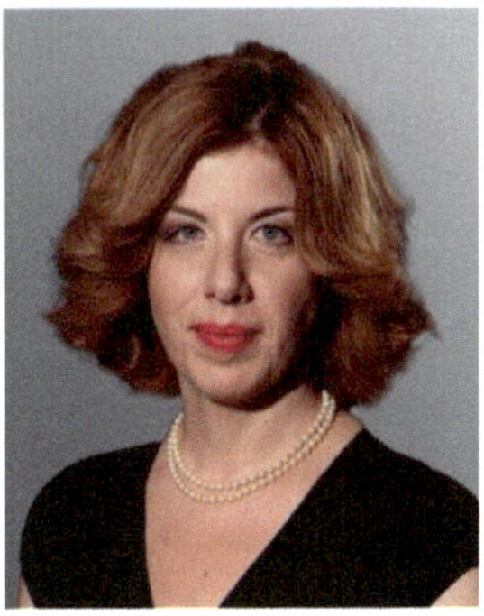

Anna Lyakhovitsky Dr. Lyakhovitsky is Associate Professor of Dermatology at the Faculty of Medicine and Health Sciences, Tel Aviv University, and Attending Physician & Head of the Hair and Scalp Disorders Clinic at Chaim Sheba Medical Center, Tel Hashomer. She trains dermatologists in hair and nail disorders and coordinates the continuing medical education program for dermatology residents. Her clinical expertise encompasses trichoscopy and the management of alopecia areata, androgenetic and cicatricial alopecias, chemotherapy-induced hair loss, pediatric hair and scalp conditions, and a range of nail disorders. Dr. Lyakhovitsky also directs both clinical and basic-science research in these areas.

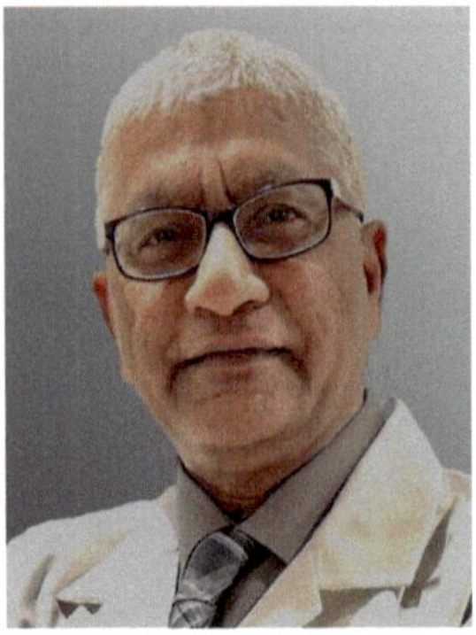

Mohammad Jafferany is Professor of Psychodermatology, Psychiatry and Behavioral sciences at Central Michigan University College of Medicine. He is Executive Secretary of Association for Psychocutaneous Medicine of North America. He has more than 172 scholarly texts and publications to his credit on various topics in psychocutaneous medicine. He has edited and authored 12 books on different topics of Psychodermatology. Psychiatric aspects of hair disorders is one of his main interests. He has conducted International Psychodermatology workshops and Master Courses in different parts of the world. He is currently the president of World Psychodermatology Day.

Contributors

Ruta Barkauskaite Faculty of Human and Social Studies, Institute of Psychology, Mykolas Romeris University, Vilnius, Lithuania

Maria Fernanda Reis Gavazzoni Dias Department of Dermatology, Fluminense Federal University, Rio de Janeiro, Brazil

Mohammad Jafferany Department of Psychiatry and Behavioral Sciences, Central Michigan University, College of Medicine, Saginaw, MI, USA

Kuzma Khobzei Department of Infectious Diseases and Clinical Immunology of the V. N. Karazin Kharkiv National University, Khobzei Clinic, Kyiv, Ukraine

Nino Lortkipanidze Department of Dermatology and Venereology at D. Tvildiani Medical University, Tbilisi, Georgia

Anna Lyakhovitsky Department of Dermatology, Sheba Medical Center, Tel Hashomer, Affiliated with the Faculty of Medicine and Health Sciences, Tel Aviv University, Tel Aviv, Israel

Yuliya Ovcharenko V. N. Karazin Kharkiv National University, University Clinic "Trichology Institute", Kharkiv, Ukraine

Lidia Rudnicka Department of Dermatology, Medical University of Warsaw, Warsaw, Poland

Inessa Serbina Department of Infectious Diseases and Clinical Immunology of the V. N. Karazin Kharkiv National University, University Clinic "Trichology Institute", Kharkiv, Ukraine

Antonella Tosti Dr. Phillip Frost Department of Dermatology and Cutaneous Surgery, University of Miami Miller School of Medicine, Miami, FL, USA

Ralph Trüeb Center for Dermatology and Hair Diseases, Wallisellen, Zurich, Switzerland

Abbreviations

AA	Alopecia areata
AA-QLI	Alopecia Areata Quality of Life Index
ACTH	Adrenocorticotropic hormone
AD	Atopic dermatitis
AD	Autosomal dominant inheritance
AE	Accumulation effluvium
AGA	Androgenetic alopecia
AR	Autosomal recessive inheritance
BPH	Benign prostatic hyperplasia
CAPB	Cocamidopropyl betaine
CCCA	Central centrifugal cicatricial alopecia
CNS	Central nervous system
CPA	Cyproterone acetate
CRH	Corticotropin-releasing hormone
DAE	Dystrophic anagen effluvium
DHT	Dihydrotestosterone
DIF	Direct immunofluorescence
DLE	Discoid lupus erythematosus
DLQI	Dermatology Quality of Life Index
DP	Dermal papilla
DS	Dermal sheath
EGF	Epidermal growth factor
FAPD	Fibrosing alopecia in a pattern distribution
FD	Folliculitis decalvans
FDA	Food and Drug Administration
FFA	Frontal fibrosing alopecia
FTG	Phototrichogram
GCS	Glucocorticosteroids
GRASS	Global Registry of Alopecia areata disease Severity and treatment Safety
HADS	Hospital Anxiety and Depression Scale
HF	Hair follicle
HGF	Hepatocyte growth factor
HPA axis	Hypothalamic-pituitary-adrenal axis

IA	Involutional alopecia
IGF	Insulin-like growth factor
IL	Interleukin
ISOQOL	International Society for Quality of Life Research
JAK-STAT	Janus Kinases-Signal Transducer and Activator of Transcription
KF	Keloid folliculitis
LLLT	Low-level laser therapy
LPP	Lichen planopilaris
MHC	Major histocompatibility complex
NGF	Nerve growth factor
NK1	Neurokinin 1
PAR-2	Protease-activated receptor 2
PAX	Paxman® PSC-2 Paxman Scalp Cooler
PCA	Prostate-specific antigen
PCOS	Polycystic ovary syndrome
PFS	Post-finasteride syndrome
PPB	Pseudopelade of Brocq
PRP	Platelet-rich plasma
PTSD	Post-traumatic stress disorder
QOL	Quality of life
SALT	Severity of Alopecia Tool
SBN	The classification of severity of Alopecia Areata—standardized system for assessing scalp hair loss—S (Scalp), body—B (Body) and nail damage—N (Nail) in patients with Alopecia Areata
SC	Scalp cooler
SC	Stem cells
SD	Seborrheic dermatitis
SHBG	Sex hormone binding globulin
SLE	Systemic lupus erythematosus
SNP	Single nucleotide polymorphism
TA	Total alopecia
TE	Telogen effluvium
TNF	Tumor necrosis factor
TTM	Trichotillomania
UA	Universal alopecia
VEGF	Vascular endothelial growth factor
WHO	World Health Organization
Wnt	Wnt signaling pathway

What Is Psychotrichology?

1

Mohammad Jafferany and Yuliya Ovcharenko

Introduction

Psychotrichology is a new emerging interdisciplinary area of modern medicine that explores psychosocial and psychiatric aspects of hair and scalp diseases.

The research of the mental component associated with trichological manifestations addresses a modern personalized patient approach, characteristic of integrative medicine. This strategy is aimed not only at managing trichological conditions, but also at assessing the most comprehensive picture of the disease, as well as at improving a patient's quality of life providing for individual perception of the pathology, dysfunctional emotional and behavioral patterns leading to and/or aggravating the hair disease symptoms.

A number of factors and observations, including a wide range of disorders characterized by trichodermatological and psychiatric symptoms interaction, have been the prerequisite for the emergence of psychotrichology. Along with primary psycological conditions, such as self-induced hair loss (trichotillomania), also prevailing are body dysmorphic or somatoform disorders, psychoimmunological disorders (alopecia areata), as well as a wide range of comorbid psychiatric pathology associated with hereditary, congenital and acquired hair diseases (androgenetic alopecia (AGA)), chronic telogen effluvium (TE), post-chemotherapy anagen alopecia, scarring alopecias, often leading to significant emotional stress accompanied by low self-esteem and worsening of patient quality of life.

M. Jafferany (✉)
Department of Psychiatry and Behavioral Sciences, Central Michigan University, College of Medicine, Saginaw, MI, USA
e-mail: jaffe1m@cmich.edu

Y. Ovcharenko
V. N. Karazin Kharkiv National University, University Clinic "Trichology Institute", Kharkiv, Ukraine

Y. Ovcharenko et al. (eds.), *Psychotrichology*,
https://doi.org/10.1007/978-3-031-64083-4_1

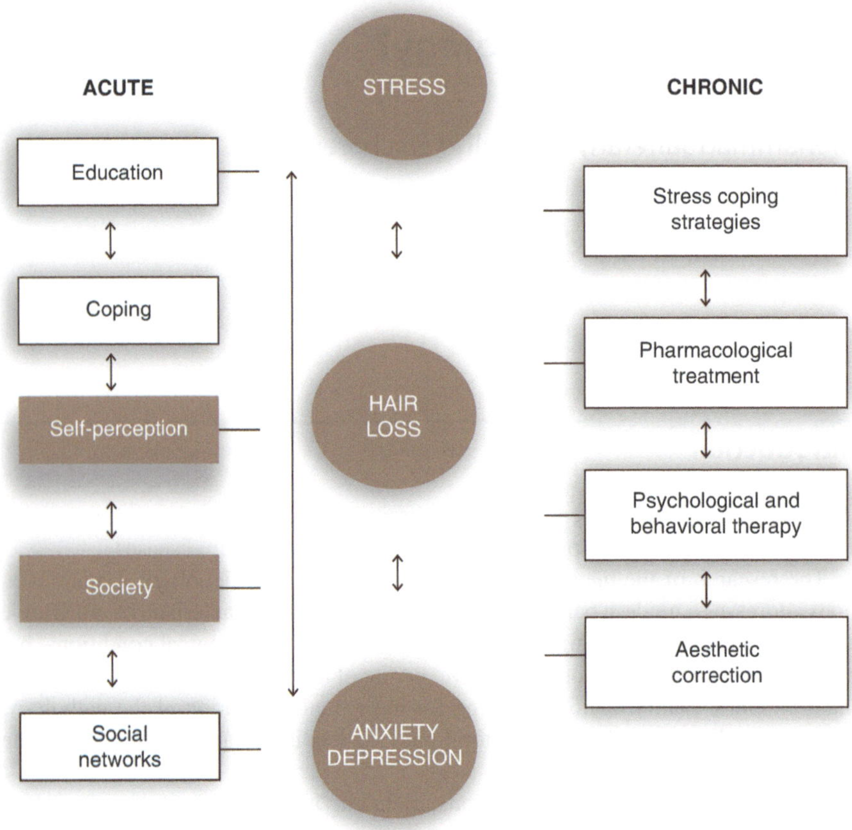

Fig. 1.1 A schematic diagram showing a self-perpetuating vicious circle of psychoemotional and psychosocial stress elements in response to previous hair loss, which contributes to the maintenance or worsening of trichological condition. *Modified from Ralph Paus, J Invest Dermatol, 2004*

Depression and anxiety disorders, as well as social isolation and stigma, are examples of secondary/reactive psychosocial diseases. Furthermore, psychosomatic comorbidity can complicate the process of adaptive psychophysiological coping with hair loss. In some patients suffering can reach a level comparable to the consequences of life-threatening diseases. This response to prior hair loss may maintain or exacerbate hair disease and create a self-perpetuating vicious cycle (Fig. 1.1).

Understanding the negative effects of stress on hair growth and incorporating stress-reduction strategies into trichopathology treatment, as well as developing new pharmacotherapeutic approaches, can help to broaden treatment modalities that offer relief of clinical symptoms and psychological sequelae.

The Role of Stress in the Development of Hair Diseases

The question of whether environmental influences or psychosocial stress may significantly affect hair growth has been debated for a very long time. The hypothalamus-pituitary-adrenals (HPA) axis is known to be activated in the classic systemic biological response to exogenous stress factors. Hypothalamic corticotropin-releasing hormone (CRH) secretion stimulates pituitary CRH receptors (CRH-R), which leads to the production and release of peptides from pro-opiomelanocortin and adrenal hormones. The systemic response to stress also involves changes in the autonomic nervous and immune systems: neuroendocrine hormones and neurotransmitters influence immune system function, which in turn influences central nervous system (CNS) activities via cytokine release. Within physiological adaptation processes, glucocorticoid secretion, such as cortisol, offers negative feedback to inhibit CRH release. Dysregulation of the HPA axis may have major ramifications for the body's functioning.

Data acquired over the last few decades indicate that the key molecular components involved in the systemic response to environmental stressors, as well as neurotransmitters and cytokines, are also expressed in the skin. Environmental influences have been found in studies to elicit a stress response not only in the body, but also in the skin, and this reaction can operate as a local counterpart of the "hypothalamus-pituitary-adrenal axis."

Although clinical studies have shown the existence of a comparable local axis in the hair follicle (HF), the molecular mechanisms behind these correlations have only recently been explored (Fig. 1.2). Cycled HF changes are known to be regulated by epithelial–mesenchymal interactions between dermal papillae, follicular keratinocytes, and fibroblasts, i.e., by a collection of molecular signals that differ across phases.

A growing body of evidence suggests that hair growth cycle may also be significantly influenced by neurohormones, neurotransmitters, and cytokines released in response to stress and largely dependent on the hair growth cycle stage. The relationship between a stressor and any subsequent changes in the hair growth cycle has resulted in the designation of a "brain–hair follicle" axis. Based on the scientific experimental data, stress causes significant changes in actively growing hair follicles and promotes their transition to the involution phase.

> Stress-induced premature cessation of HF development is related with keratinocyte apoptosis, increased mast cell degranulation, and the accumulation of perifollicular inflammatory infiltrates containing activated macrophages. A variety of trichodermatological disorders fit the conventional stress model and exhibit a pathological paradigm.

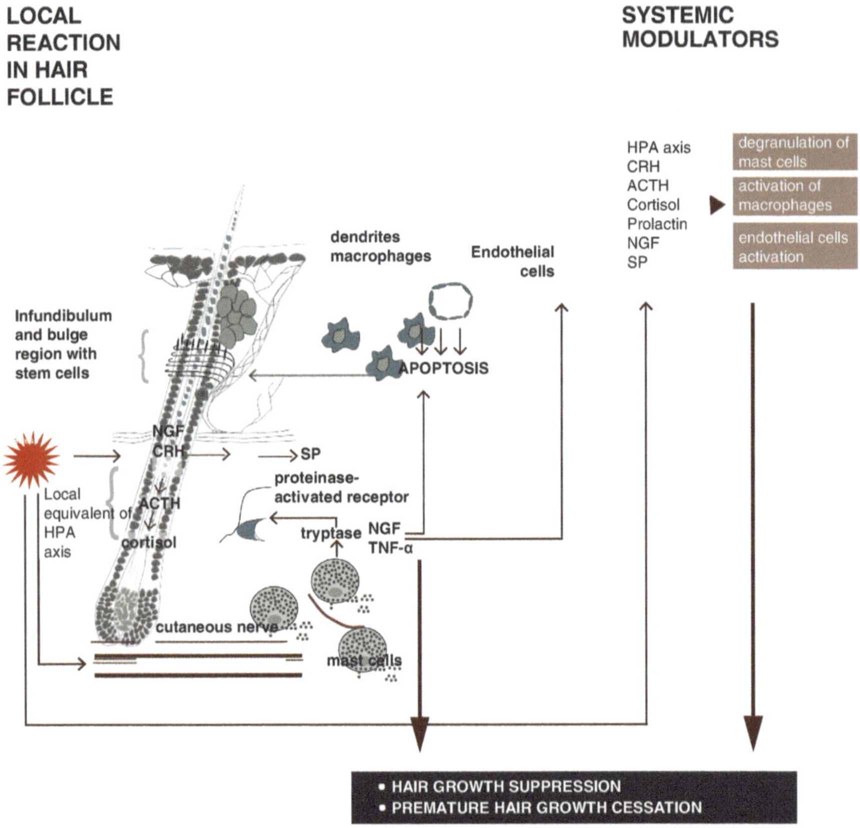

Fig. 1.2 Possible pathways of neuroimmunoendocrine stress exposure leading to inhibition of hair growth. Inflammatory neuropeptides released by nerve fibers promote mast cell degranulation, which causes the production of histamine, proteases, and neuropeptides. Substance P (SP) and nerve growth factor (NGF) control this neurogenic inflammation (NGF). These neuroimmune interactions causes the premature cessation of hair growth. *Modified from Eva Peters* et al., *Exp Dermatol, 2006*

Normally, the HF epithelium is immunoprivileged, with extremely low expression of major histocompatibility complex (MHC) class I and II antigens and local secretion of potent immunosuppressors.

The research of the neuroimmunoendocrine regulation of phase change in the hair follicle growth cycle discovered that peptidergic nerve fibers regulate their activity through the release of neurotransmitters by building intimate relationships with mast cells. It has been proven that these interactions are characterized by modifications that are dependent on the phase shift in the hair development cycle, demonstrating the importance of communication between nerve fibers and mast cells in the control of hair growth. Mast cell mediators, in fact, can both increase the initiation and progression of the anagen phase, as well as promote HF regression [1].

Due to surrounding dense perifollicular networks of sensory nerve endings, which are closely associated with mast cells and exhibit plasticity during chronic stress, follicles are the target of neuroimmunomodulatory and neuroinflammatory mediators. This interaction scenario postulates that stress-related hair growth inhibiting induction of catagen and hair-damaging pro-inflammatory effects likely occur because of a key role of substance P, CRH, and nerve growth factor (NGF) released in response to stress both systemically and locally from perifollicular nerve fibers. This leads to activation and degranulation of mast cells, releasing a variety of proinflammatory mediators such as histamine and tumor necrosis factor-alpha (TNF-a) that provoke the induction of neurogenic inflammation with the release of reactive oxygen species, premature transition to catagen, and hair growth arrest. Furthermore, substance P was found to activate follicular MHC expression leading to the collapse of the MHC-based immune privilege of the HF. The biochemical imbalance driving the evolution of alopecia areata (AA) is stress-mediated immune privilege collapse, which leaves the follicle defenseless against activation of inflammatory cascades and consequent hair loss. Low cortisol levels found in chronic stress or chronic inflammation boost keratinocyte synthesis of substance P.

The current focus on substance P is supported not only by its previously documented involvement in suppressing stress-induced hair growth in mice, but also by its influence on stress-sensitive clinical hair loss diseases. There is evidence that HF and human scalp keratinocytes contain neurokinin 1 (NK1) receptors (a specific SP receptor antagonist).

In 2007, a group of scientists led by Ralph Paus conducted a clinically relevant organ culture analysis to study the direct effects of stress mediators on a complex mini-organ. They demonstrated the sensitivity of the human HF to substance P—a key neuropeptide associated with stress. The experiment showed NK-1 inhibition and early induction of catagen by substance P in the human HF epithelium, which is similar to the substance P-dependent stress response previously described in vivo inside or surrounding hair follicles in mice.

In vitro response of human HF to stimulation with this essential stress-related neuropeptide was associated with signs of neurogenic inflammation. Furthermore, substance P was found to increase intrafollicular expression of NGF and its receptor

Table 1.1 Hypothetical scenarios of human hair growth inhibition due to substance P-mediated psycho-emotional stress

Suppression of substance P pro-proliferative signaling in HF keratinocytes
Harmful neurogenic inflammation caused by substance P activation of perifollicular mast cells
Activation of catagen-inductive growth factor cascades
Enhanced immune attack on HF that have lost their immune privilege

p75NTR, both of which promote apoptosis and catagen, while decreasing TrkA receptor expression, which is known to contribute to hair growth.

Another important response was demonstrated: substance P activates ectopic expression of MHC class I and 2 microglobulin complex, regarded as evidence of stress-related collapse of HF immune privilege based on MHC class I. These findings allowed scientists to create hypothetical scenarios of human hair growth suppression caused by substance P-mediated psychoemotional stress (Table 1.1). The evidence that systemic treatment of NK1, NGF neutralizing antibodies, or topical minoxidil can prevent local inflammatory response, apoptosis, decreased proliferation, and hair growth cessation emphasizes the therapeutic importance of these findings. The authors of this study were the first to provide a scientific, evidence-based explanation of how stress can cause or exacerbate telogen effluvium, alopecia areata, and several types of scarring hair loss.

In addition to substance P, a variety of additional stimuli and mediators (such as neurotransmitters, neuropeptides, neurohormones, and neurotrophins) should be taken into account as possible local or systemic mediators of stress-induced hair growth inhibition, since HF has been identified as a marked peripheral organ-target and source of many bioregulatory molecules known for being mediators of stress responses [2–5].

For example, in telogen effluvium, hair follicle cycling in mice and/or humans is controlled by three conventional bioregulators of systemic stress responses: catecholamines, prolactin, and nerve growth factor [2].

By interacting and interrupting the production of different neuropeptides, common stress hormones such catecholamines, prolactin, adenocorticotropic hormone (ACTH), CRH, ß-endorphins, glucocorticoids, and substance P can either directly or indirectly alter hair growth [5, 6].

Additionally, research has revealed that HF has the unusual capacity to produce its own stress hormones (ACTH, CRH, and cortisol) via the analog of the HPA axis with established regulatory feedback loops (Fig. 1.2). Systemic CRH binds to follicular receptors at times of extreme stress, stimulating the follicle's internal hormonal axis to release local amounts of ACTH, cortisol, and CRH. This causes the degranulation of mast cells [6]. Inflammatory stimuli, particularly those linked to neurogenic inflammation, have recently come to light as having the potential to significantly influence hair growth [3–5]. The finding that prolonged exposure to psychological stress inhibits hair growth and is associated by significant variation in TH1/TH2 ratio provides more evidence for the function of stress in follicular immune dysregulation and perifollicular inflammation.

In conjunction to earlier research conducted in vitro, a recent study found that stress has a role in the pathogenesis of hair disorders in vivo. This study showed that CRH stimulates the HPA stress axis in skin samples taken from men with androgenetic alopecia. Additionally, it was demonstrated that the neurogenic stress axis is distinct from the HPA. Additionally, researchers found that caffeine has the ability to prevent stress-related hair damage by blocking both stress axis in vivo, as had been shown to be the case in vitro.

Although more research is required to fully understand how these factors interact in the biology of human HF, as well as the effects of acute and chronic psychoemotional stress on neuropeptide release and their impact on human hair growth, these stimuli should now be considered when discussing the approach to treating hair loss.

Epidemiology

The epidemiological characteristics and psychological aspects of the trichologist's work are particularly noteworthy since individuals seeking our medical guidance need a thorough, compassionate, and careful approach. Only a few dermatological problems have as strong an emotional impact as complaints about hair-related conditions.

Studies show that psychiatric disorders are significantly more common among patients with dermatosis than in the general population: approximately 30% of patients in this group have symptoms from the spectrum of depressive and anxiety disorders, as well as delusional disorders or suicidal tendencies. According to Picardi [7], the largest number—35%—was found in patients with hair loss.

A dermatologist who practices in the field of clinical trichology is well aware that, compared to a classic dermatological appointment, there are disproportionately more patients with biopsychosocial disorders at a trichological consultation, who are often referred to at first glance as "problematic" or "difficult" patients.

Approximately 30% of individuals who present with complaints of hair loss have no evidence of an abnormality or merely age-appropriate normal changes. The common characteristic for this group of patients is a significant deterioration in quality of life as a result of a strong conviction in the presence of a hair disease. The exact prevalence of such complaints in any given dermatological practice is likely to be dependent on the dermatologist's attention to the complex problem.

For a clinician, changes in hair condition are often markers of pathological processes. Data from clinical practice, on the other hand, confirm that patients who seek trichological consultations, despite having medical conditions involving more than just hair, frequently notice only hair-related symptoms, making the trichologist both the primary link in medical care and a "medium" among colleagues. Even though the primary illness is psychological, the dermatotrichologist is frequently the first expert to whom the patient seeks for assistance in dealing with their principal complaint. Often, patients are driven by a fear of being stigmatized if they seek therapy with a psychiatrist.

Data from retrospective clinical investigations of individuals with body dysmorphic disorder show that any part of the body can cause discomfort, but the most prevalent troublesome regions are skin (73%) and hair (56%), with 30% of patients reporting hair loss.

Alopecia is traditionally classified as a socially significant disease, but among its important characteristics is the discrepancy between the clinical severity of the condition and the impact on the patient's quality of life, which, according to the results of published reports, does not allow to reliably predict changes in its level for patients with alopecia areata, androgenetic alopecia, and telogen effluvium [8].

> Despite the benign process of hair loss, patients experience severe psychoemotional stress, often leading to a decrease in the quality of life and secondary psycho-comorbidity. In some patients the distress can reach a level comparable to the burden caused by much more severe chronic or life-threatening diseases.

According to published studies, there is a considerable negative correlation between male pattern baldness and quality of life, which can lead to major emotional problems. Reduced self-esteem, perceptions of physical unattractiveness, depression, emotional distress, heightened feelings of embarrassment, anxiety, and psychosocial maladjustment have all been documented as negative outcomes. Furthermore, many patients express dissatisfaction with their own appearance, obsession with hair loss, anxiety about other people's thoughts and judgments, and fear of social rejection [9].

For a subgroup of patients with alopecia areata, a multifactorial biopsychosocial pathogenesis is discussed, when life events can cause the onset, development, and exacerbation of the disease, and the disorder's "disfiguring effect" is regarded as a provoking factor to a whole range of secondary mental disorders. It is known that alopecia areata leading to relatively minor changes in physical condition significantly worsens the emotional and social components of the quality of life, often being the cause of depression, dysmorphophobia, and in some cases, suicidal attempts [10].

These findings show and emphasize hair's indisputable psychological significance, which extends well beyond its biological function.

Hair Symbolism, Social and Cultural Factors

For centuries, hair has been considered a symbol of fertility, as well as the source of concentration of mental, physical, and sexual strength. Trends in hair are constantly changing and in today's world are heavily influenced by the media. Nowadays the psychological preoccupation with hair is even more intense, as an increase in life expectancy inevitably provokes the desire to prolong our youth [11].

Hair growth and hair styling have become important elements of both self-identification and perception by others. Face and hair directly convey information about our age, gender, individual, and group affiliation. The most prevalent cultural hair norm, according to American sociologist Rose Weitz, is that men's and women's hair should be distinct from one another.

It is the condition of hair that largely influences whether a person is perceived as physically attractive. This is not surprising, since throughout history hair has had major symbolic significance. The biblical account of Samson losing his remarkable physical strength after having his hair cut off, and the scalping of defeated enemies practiced in some cultures, are both frequently cited examples.

Charles Berg studied the anthropological literature on hair in his 1950 book, "The Unconscious Significance of Hair," and emphasized its significance in several rituals in various primitive cultures. Hair has two subjectively perceived symbolic implications in spiritual contexts: on the one hand, uncut hair is considered as a release from materialistic anxieties and concerns; while on the other hand, shaven hair is a symbol of celibacy and chastity. In truth, many religions, and civilizations, including Buddhism, Hinduism, and Christianity, use shaving of the head as a symbol of devotion to God. Similarly shaving head after specific religious rituals in Islam is regarded as getting rid of previous sins.

The author also suggested that for a modern individual, their hair has almost no other significance than sexual, and that any normal person has some degree of hair fetishism. From a sexual perspective, letting one's hair down is viewed as a seductive ritual, frequently perceived as a symbol of unrestricted libido. Cutting one's hair off is often perceived as a sign of submission or humiliation.

Because the appearance of our hair affects our self-perception, it also influences our social behavior. For millennia, individuals have used their hair to express their identity in relation to a wide range of social phenomena: religious, political, sexual, professional, and so on. Short hair is regarded a sign of sophistication and readiness to live by the laws of a civilized society, whereas wild hair is generally viewed as a reflection of rudeness, disobedience, and lack of constraint. It may also be used to symbolize fearlessness and danger, as in the case of the skinhead subculture; a shaved head shows that a person has nothing to lose or that this person is invincible.

The significance that many militaries accord short hair reinforces the widely held belief that short hair is a sign of authority and discipline. In contrast, investigations of male students whose hair length was "out of the norm" revealed that these individuals valued independence highly and were less concerned with approval and conventions [11].

Being a physical component of our bodies, hair also denotes personality qualities, and the state of our hair indicates our physical and mental health. Therefore, any alteration in our hair is anticipated to have a significant effect on how people see us, how we view ourselves, and ultimately how we feel about ourselves.

From a biopsychosocial perspective, the issue of hair loss is heavily influenced by society and social factors. Modern research has confirmed that in most human relationships the most advantageous has been the perception of a person as "attractive" by the standards of a particular culture. In contrast, a negative social standing is linked to a person's perception of themselves as "unattractive," particularly if this perception is brought on by a dermatological condition. Such an attitude can have far-reaching effects that go beyond simple personal isolation, such as outright discrimination in employment.

Nowadays the urge to avoid baldness is not new. There are almost as many references to hair in literature as there are myths and legends related to it. Beginning with the papyrus records of Ancient Egyptians dating back 4000 years, throughout the Greek and Roman civilizations and up to our own time, the growth and color of human hair has been the object of superstition and mystery, as well as cosmetic and medical interest. And even though the oldest mention of hair is about 30,000 years old, the story still continues [11].

Today, the desire to avoid becoming bald is evident in a wide range of medical and cosmetic goods, treatments, and imitations, including stimulating lotions, vitamins, physiotherapy devices, hairpieces, wigs, hair replacement systems, synthetic fiber implantation, and surgical hair transplantation. In the 1980s, there were over 300,000 over-the-counter treatments in the United States that purported to reverse hair loss. Nowadays, the psychological obsession with hair is much stronger, as increased life expectancy necessarily leads to a desire to maintain youth. The same desire is fueling the rapid expansion of the hair care sector, which is estimated to be worth billions of Euros globally (data from Euromonitor) [11].

Given the psychological and symbolic value of hair, as well as the fact that hair removal is used as a punishment in many cultures, it is not unexpected that baldness may have an impact on a person's quality of life. Unfortunately, this negative impact is often downplayed or even ignored by those not affected. Analyzing varied symptoms of hair loss requires considering the patient's socioeconomic and cultural background [12].

Goals and Objectives of Psychotrichology

The joint efforts of dermatologists and psychiatrists have been evident throughout history and reflect the continued growth of cross-specialty research. The emergence of psychotrichology, the interdisciplinary field, was also facilitated by the introduction of the main trends in modern medicine, namely, improving patients' quality of life and personalized medicine. A comprehensive understanding of individual diseases within the framework of psychotrichology is an important initial step for potential clinical strategies. Building a solid understanding of the psychosocial and stress-related factors involved in the development of specific hair disorders can further improve and create effective therapeutic interventions for patients.

Psychotrichology therapy focuses on the role of stress in hair illness and prioritizes the development of appropriate coping skills and the improvement of patients' quality of life. Recent research has focused on the influence of hair diseases on patients' quality of life, as well as the development and validation of rating scales for diverse trichopathologies in different populations [13].

According to published research, there is a considerable unfavorable association between irreversible and recurring trichopathies and quality of life. According to the authors, assessing the quality of life in hair disorders is significant as an integrated indicator characterizing the most important human functions and allowing for a comprehensive complex investigation of changes in these functions throughout the disease development and normalization with therapy.

Data form studies conducted in Ukraine revealed that, the degree of alopecia areata-related negative impact on quality of life may not correlate with the objective severity of patient's condition, which is often not taken into account in the diagnosis and treatment of the disease. These observations substantiated the need to expand the criteria for selecting and monitoring the therapy effectiveness in the national clinical guidelines for management of patients with AA, developed by the Ukrainian Hair Research Society (see Chap. 6). Low quality of life (QoL) indexes in patients with objectively mild and/or moderate AA serve as a rationale for managing these patients as having severe AA. In Ukrainian protocols, along with clinical and trichoscopic evaluation, measuring QoL index as a therapy efficacy criterion is recommended after 6 months of treatment. These data motivate further efforts to explore the effect on the QoL in other nosologies in order to develop individual therapeutic routes, where the QoL index is a criterion for complex therapy selection [10].

From the standpoint of the health risk, AA is known to be a benign condition, nevertheless, its psychological percussion can reach a level comparable to the consequences of life-threatening or disabling diseases that significantly worsen the QoL of adults, children, and their family members. Adaptation in society and adaptation of society to people with alopecia is another difficult and very important task in the scope of modern psychotrichology. Support groups offering regular meetings of AA patients and their families can become invaluable resource for this group of people. Patients receive emotional support and information to help with forming positive coping strategies, improving quality of life and treatment effectiveness. This means that the advancement of psychotrichology and using psychotherapeutic measures are a source of support for patients with hair problems.

Today various pharmacological agents and psychotherapeutic approaches have been implemented in the treatment of psychotrichological disorders; however still further research is required to identify specific mediators in the pathogenesis of conditions resulting in hair pathologies. A comprehensive understanding of individual disorders within psychotrichology is an important basis for potential clinical applications in the future.

To successfully manage the psychodermatologic and psychothrichologic cases in their practice, dermatologists who treat these patients must increase their clinical expertise and treatment armament.

Summary

- The role of stress in the etiology of various types of hair loss remains in focus of active research. Recent in vivo experiments have confirmed the belief that stress may have an inhibitory effect on hair growth by catagen induction and hair-damaging pro-inflammatory effects, with substance P, CRH, and NGF likely playing a key role.
- Hormones, the "brain-HF" axis, and the "environment-HF" axis all have an influence on the hair follicle by working against its regulatory cascades and, in the absence of countermeasures, may eventually overpower the internal HF

regulation mechanisms. As a result, a detrimental self-perpetuating inflammatory cascade may become the new status quo. The HF recovery to a homeostasis state requires a new approach to therapy.

- Understanding the negative effects of stress on hair growth and incorporating stress-reduction strategies into trichopathology treatment, as well as developing new pharmacotherapeutic approaches, can help to broaden treatment modalities that offer alleviation of clinical symptoms and associated psychological sequelae.
- A comprehensive understanding of individual diseases within the framework of psychotrichology is an important initial step for developing new therapeutic strategies.
- Summing up, we can say that Hippocratic medicine concept of "Treating the Patient, Not Just the Disease" laid both the foundation for the traditional clinical school, and, perhaps, became a new symbol of the modern integrative medicine era.

References

1. Peters EMJ, Arck PC, Paus R. Hair growth inhibition by psychoemotional stress: a mouse model for neural mechanisms in hair growth control. Exp Dermatol. 2006;15:1–13.
2. Paus R, Cotsarelis G. The biology of hair follicles. N Engl J Med. 1999;341:491–8.
3. Arck PC, Handjiski B, Hagen E, Joachim R, Klapp BF, Paus R. Indications for a 'brain-hair follicle axis (BHA)': inhibition of keratinocyte proliferation and up-regulation of keratinocyte apoptosis in telogen hair follicles by stress and substance P. FASEB J. 2001;15:2536–8.
4. Arck PC, Handjiski B, Peters EMJ, Peter AS, Hagen E, Fisher A, Klapp BF, Paus R. Stress inhibits hair growth in mice by induction of premature catagen development and deleterious perifollicular inflammatory events via neuropeptide substance P-dependent pathways. Am J Pathol. 2003;162:803–14.
5. Botchkarev VA. Stress and the hair follicle: exploring the connections. Am J Pathol. 2003;162(3):709–12.
6. Slominski A, Wortsman J, Luger T, Paus R, Solomon S. Corticotropin releasing hormone and proopiomelanocortin involvement in the cutaneous response to stress. Physiol Rev. 2000;80:979–1020.
7. Picardi A, Abeni D, Melchi CF, Puddu P, Pasquini P. Psychiatric morbidity in dermatological outpatients: an issue to be recognized. Br J Dermatol. 2000;143(5):983–91. https://doi.org/10.1046/j.1365-2133.2000.03831.x.
8. Harth W, Blume-Peytavi U. Psychotrichology: psychosomatic aspects of hair diseases. J Dtsch Dermatol Ges. 2013;11(2):125–35. https://doi.org/10.1111/j.1610-0387.2012.08034.x. Epub 2012 Nov 26. PMID: 23176605.
9. Grimalt R. Psychosocial impact of androgenetic alopecia. In: Koo J, Lee CS, editors. Psychocutaneous medicine. New York: Dekker; 2003. p. 251–66.
10. Serbina I, Andrashko Y, Galnykina S, Kadigrob I, Khobzei K, Liadova T, Litus O, Sviatenko T, Svistunov I, Syzon O, Vozianova S, Ovcharenko Y. Clinical guidelines of the Ukraine Hair Research Society. Diagnosis and treatment of alopecia areata. Actual problems of modern medicine. 2023;12:45–67. https://doi.org/10.26565/2617-409X-2023-12-06.
11. Trüeb RM, Gieler U. Pschychocutaneous disorders of hair and scalp. In: Blume-Peytavi U, Tosti A, Whiting D, Trüeb RM, editors. Hair growth and disorders. New York: Springer; 2008. p. 407–26.
12. Grimalt R. Trichopsychodermatology. Dermatol Psychosom. 2001;2:41–50.
13. Jafferany M, Patel A. Trichopsychodermatology: the psychiatric and psychosocial aspects of hair disorders. Dermatol Ther. 2020;1:e13168. https://doi.org/10.1111/dth.13168. Epub 2019 Nov 25

Diagnosis of Psychotrichological Disorders

2

Mohammad Jafferany and Yuliya Ovcharenko

Introduction

The research on the psychological components associated with hair disorders addresses a modern personalized patient-centered approach. This strategy aims to understand the disease in its complexity taking into account patients' unique characteristics, dysfunctional emotional and behavioral patterns that contribute to or aggravate the hair condition or result from the effect of trichopathology on patients' mental sphere and quality of life. Patients frequently seek assistance from a trichologist in the treatment of their primary complaint (even if it is a psychiatric one), out of fear that receiving therapy from a psychiatrist may stigmatize them. Trichologists face a significant challenge in managing these individuals.

Therefore, for effective treatment of psychotrichological cases it is important for specialists working with these patients to expand their clinical horizons and improve their practical skills. See chapters devoted to individual nosologies for detailed description of clinical and trichoscopic diagnostics. The purpose of this chapter is to present a practical approach to assess the psychological component of psychotrichological disorders and the relationship between psychiatric and trichological manifestations.

M. Jafferany (✉)
Department of Psychiatry and Behavioral Sciences, Central Michigan University, College of Medicine, Saginaw, MI, USA
e-mail: jaffe1m@cmich.edu

Y. Ovcharenko
V. N. Karazin Kharkiv National University, University Clinic "Trichology Institute", Kharkiv, Ukraine

Y. Ovcharenko et al. (eds.), *Psychotrichology*,
https://doi.org/10.1007/978-3-031-64083-4_2

Classification of Psychotrichological Disorders

The connection between trichology and psychiatry is so multifaceted that trichologists and other healthcare professionals need a proper classification system in order to correctly understand and address patients' problems, as well as choose the best therapeutic strategy.

There are two approaches to categorize psychotrichological conditions: by the type of dermatotrichological symptoms (such as trichotillomania) and by the characteristics of the underlying psychopathological disease (e.g., depressive disorder, generalized anxiety disorder, or obsessive-compulsive disorder). Different classifications and opinions that represent the dermatologists' and psychiatrists' perspectives—points of view that frequently have fundamental differences—present a particular dilemma. In addition to terminological discrepancies reflecting the dominance of the "dermatological paradigm," there are a number of conflicting interpretations of this pathology in the official classifications of mental disorders.

Currently, no well-documented classification system with international consensus exists to classify psychotrichological disorders. Authors in this review attempted to create a new classification system based on primary and secondary disorders, reflecting the relationship of trichodermatological and psychiatric symptoms (Table 2.1).

Primary psychiatric disorders. This category includes self-inflicted hair and skin diseases, somatoform disorders, and somatopsychosis, when there is no actual hair or skin disease. These conditions are known as psychotrichodermatological disease stereotypes. The spectrum of nosologies encountered in the practice of a trichologist includes trichotillomania and its variants, neurotic excoriations, dermatitis artefacta (see Chap. 5); cutaneous sensory syndromes, psychogenic pruritus, delusions of parasitosis (see Chap. 12); psychogenic pseudoeffluvium, accumulated effluvium, ecosyndromes, telogenomania (see Chap. 7). Despite the stereotypical clinical picture, the underlying psychopathology varies, so efforts in establishing the nature of the underlying psychopathological condition represents a critical step in psychotrichology. This group of patients may suffer from a variety of psychopathologies, including anxiety disorder, depressive disorder, obsessive-compulsive disorders, multiple symptoms of somatization disorder, hypochondriacal disorder, dissociative disorders, delusional disorder, and personality disorders.

Secondary psychiatric disorders. Secondary psychiatric disorders are characterized by hair diseases leading to psychological condition. Even though most patients with hair disorders experience significant psychological impact, it does not meet the criteria for the diagnosis of mental illness. Nevertheless, the impact that hair disorders have on body image significantly contributes to the overall impact on the patient's quality of life. This is especially true for patients who are discriminated against because of an objective change in their body image caused by hereditary, congenital, or acquired hair loss, and who suffer from psychological complications in addition to the plethora of factors that implicitly affect the course of the disease.

Secondary psychiatric disorders mainly include adjustment disorders, depression, and anxiety disorders. They may lead to social isolation, loss of self-esteem,

Table 2.1 Classification of psychotrichological disorders

PRIMARY PSYCHIATRIC DISORDERS	
Major psychiatric disorder	Trichodermatological clinical phenomenology
• Anxiety disorders • Depressive disorders • Delusional disorder • Obsessive compulsive disorders and related conditions • Personality disorders • Somatoform disorders and related condition – Somatic symptom disorder – Chronic somatoform pain disorder – Hypochondriacal disorder – Body dysmorphic disorder – Conversion disorder	• Trichotillomania • Trichotemnomania • Trichoteiromania • Trichodaganomania/ Trichodaknomania • Trichorhizophagia/Trichophagia • Neurotic excoriations • Dermatitis artefacta • Telogenomania • Delusions of parasitosis • Psychogenic pruritus • Dysesthesia • Psychogenic Pseudoeffluvium • Chronic telogen effluvium • Accumulated effluvium • Ecosyndromes
SECONDARY PSYCHIATRIC DISORDERS	
Psychiatric comorbidity	Hair and scalp diseases triggering mental disorders
• Adjustment disorders • Acute reaction to stress • Post-traumatic stress disorder • Depressive disorders • Anxiety disorders • Mixed anxiety-depressive reactions • Body dysmorphic disorder/ dysmorphophobia • Personality disorders	• Alopecia areata • Androgenetic alopecia • Chronic telogen effluvium • Anagen effluvium • Involutional alopecia • Cicatricial alopecia • Congenital/hereditary atrichia and hypotrichosis • Scalp neoplasia • Hair shaft abnormalities • Hirsutism/hypertrichosis
PSYCHOSOMATIC DISORDERS	
Psychiatric comorbidity	Stress-reactive hair and scalp diseases
• Disorders associated with stress • Disorders associated with anxiety or fear, emotional conflicts	• Seborrheic dermatitis • Psoriasis • Hyperhidrosis • Atopic dermatitis • Chronic telogen effluvium • Alopecia areata

stigmatization, and significant impairment in patient's quality of life. This condition may seriously complicate treatment outcomes, therapy compliance, and the process of adaptation to the disease. According to Niemeier et al. [1], among the total number of persons with cutaneous diseases, the highest level of helplessness is registered in patients with hair conditions. In some patients, the level of suffering can be comparable to the consequences of life-threatening or disabling condition and contribute to the persistence and/or aggravation of hair disease and create a self-perpetuating vicious cycle.

Among **psychosomatic disorders** are a variety of psychotrichological conditions in which emotional and psychological stress is a trigger for the recurrence of certain hair and scalp diseases in a substantial proportion of patients.

Examples of these nosologies include hyperhidrosis, psoriasis, seborrheic dermatitis, atopic dermatitis, chronic telogen effluvium, and alopecia areata. Patients suffering from any of these disorders may be divided into two groups: those whose emotional state has no effect on the natural course of the disease and those who have a clear temporal association between stressful situations and dermatotrichological condition worsening. The second category of patients is referred to be "stress-responsive." Psychosomatic disorders, which are characterized by physical manifestations of unresolved emotional problems, are also included in this group. For example, chronic telogen effluvium in women, which cannot be explained by any other reason, may be linked to personal life problems.

Primary Psychiatric Disorders

Anxiety Disorders

Generalized anxiety disorder (ICD 10 F41.1) is marked by excessive, exaggerated anxiety and worry for no obvious reason that is not directed at a specific object or situation. To confirm a diagnosis, the patient must present with primary symptoms of anxiety for at least 6 months. Most often they include: fears (anxiety about future failures, a feeling of excitement, difficulty concentrating, etc.); motor tension (fussiness, tension headaches, tremors, inability to relax); autonomic hyperactivity (sweating, tachycardia or tachypnea, epigastric discomfort, dizziness, dry mouth, etc.). The comorbidity of generalized anxiety with other anxiety disorders is high: with panic attacks (56%), obsessive-compulsive disorder (35%), and social phobia (32%–42%). According to different authors, comorbidity with depression reaches 23%–87%.

Among possible manifestations of generalized anxiety disorder in trichological practice are:

- Neurotic excoriations of the scalp
- Dysesthesia of the scalp

Depressive Disorders

In depressive disorder (ICD-10 F32, F33), the dominant symptom is a subjective feeling of low mood, which may alternate with shorter or longer periods of normal mood. The spectrum of depression ranges from mild, temporary disturbances up to severe psychotic disorders with suicidal ideation.

Depression is characterized by subjective symptoms such as:

- Depressed mood
- Feeling tired and losing energy
- Decreased interest in usual activities
- Feeling suddenly tearful
- Anhedonia (inability to experience pleasure)
- Feeling hopeless, helpless, and worthless
- Underlying excessive feeling of guilt, inferiority
- Suicidal ideation

Common physiological interrelated variables include:

- Psychomotor retardation or agitation
- Insomnia or hypersomnia
- Loss of appetite or hyperphagia
- Constipation (especially in older patients)

Depression causes significant problems on a personal, family, work, and interpersonal level. The prior medical history of those who suffer from depression may include suicidal attempts. In most cases, it is difficult for the patient to admit that their depressed state is caused by social stigma associated with psychiatric diagnoses. In turn, somatization of mental disorders in the form of certain physical symptoms is possible.

Possible manifestations of a depressive disorder in trichological practice include:

- Neurotic excoriations of the scalp
- Dysesthesia of the scalp
- Psychogenic pseudoeffluvium

Delusional Disorder

Hypochondriacal psychosis is characterized by a delusional ideation revolving around one particular hypochondriacal concern, while in schizophrenia, in addition to the presence of delusional ideation, many other affective and cognitive functions are also compromised.

Delusion is understood as a set of false ideas, reasonings and conclusions in patient's mind, that distortedly reflect reality and are not amenable to correction from the outside. A delusion is a false idea on which the patient is absolutely fixed. Delusional ideas are closely associated with personality changes, they dramatically change the patient-inherent system of ego–environment relations.

As for delusions in dermatological practice, the most common type is delusional infestation, delusions of parasitosis or Ekbom's disease. It is associated with an unshakable conviction by patient that the skin is infested by parasites. From a nosological point of view, delusions of parasitosis are classified as a delusional disorder of the somatic type with predominantly somatic delusions (ICD-10 F22.0). According to medical literature, the typical patient with delusions of parasitosis is a middle-aged woman, although there appears to be a bimodal age group distribution. The condition can also be present in individuals 20–30 years of age of either sex, with fairly low socioeconomic status and often linked to marginalized social, work, and interpersonal groups. Patient-reported skin sensations include crawling, biting, and tingling, which they strongly attribute to parasite infestation. In an attempt to prove the existence of parasites, patients often bring along bits of dry skin and other specimens to the physician (Match Box sign). Sometimes as a result of excessive scratching comorbid skin damage or infection occurs.

Possible manifestations of a delusional disorder in trichological practice include:

- Delusions of parasitosis
- Psychogenic pseudoeffluvium

Obsessive Compulsive Disorders and Related Conditions

An obsession is a persistent idea, thought, impulse, or image that spontaneously arises and uncontrollably intrudes into a person's consciousness causing distress and anxiety. By definition, unlike patients with delusions, patients suffering from obsessive-compulsive disorder have insight into their condition. They realize that the obsession is inappropriate and irrational but cannot resist. Compulsions are repetitive, stereotyped motor acts, often ritualized and designed to reduce intolerable anxiety or distress. Patients may feel the urge to act in response to the obsessions.

Obsessive compulsive symptoms are often seen across the whole spectrum of psychopathology. In early childhood, they may occur as a temporary phenomenon in response to stress or anxiety, e.g., trichotillomania, as a psychoneurotic symptom in a person with some obsessive-compulsive personality traits, e.g., onychophagia or skin trauma (acne excoriée), as a feature of the obsessive-compulsive disorder, or in patients with psychosis. Obsessive and compulsive symptoms connected to hair may arise during or shortly after drug intoxication or medication exposure.

Obsessive-compulsive disorders (ICD-10 F42) include either predominantly obsessive ideas, obsessive actions, or mixed symptoms.

Obsessive topics may involve aggression and violence (harming self or others), contamination, sex, religion, or somatic concerns. Patients sometimes complain of constant preoccupation with their appearance due to hair loss (body dysmorphic disorder (classified as obsessive-compulsive and related disorders in the Diagnostic and Statistical Manual of Mental Disorders 5th edition (DSM-5)). In this case, obsessive thoughts are defined as constantly recurring ideas related to hair loss and causing significant anxiety. Compulsions are repetitive behaviors, including almost non-stop self-care activities (telogenomania). Among these activities:

- Hair combing for several hours
- Looking at or touching their hair in front of mirror for longer times (to make sure that hair is right and the alopecia areas are covered)

Possible manifestations of obsessive-compulsive disorder in trichological practice include:

- Trichotillomania
- Neurotic excoriations of the scalp
- Dermatitis artefacta of the scalp
- Telogenomania

Personality Disorders

Some patients with psychotrichological symptoms may suffer from underlying personality disorders (ICD 10 F60) that negatively affect the course and prognosis of the disease. Personality disorders are enduring patterns of behaviors deviating from those generally accepted in society. These patterns are persistent, rigid, and affect interpersonal functioning, emotional and behavioral response, compulsivity, and cognition. As a rule, personality disorders begin in adolescence or early adulthood and must have a significant impact on patients' social and occupational functioning.

This pattern consists of:

- Ways of perceiving and interpreting self, other people, and events
- Interpersonal functioning
- Impulse control and the range, intensity, and appropriateness of emotional response

Among the psychotrichological conditions, the most frequently observed personality disorders are obsessive-compulsive, narcissistic, and histrionic personality disorders.

Obsessive Compulsive Personality Disorder. Individuals with an obsessive-compulsive personality are rigid, perfectionistic, and indecisive for fear of making a mistake; they lack self-confidence, are sensitive to criticism, and are socially reserved. They have a profound difficulty in handling negative emotions—anger and aggression, which sometimes are explosive and at other times are displaced into self-manipulation rather than being expressed directly in a modulated fashion.

Narcissistic Personality Disorder. The most common elements of this personality are grandiosity, need for admiration and lack of empathy. These patients have grandiose sense of self-importance and are preoccupied with fantasies of unlimited success and power. Patients believe that they are special or unique and have a sense of entitlement, take advantage of others to achieve their own goals, lack empathy, and are envious of others. These patients feel their entitlement is threatened when they develop hair disorder.

Histrionic Personality Disorder. Excessive emotionality and constant attention-seeking actions are characteristics of it. These individuals exhibit self-dramatization, impressionistic speech that lacks specifics, labile and superficial emotional expression, and a need to be the focus of attention. This common personality disorder has an impact on the relationship between the doctor and patient as well as the course of therapy for numerous hair disorders.

Somatoform Disorders and Related Conditions

In dermatotrichology, somatoform disorders are characterized by heterogeneous pattern of various clinical features, which is based on comparable emotional distress accompanied by frequent physical symptoms in combination with patient's insistence on medical examination despite repeated negative results and reassurance by the physician that the symptoms are not caused by physical abnormalities. For this disorder the term "dermatologic nondisease" has been coined [2, 3].

The classification of somatic psychiatric disorders is far from complete, and the diagnostic rubrics in the somatoform disorders section of ICD-10 are quite controversial. The main somatoform and somatopsychic disorders in the field of trichology include subgroups of multiple somatization disorder (ICD-10 F45.0), somatoform pain disorder (trichodynia) (ICD 10 F45.4), hypochondriacal disorder, including body dysmorphic disorder (ICD 10 F45.2), and conversion disorder, also known as conversion hysteria (ICD-10 F44.xx)

Somatization disorder (ICD-10 F45.0) presents itself as repeated multiple somatic unsubstantiated complaints. Adult patients typically develop physical complaints and seek treatment within a few years, with their complaints associated with a significant deterioration in social, occupational, or personal functioning. Pain symptoms in various areas of the body or changes in bodily functions, gastrointestinal symptoms, sexual dysfunction, and pseudo-neurological symptoms are common. These symptoms are not limited to pain (as in somatoform pain disorder). Physical examination or laboratory findings show that none of the symptoms are fully explained by somatic illness or substance abuse, or, when somatic illness is present, the observed disorder or complaint is more severe than would be expected based on the history, laboratory findings, and physical examination results.

In trichodermatology, complaints about physical conditions associated with the environment, known as **ecosyndromes** (ICD-10 F45.0), should be ruled out. Despite the absence of objective evidence of any direct toxicity exposure, patients present with a variety of multi-organ system complaints that raise the possibility of being caused by environmental toxins. An example in the context of trichology would be a complete rejection of sulfate shampoos, and sometimes any cosmetics, in favor of "natural products" (see Chap. 7). Patients usually also have symptoms of depression [12].

Chronic somatoform pain disorder (ICD-10 F45.4). Some patients complain only of sensory sensations, in particular itching, burning, stinging, etc., in the absence of any dermatological, neurological, or medical diagnosis.

A special term ending with the suffix "dynia" is used to describe cutaneous sensory disturbances (sensation of pain) that occur in certain parts of the body, such as "glossodynia" for a burning mouth syndrome or "vulvodynia" for a pain syndrome in the vulvar area. Patients with trichodynia (see Chaps. 5 and 11) complain of painful dysesthesia in hair and hair roots, especially if hair is touched. According to Rebora et al. [4], soreness of the scalp without any visible pathological somatic manifestations is observed in 34% of patients with hair loss, including patients with:

- Chronic telogen effluvium
- Androgenetic alopecia
- Chemotherapy-induced alopecia

Possible causes that are the subject of controversy and the focus of current research include the role of the perifollicular inflammatory infiltrate in trichodynia, as well as neuroendocrine/neuroimmune factors.

Patients with chronic cutaneous sensory disturbances of unknown etiology are classified as having or not having medically diagnosed psychiatric symptoms like depression or anxiety. It is believed that the latter group of patients suffer from somatoform pain disorder. Most common psychiatric associations include:

- Depression
- Anxiety
- Obsessive compulsive spectrum disorders
- Other somatic symptom-related disorders

Somatoform pain disorder, by definition, brings pain to the forefront. When compared to clinical presentation, this condition is characterized by disproportionate and excessive thoughts, feelings, or behaviors related to a somatic symptom. This disorder manifests itself psychopathologically as a syndrome of limited hypochondria (hypochondria circumscripta) characterized by persistent monomorphic algias. Self-destructive behavior is also possible when there is a desire to eliminate the "affected" area (self-harm) or when the "trusted" self-harm is present (surgical interventions). These somatoform disorders are frequently spontaneous, lasting from 6 months to several years. Most cases result in a complete resolution of the algic syndrome. Some patients also experience somatic depression.

Possible manifestations of a somatoform pain disorder in trichological practice include:

- Dysesthesia of the scalp (trichodynia)

Hypochondriacal disorder (ICD 10 F45.2). When there are normal bodily functions, the patient looks for signs of a dangerous disease. The patient is seriously preoccupied with thoughts or fears of a serious illness, which do not go away even after receiving the results of relevant medical examinations and assurances from doctors. These thoughts either cause clinically significant stress or have a negative impact on professional, social, or interpersonal functioning. Such patients are not delusional (as in delusional disorder), and their preoccupation with appearance is not limited (as in body dysmorphic disorder). Hypochondriac disorder typically manifests in adulthood or later in life and is chronic. Patients usually go to the doctor to request a series of tests and to get reassurances

Possible manifestations of a hypochondriacal disorder in trichological practice include:

- Psychogenic pseudoeffluvium

Body dysmorphic disorder, which is classified as a kind of hypochondriacal disorder by ICD 10 (F45.2) and in obsessive-compulsive and related disorders in DSM-5 is a common diagnosis in dermatological practice and accounts for a sizable portion of difficult patients, many of whom are young. Such individuals frequently seek medical attention in an attempt to address a minor or nonexistent cosmetic problem. Body dysmorphic disorder cases can range in severity from moderate to extremely severe. The patient is preoccupied with an imaginary defect in appearance or has an excessive concern about a slight physical defect.

Such concentration can have a negative impact on one's ability to operate professionally, socially, or interpersonally.

The focus of the preoccupation and concern is on those parts of the body that are important in body image. According to Fontenelle et al. [5], approximately 30% of patients with body dysmorphia complain of hair loss. Patients with imaginary hair loss, also known as **psychogenic pseudoeffluvium** (see Chap. 7), are afraid of going bald or believe they are going bald despite no objective evidence of hair loss. Despite the fact that female patients predominate, men can sometimes blame their inability to communicate and form relationships with the opposite sex on anxiety about hair loss. Body dysmorphic disorder may be misdiagnosed as androgenetic alopecia or involution alopecia (see Chap. 9).

One theory that attempts to explain the development of body dysmorphic disorder is the "self-discrepancy theory," in which patients experience conflicting beliefs against the background of discrepancies between their actual and desired selves. Patients have unrealistic physical appearance expectations. It is believed that social media and the TV contribute to the development of body dysmorphic disorder by setting beauty standards for people to follow. The good example is the recently described Dorian Gray syndrome syndrome [6], in which patients seek means and methods to slow the natural aging process in order to remain forever young.

Among possible manifestations of body dysmorphic disorder in trichological practice is:

- Psychogenic pseudoeffluvium

Conversion and dissociative disorders are characterized by a loss of body functions (loss of memory for recent events; loss or decrease in motor functions;

loss of sensitivity and sensations; inability to recognize oneself as an individual; and loss of connection with reality).

Some types of dissociative disorders are referred to as "conversion." It occurs when a person develops an affective state as a result of an unresolvable life situation or a serious conflict. A person suffering from conversion disorder is frequently hesitant to acknowledge their problems and instead blames them on somatic symptoms.

Unlike hypochondria, where the patient is often not ill but is overly obsessed with normal bodily functions, the patient with conversion disorder is aware of the functional impairment and simply uses it to avoid uncomfortable situations. This is an involuntary state.

Patients with conversion disorder are subjected to an acute stressor that creates a psychological conflict, and physical symptoms serve as a tool for resolving the conflict, even if the patients are unaware of the stressor's presence. Conflicts or other stressors that occur prior to the onset or worsening of symptoms indicate a link with psychological factors. The best approach would be to regard the disorder as a disturbance in one's perception of an illness or need.

According to psychodynamic theory, the cause of symptoms is a defense mechanism that neutralizes anxiety caused by an unacceptable urge or desire. The patient does not consciously imitate illness symptoms in order to gain material gain or to make others believe that they are sick.

Possible manifestations of a conversion disorder in trichological practice include:

- Dysesthesia of the scalp
- Chronic telogen effluvium

Secondary Psychiatric Disorders

Psychogenic reactions (depressive reactions, reactions with somatic phobias) are caused by the psycho-traumatic effect of a somatic disease associated with its subjectively severe manifestations, widespread opinion about the danger of the diagnosis, restrictions imposed by somatic suffering on personal, domestic, and professional activities.

Long-lasting disease, accompanied by massive hair loss, often has a psycho-traumatic effect and can lead to psychogeny. Most often, nosogenic reactions occur in hair diseases characterized by progressive, relapsing course. However, given the social significance of the scalp area, even reversible alopecia can trigger a secondary mental disorder.

Researchers consider **depression** as the most common reaction to hair disease. A number of authors emphasize the importance of genetic predisposition, pointing out that chronic hair and scalp diseases can exacerbate abnormalities, leading to decompensation of an existing personality disorder. Depressive nosogenic reactions can occur when the dominant anxious, hypochondriacal, or hysterical symptoms are present. A combination of depressed mood, sudden tearfulness, irritability, and sleep disturbances caused by ideas of a physical disability that is unpleasant for others determines the psychopathological structure of affective pathology. This condition can cause depressive symptoms such as anhedonia, sadness, low self-esteem, and feelings of hopelessness, helplessness, and worthlessness.

Patients with alopecia areata have a significant worsening of social-emotional aspects of their quality of life, with an increased rate of depression, dysmorphophobia, and, in some cases, suicidal ideation.

According to published studies, there is a significant negative correlation between male pattern baldness and quality of life, which is frequently associated with psychological issues [7]. Depression, emotional distress, decreased self-esteem, feelings of physical unattractiveness, increased feelings of embarrassment, anxiety, and psychosocial maladjustment have all been reported as negative effects. Postmenopausal effluvium and senile alopecia are typical symptoms that fall on a spectrum between clinically detectable and often mild effluvium with perimenopausal depression and worsening of a minor problem due to perimenopausal depression exacerbation. These patients require psychoeducation, psychotherapy, and psychopharmacotherapy in addition to traditional hair disorder treatment.

There is a strong predisposition to the development of social **anxiety disorder** among patients with hair disease. These patients engage in avoidance behaviors in order to avoid perceived scrutiny from others. They are afraid of other people's criticism and try to avoid situations involving public contact. These patients are excessively concerned with having or developing a serious hair disorder. They are anxious and perform repeated hair checks, exhibit maladaptive avoidance, or even avoid medical treatment.

This illness preoccupation should be present for at least months in order to be diagnosed. There are two types of patients: those who seek care (frequently use medical services) and those who avoid care (avoiding medical help). They isolate themselves and eventually develop interpersonal relationship problems. Other psychiatric comorbidities may be associated with social anxiety.

Common conditions associated with social anxiety, isolation, and withdrawal include:

- Androgenic alopecia at younger age
- Alopecia areata
- Trichotillomania

A long-term hair disease can result in the development of **social phobia,** which is clinically characterized by acute shyness associated with a loss of external attractiveness, painful perception of a cosmetic defect, feelings of inferiority, and avoidant behavior. The circle of communication is limited to the patients' closest relatives, who are already accustomed to disfiguring changes in their appearance. Social visits cause significant discomfort, exacerbate social phobia events, and increase anxiety and self-doubt, with various attempts made to hide alopecia zones.

Personality disorders may develop when a hair disease takes protracted or chronic course. Although, according to researchers, a constitutional predisposition along with the permanent impact of psycho-traumatic factor represent the ground for pathological development. Premorbid abnormalities are dominated by paranoid and schizoid personality disorders. In hypochondriacal development of a personality, inflated self-esteem and an overvalued attitude toward one's appearance come to the fore. Such patients, not satisfied with the results of medical examination, roam from one doctor to another, often practicing self-medication, which further aggravates the course of the hair disease. Sensitive personality type is characterized by the development of a complex of inferiority, timidity, and shyness.

Progressive hair disorders may lead to significant stress, emotional reactions, and behavioral symptoms in response to visible hair pathology. An **adjustment disorder** is a debilitating emotional or behavioral reaction to a stressful event or situation. Symptoms or behavior are clinically significant, manifesting as distress that is significantly greater than expected, or severe impairment of social, occupational, or educational functioning.

From diagnostic standpoint, these symptoms should present within 3 months of the stressor onset. From a psychopathological point of view, adjustment disorders may result from the stressful event of hair loss, depending on its acuteness, severity, and prognosis.

Adjustment disorders caused by hair pathology may be accompanied by depression, anxiety, a combination of anxiety and depression, a disturbance of conduct, or a combination of disturbance of emotion and conduct.

Hair loss related to a traumatic event can result in **acute stress disorder** or **post-traumatic stress disorder (PTSD),** depending on the time period from exposure to development of pathology. Acute stress disorder is defined by exposure to a traumatic event or direct encounter with a life-threatening situation within 1 month duration.

Depending on the duration, hair loss due to any cause and related to traumatic event may cause acute stress disorder or **acute or post-traumatic stress disorder (PTSD)**. Acute stress disorder is characterized by exposure to actual traumatic event or direct encounter with a life threat. There are several categories of symptoms, including:

- Intrusive symptoms
- Negative mood
- Dissociative symptoms
- Avoidance and arousal symptoms

Three days to 1 month following trauma exposure is the time frame for acute stress disorder symptoms, and more than 1 month for PTSD symptoms.

Psychosomatic Disorders

Disorders of a psychosomatic spectrum include a group of disease states that manifest as exacerbation of somatic pathology and are characterized by the development of symptom complexes arising from the interaction of mental and somatic factors, namely, somatization disorders, as well as mental disorders reflecting different individual response to a somatic disease. Psychosomatic diseases develop in response to a conflict experience (due to the interaction of "predisposition-personality-situation") in the form of a primary bodily reaction with the subsequent appearance of morphologically established changes in organs. The corresponding predisposition can influence the affected organ or system.

It was hypothesized that a number of factors contribute to an increase in the vulnerability of organ systems to psychosomatic diseases. Emotional central nervous system-mediated factors, intrapsychic processes, specific interdependence between emotional drive and target organ, and systemic vulnerability of the target organ are among these factors. The ICD-10 code F54 "Psychological and behavioral factors associated with disorders or diseases classified elsewhere" denotes the presence of a distinct psychosomatic component in the structure of a somatic disease.

Psychogenic factors have long been recognized for their role in causing skin and hair diseases. The occurrence and recurrence of a number of chronic diseases encountered in dermatotrichological practice are clinically and evidently influenced by psychogenic influences. Atopic dermatitis, psoriasis, seborrheic dermatitis, hyperhidrosis, chronic telogen effluvium, and alopecia areata are examples of this link.

However, modern research data show that the majority of hair and scalp diseases, which were previously classified as psychosomatic, have a genetic and immunological basis.

The influence of psychogenic factors on a sequence of subsequent immunological events that cause a worsening of dermatotrichopathy can be interpreted as indicating a close relationship between these psychogenic factors and the major pathogenetic pathways.

According to a study by Griesemer [8], all patients with hyperhidrosis, 70% of those with atopic dermatitis, 62% of those with psoriasis, and 41% of those with seborrheic dermatitis have emotional triggers.

Despite the fact that the role of stress in the occurrence and recurrence of some chronic dermatoses was previously considered, the modern paradigm calls for revision. Based on the experience of the war in Vietnam, the Persian Gulf, Bosnia, and Afghanistan, the structure of the dominant dermatological nosology in military personnel and civilians in combat environment was analyzed. It is obvious that among these diseases, nosologies caused by external actions, as well as dermatoses caused by psychotrauma, were identified [9]. According to preliminary statistical data of specialized dermatotrichological clinics of Ukraine, it is possible to notice an increase in the incidence of five nosological diseases in military personnel and civilians in the war zone compared to the previous year: psoriasis, seborrheic dermatitis, telogen effluvium, alopecia areata, and pressure alopecia [13].

In trichology, chronic idiopathic telogen effluvium is a classic example of somatic manifestations of unresolved emotional conflicts. Previous research indicates that approximately 40% of women with telogen effluvium had marital problems, and approximately 63% had professional career problems.

Psychogenesis play an important role in the genesis of alopecia areata (in 44.7% of cases). There have been cases where psycho-emotional stress clearly preceded disease onset or relapse. However, it is difficult to objectively distinguish stress as a true disease trigger from distress caused by the disease itself, which can be identified retrospectively and incorrectly as the cause of hair loss in alopecia areata. It was also suggested that, in addition to playing a role in the onset of alopecia areata, anxiety and depression caused by the disease itself may affect the course of the disease through the release of stress mediators.

There is evidence of neurohumoral changes in alopecia areata. A recent study discovered that the disease is associated with a change in the hypothalamic-pituitary-adrenal system's functioning. Furthermore, high activity of the corticotropin-releasing hormone receptor, as seen in active alopecia areata lesions, can cause mast cell differentiation from hair follicle mesenchyme. It has been observed that the progression of alopecia areata alters the expression of substance P, resulting in mast cell degranulation, accelerated hair follicle catagen regression, and an increase in the number of compounds expressing CD8 + T cells.

Studies conducted in Ukraine presented data, which was based on the study of adaptive hormones—cortisol and insulin, as well as the adaptive potential stress coefficient K, on the role of stress and maladjustment disorders in patients with alopecia areata. As a result, scientists came to the conclusion that under conditions of inflammation in alopecia areata, an acute protective inflammatory reaction is transformed into a chronic uncontrolled pathological process, manifested by a change in the corresponding phases from an increase to a decrease in the level of cortisol and insulin, as well as a similar change in the K index with tension and disruption of adaptive capabilities, which can lead to structural and functional disorders at all levels, and especially in the neuroendocrine and immune systems [14].

However, it should be noted that there is a whole range of nosogenic reactions aggravating the course of the disease in patients with psychosomatic hair and skin pathology. It can be explained by socially and cosmetically significant localization of the disease, as well as by its recurrent nature and resistance to therapy. At the same time, dermatotrichological symptoms and induced psychogenesis themselves have a psycho-traumatic effect, triggering a torpid course of the disease as well as forming new waves of exacerbations during the relapse itself. This cascade of reactions provokes a self-perpetuating vicious cycle. Thus, psychiatric disorders are closely integrated into the overall clinical presentation of hair and skin diseases.

Diagnosis Methods and Questionnaires Used in Psychotrichology for Psychiatric Screening

Some patients lack insight about the recognition of a psychological component associated with their hair disease. Therefore, the clinician is primarily responsible for diagnosing and treating these patients. In these cases, a thorough trichodermatological and psychiatric assessment should both be part of the clinical interview. Focusing on the psychological distress brought on by hair disease is crucial, as is determining the effect it has had on the patient's general functioning and wellness. Thus, the first step in the treatment is to establish a good rapport with the patient.

Table 2.2 Common psychiatric screening questionnaires used in psychotrichology

Assesment tool	No. of questions	Diagnosis
PHQ-9	9	Depression
PHQ-15	15	Somatic symptom disorders
PHQ	59	Depression, anxiety, somatic symptoms disorder, alcohol abuse, eating disorder
HADS	14	Anxiety, depression
BDI-II	21	Depression
Y-BOCS	10	Obsessive compulsive disorder
CAGE questionnaire	4	Alcohol and substance abuse
GAD-7	7	Generalized anxiety disorder
SCARED	41	Childhood anxiety
MGHHPS	7	Trichotillomania
MIST-C	25	Trichotillomania
PITS	6	Trichotillomania
THDIS	27	Trichotillomania

PHQ Patient Health Questionnaire, *HADS* Hospital Anxiety and Depression Scale, *BDI* Beck Depression Inventory, *Y-BOCS* Yale-Brown Obsessive-Compulsive Scale, *GAD* Generalized Anxiety Disorder Questionnaire, *SCARED* Screen for Child Anxiety Related Disorders, *MGH-HPS* Massachusetts General Hospital Hairpulling Scale, *MIST-C* Milwaukee Inventory for Subtypes of Trichotillomania-Child Version, *PITS* Psychiatric Institute Trichotillomania Scale, THDIS Scale for severity of distress and damage caused by hair pulling.

Rather a gentle nonjudgmental and friendly approach yields trust and helps develop a therapeutic bond with the patient.

A psychotrichological assessment should be conveyed to the patient in simple language that is not laden with medical terms. Except where required by law, the patient must be informed of the confidentiality. It is beneficial to obtain collateral information from family, friends, and relatives when assessing personality structure, rather than relying solely on information provided by the patient. During the interview, the impact of hair disease on the patient's life should be thoroughly investigated, including detailed questions about anxiety, mood, and suicidal ideation. If the trichologist suspects that the risk of self-harm is high and there is a safety concern, a referral to psychiatry may be warranted.

In clinical practice, a variety of psychiatric screening tests are employed. The majority of them primarily concentrate on anxiety and depression, which are the most prevalent psychopathologies connected to hair diseases (Table 2.2). Stress, both psychological and physical, has been shown to impact the development of a variety of skin and hair disorders. Hair cortisol analysis has recently been established as a useful tool for evaluating hypothalamic-pituitary-adrenal axis abnormalities [10]. Hair cortisol levels vary with physical and mental stress and have proved to be more reliable than cortisol levels measured in blood, saliva, and urine [11]. Hair cortisol may be useful in research and healthcare since it indicates chronic stress, which is a contributor to various skin and hair alterations.

Dermatological and hair problems can have a substantial impact on one's emotional and social well-being, resulting in a decrease in quality of life (QoL). General medical scales, dermatological scales, including those for specific dermatological illnesses, are used to measure QoL in dermatology. To acquire trustworthy and full information while measuring QoL, questionnaires with high validity, reliability, and sensitivity that relate to the study's aims and objectives are required.

The evaluation of QoL at disease onset and throughout the disease course is critical. It can be used to characterize the severity of the disease process, its dynamics, and the efficacy of treatment approaches from the perspective of the patient. As a result, the QoL evaluation should become a requirement in patient management (see Chap. 3).

Summary

- The skin, its appendages, and the nervous system all have the same embryonic origin. Hair disorders, like many other psychocutaneous disorders, have significant emotional effects, and are associated with impaired quality life and low self-esteem.
- Psychotrichology and the psychiatric elements of hair disorders are linked to a wide range of psychological outcomes, including, but not limited to, depression, anxiety, low self-esteem, and a reduced quality of life. The treatment and management of these individuals is a challenge for dermatologists and trichologists. Due to the stigma involved with visiting a psychiatrist, the majority of patients refuse to be referred to a psychiatrist or psychologist.
- Many patients are unaware of the existence of a psychological component linked with their hair diseases. In these cases, the attending physician is charged with the additional task of diagnosing and managing these challenging patients.
- Having a thorough grasp of the psychopathological elements that play a role in psychotrichological diseases will enable the clinician to develop a care strategy that is tailored to the patient's needs. In these cases, a thorough trichodermatological and psychiatric examination should be included of the clinical interview.
- The intensity of stress experienced by a patient should be part of the equation when a physician decides how aggressively to treat a hair condition.
- Consultations with psychiatrists will be beneficial in the care of psychotrichological patients since dermatotrichologists and psychiatrists analyze clinical situations differently, employing distinct ways of communication and therapeutic approaches.

References

1. Niemeier V, Harth W, Kupfer J, Mayer K, Linse R, Schill WB, Gieler U. Prevalence of psychosomatic disorders in dermatologic patients. Experiences in 2 dermatology clinics with a liaison therapy model. Hautarzt. 2002;53:471–7.
2. Cotterill JA. Dermatologic nondisease. Dermatol Clin. 1996a;14:439–45.

3. Cotterill JA. Body dysmorphic disorder. Dermatol Clin. 1996b;14:457–63.
4. Rebora A, Semino MT, Guarrera M. Trichodynia. Dermatology. 1996;192:292–3.
5. Fontenelle LF, Telles LL, Nazar BP, de Menezes GB, do Nascimento AL, Mendlowicz MV, Versiani M. A sociodemographic, 31 phenomenological, and long-term follow-up study of patients with body dysmorphic disorder in Brazil. Int J Psychiatry Med. 2006;32(36):243–59.
6. Brosig B., Kupfer J., Niemeier V. et al. The "Dorian Gray Syndrome": psychodynamic need for hair growth restorers and, other "fountains of youth". Int J Clin Pharmacol Ther 2001; 39: 279–283.
7. Cash TF. The psychological effects of androgenetic alopecia in men. J Am Acad Dermatol. 1992;26:926–31.
8. Griesemer RD. Emotionally triggered disease in a dermatology practice. Psychiatr Ann. 1978;8:49–56.
9. Gelman AB, Norton SA, Valdes-Rodriguez R, Yosipovitch G. A review of skin conditions in modern warfare and peacekeeping operations. Mil Med. 2015;180(1):32–7. https://doi.org/10.7205/MILMED-D-14-00240.
10. Gow R, Thomson S, Rieder M, Van Uum S, Koren G. An assessment of cortisol analysis in hair and its clinical applications. Forensic Sci Int. 2010;196(1–3):32–7. https://doi.org/10.1016/j.forsciint.2009.12.040. Epub 2010 Jan 21.
11. Wester VL, van Rossum EF. Clinical applications of cortisol measurements in hair. Eur J Endocrinol. 2015;173(4):M1–M10. https://doi.org/10.1530/EJE-15-0313. Epub 2015 Apr 29.
12. Trüeb RM, Gieler U. Pschychocutaneous disorders of hair and scalp. In: Blume-Peytavi U, Tosti A, Whiting D, Trüeb RM, editors. Hair growth and disorders. New York: Springer; 2008. p. 407–26.
13. Ovcharenko Y, Serbina I, Liadova T, Kadigrob I, Kachuk Y, Vozianova S, Syzon O, Andrashko Y, Galnykina S, Khobzei K, Litus O. Prevalence of dermatotrichological pathology among civilian and military population in Ukraine during wartime: a cross-sectional study. 2025. (in press)
14. Serbina I, Andrashko Y, Galnykina S, Kadigrob I, Khobzei K, Liadova T, Litus O, Sviatenko T, Svistunov I, Syzon O, Vozianova S, Ovcharenko Y. Clinical guidelines of the Ukraine Hair Research Society. Diagnosis and treatment of alopecia areata. Actual problems of modern medicine. 2023;12:45–67. https://doi.org/10.26565/2617-409X-2023-12-06.

Assessment of the Quality of Life in Various Trichopathologies

3

Inessa Serbina

Introduction

A person's subjective sense of their quality of life (QoL) is a complex characteristic of their physical, psychological, emotional, and social functioning. There is currently a significant surge in the interest in researching patient's QoL, both for acute and chronic illnesses.

The World Health Organization (WHO) defines QoL as "an individual's perception of their position in life in relation to their goals, expectations, standards, and concerns in the context of the culture and value systems in which they live." QoL reflects an individual's emotional state, level of life satisfaction, and the sense of well-being. The integral QoL indicator can be viewed as an objective way to assess subjective factors. This is a reliable and informative method for assessing patient's health, both individually and at group level. The International Society for Quality of Life Research (ISOQOL) is an important player in shaping specialist knowledge and unified approaches.

Standardized questionnaires based on psychometric methods are the primary research instruments for examining QoL. According to WHO recommendations, QoL questionnaires primarily address three topics: social functions, mental/psychological health, and physical health. It is important to note that these questionnaires only reflect how patients are coping with their condition and do not assess the severity of the disease or the degree of health impairment.

Criteria for Quality of Life Rating Scales

There are certain requirements for QoL rating scales (questionnaires):

I. Serbina (✉)
Department of Infectious Diseases and Clinical Immunology of the V. N. Karazin Kharkiv National University, University Clinic "Trichology Institute", Kharkiv, Ukraine

Y. Ovcharenko et al. (eds.), *Psychotrichology*,
https://doi.org/10.1007/978-3-031-64083-4_3

- Universality (integrality)—each aspect of QoL is transferred on a certain scale of the questionnaire, that comprised of a set of questions
- Multidimensionality—the ability to reflect several main components of QoL
- Reliability—internal consistency and reproducibility.
- Validity (criterial; constructive—convergent and discriminant)
- High sensitivity to changes
- Conciseness and ease of understanding, regardless of the respondent age and the level of education; rapidity of completion and ease of interpretation; compliance to international standard questionnaires; availability of an adapted language versions

Additionally, the following factors should be considered while choosing a questionnaire to examine health-related QoL:

- The study objectives (assessment of population health quality and effectiveness of medical care, assessment of effectiveness of treatment/diagnosis/rehabilitation/prevention program)
- The study object and scope (population as a whole or different age groups, healthy or unhealthy, patients with a specific nosological form of the disease, etc.)
- The study subject and level: health state (individual, group, regional, population), efficacy of a specialist, structural factors; structural subdivision, healthcare institution, healthcare system.

The existing QoL questionnaires are classified by purpose (field of application and degree of specialization) and structure, which are further subdivided into two broad categories: generic and disease-specific. Generic questionnaires can be used to assess general health and can be used for a variety of diseases, but they cannot identify changes that are specific to a condition. The advantage of disease-specific questionnaires is the ability to consider factors specific to a given disease in addition to general QoL factors, as well as higher efficacy in differentiation and high sensitivity to changes.

Generic Quality of Life Questionnaires

To date, the following generic questionnaires have been widely used in medical practice to assess patients' QoL regardless of disease type: SF-36 (36 Item Short Health Status Survey), SF-12 (Short Form Health Survey, SF-12v2), and EuroQoL. (EQ-5D). The advantage is the high validity and universality, as well as the widespread prevalence and ease of questioning.

The SF-36 questionnaire consists of 36 items grouped into 8 scales and includes the following sections:

- General Health (GH)—an individual assessment of current health state, as well as resistance to disease and aging, the prospect of treatment

- Physical Functioning (PF), reflecting the degree to which the physical condition limits physical activities (self-care, walking, climbing stairs, carrying weight, etc.), as well as the tolerance to strenuous exercise
- Role-Physical Functioning (RP)—the impact of physical condition on daily role-playing activities (work, daily duties)
- Role-Emotional Functioning (RE) involves an assessment of the degree to which the emotional state interferes with ability to perform daily tasks or other daily activities (including increase in time to perform a task, decrease in volume and quality of activity, etc.)
- Social Functioning (SF) is determined by the degree to which the physical or emotional state limits social activity (communication)
- Bodily Pain (BP) and its impact on the ability to engage in daily activities, including work at home and outside
- Vitality (VT)—feeling full of strength and energy or, on the contrary, exhausted, tired
- Mental health (MH) characterizes mood, presence of depression, anxiety, general indicator of positive emotions

Scales allow evaluating two integral indicators of QoL: physical (Physical health— PH) and psychological (Mental health—MH) component of health. The indicator score in each scale varies from 0 to 100, a higher score indicates a higher quality of life, i.e., a score of 100 represents complete health.

Currently, the SF-12v2 questionnaire, which is a shortened version of the SF-36, is widely used. SF-12v2 consists of 12 questions, requiring a patient to choose one of five response options to assess the health impacts on various life aspects. To evaluate the results, answers given are also grouped into eight individual scales, which then are used to calculate values characterizing QoL on the integral scales of the physical and mental components of health (PH and MH, respectively). The questionnaire scales have a minimum value of 0 and a maximum of 100. As indicators of physical and mental health, the score from 0 to 20 corresponds to a poor; 21–40—mediocre; 41–60—high; 61–80—very high; 81–100—excellent quality of life.

A group of European researchers created the EQ-5D questionnaire, which is a standardized tool with the following characteristics: versatility, ease of completion, and wide application in various countries. Following the processing of the collected data, a single score is calculated and used to evaluate the state of health, the efficacy of treatment, rehabilitation, and various types of medical care.

The first and basic part of the EQ-5D questionnaire is designed to assess the health status of an individual in five components, reflecting: mobility (movement in space), self-care, activity in daily life, presence of pain/discomfort, and anxiety/depression. These components are presented as separate items (questions), for each of which the respondent must indicate the severity of the problem on the proposed scale. The scale assessing each component has three levels depending on the severity of the problem: 1—no abnormalities; 2—moderate abnormalities present; 3—severe abnormalities present. The level chosen for this measurement is expressed by a single-digit number that is the result of the patient's assessment of his or her health. Five components' combined values describe 243 variants of the patient's health state.

The second part of the questionnaire is a visual-analogue scale, the so-called “health thermometer,” on which the subject makes a mark corresponding to their health state at the time of completion. It's a vertical graduated ruler of 20 cm where 0 is the best imaginable health state and 100 is the worst imaginable health state.

Assessment of the Quality of Life in Trichodermatological Diseases

The most well-known generic methods for assessing QoL in dermatological diseases include: Dermatology Quality of Life Scale (DQOLS), Dermatology Life Quality Index (DLQI), Dermatology-specific Quality of Life Instrument (DSQLI), Skindex (Life Quality Index for Dermatology Patient), Children's Dermatology Life Quality Index (CDLQI).

The most well-known disease-specific methods for assessing QoL in dermatological diseases include: Acne Disability Index (ADI), Psoriasis Disability Index (PDI), Psoriasis Life Stress Inventory (PLSI), Atopic Dermatitis Disability Index (ADDI), etc.

The Dermatological Quality of Life Index (DLQI) is a widely used method for assessing dermatological quality of life, both in general and for the majority of individual skin diseases (Table 3.1). Because of its high degree of objectivity and reliability, the DLQI is the most commonly used tool for assessing QoL. DLQI is intended for adult use. This questionnaire assesses the impact of a skin disease on a patient's QoL over the previous 7 days. The questionnaire is simple to complete and does not necessitate additional detailed explanations from the physician. Completion of the form usually takes 1–2 min. The numerical indicator derived from the response analysis reflects the level of the disease's negative impact on the patients' QoL.

DLQI comprises of ten questions relating to the following six categories: symptoms and feelings, daily activities, leisure, work and learning, personal relationships, and treatment. There are four variants of answers:

«Very much»—3 points, «Quite a lot»—2 points, «A little»—1 point, «Not at all»—0 point. The DLQI is calculated by adding the score of each question, resulting in a maximum of 30 and a minimum of 0. The higher the score (number of points), the more quality of life is impaired. A score of 0–1 indicates that the patient's quality of life is not affected by their skin disease; 2–5—slightly affected; 6–10—moderately affected; 11–20—severely affected; 21–30—very severely affected.

Skindex is a 61-item instrument to measure the effects of skin disease on patients' quality of life. Skindex shortened versions with 29 and 16 items were recently created. The Skindex questionnaire has been used in a variety of studies, ranging from general dermatology to botulinum toxin injections and skin cancer. The Skindex-61

Table 3.1 Dermatology Life Quality Index (DLQI), Finlay A. Y., Khan G. K., 1994

QUALITY OF LIFE ASSESSMENTS IN DERMATOLOGY PATIENTS

Hospital No:	**Date:**	**DLQI**
Name:	**Diagnosis:**	**Score:** ☐
Address:		

The aim of this questionnaire is to measure how much your skin problem has affected you OVER THE LAST 7 DAYS. Please tick✓ one box for each question.

1. Over last 7 days, how **itchy, sore, painful** or **stinging** has your skin been?	Very much	☐		
	Quite a lot	☐		
	A little	☐		
	Not at all	☐		
2. Over last 7 days, how embarrassed or self-conscious have you felt about your skin?	Very much	☐		
	Quite a lot	☐		
	A little	☐		
	Not at all	☐		
3. Over last 7 days, how much has your skin interfered with you **going shopping** or looking after your **home** or **garden**?	Very much	☐		
	Quite a lot	☐		
	A little	☐		
	Not at all	☐	Not relevant	☐
4. Over last 7 days, how much has your skin influenced the clothes you've worn	Very much	☐		
	Quite a lot	☐		
	A little	☐		
	Not at all	☐	Not relevant	☐
5. Over last 7 days, how much has your skin affected any **social Activities** or **leisure** activities?	Very much	☐		
	Quite a lot	☐		
	A little	☐		
	Not at all	☐	Not relevant	☐
6. Over last 7 days, how much has your skin made it difficult for you to do any **sport**?	Very much	☐		
	Quite a lot	☐		
	A little	☐		
	Not at all	☐	Not relevant	☐
7. Over last 7 days, has your skin prevented you from **working** or **studying**?	Yes	☐		
	No	☐	Not relevant	☐
If "No", over last 7 days, how much has your skin been a problem at **work** or **studying**?	Quite a lot	☐		
	A little	☐		
	Not at all	☐		
8. Over last 7 days, how much has your skin created problems with your **partner** or any of your **close friends** or **relatives**?	Very much	☐		
	Quite a lot	☐		
	A little	☐		
	Not at all	☐	Not relevant	☐
9. Over the last week, how much has your skin caused any **sexual difficulties**?	Very much	☐		
	Quite a lot	☐		
	A little	☐		
	Not at all	☐	Not relevant	☐
10. Over the last week, how much has the treatment of your skin condition caused a problem, such as making your home messy or taking up time?	Very much	☐		
	Quite a lot	☐		
	A little	☐		
	Not at all	☐	Not relevant	☐

version includes seven paragraphs and two parts on patients' physical condition and three parts on their psychosocial state: "Negative effect," "Self-Esteem," "Anxiety," "Physical Discomfort," "Physical Limitations," "Self-consciousness," "Intimate Relationships." Skindex-29, the 29-item version, also performs well psychometrically and covers three areas: "Emotions," "Symptoms," and "Physical Activity." Skindex-16's efficacy was confirmed in a study involving 541 patients. The paragraphs in this questionnaire are the same as those in Skindex-61. This shortened version was created to reduce the patient's workload.

Assessing children's QoL has always been a challenging task. The CDLQI was created to assess QoL in children aged 4 and up with skin disorders. The CDLQI has been translated into several languages and used in numerous studies, and it continues to be the only dermatological tool for assessing QoL in this age group. The questionnaire consists of ten questions with four possible answers that reflect the impact of skin diseases on children's lives over the previous 7 days. Children self-administer the questionnaire. Each question's answers are graded on a scale of 0–3. The following parameters were evaluated: "Symptoms/Well-Being," "Daily Activity," "Personal Relationships/Communication with Friends," "Learning/Leisure," and "Therapy." The CDLQI score is calculated by summing the scores giving a maximum of 30 and a minimum of 0. There is an inverse relationship between the CDLQI score and QoL: the higher the score, the lower the patient's QoL. The CDLQI score is assessed as follows: 0–1 point—no effect on the patient's QoL; 2–5 points—small effect; 6–10 points—moderate effect; 11–20 points—pronounced effect; 21–30 points—a very pronounced effect on the patient's QoL. InToDermQoL (The Infants' and Toddlers' Dermatology Quality of Life) was recently designed and is currently undergoing an initial evaluation. It is a dermatological questionnaire for measuring QOL in infants and toddlers with skin conditions aged 0–4 years.

In order to assess psycho-emotional disorders in hospitalized patients, the Hospital Anxiety and Depression Scale (HADS) is utilized. This assessment gauges the severity of impairment and enables prompt correction (Table 3.2). The popularity of the scale is largely attributable to its simplicity, quickness, and usability (filling out the questionnaire is not time consuming and not difficult for the patient).

There are four different answer options for each statement. The choice that best summarizes the respondent's situation and condition should be selected. Subclinical anxiety/depression is diagnosed with a score of 8–10, and clinically obvious anxiety or depression with a score of 11 or higher. More sensitive evaluation techniques, including the Hamilton Depression Scale, Beck Depression Inventory, etc., are advised for a more thorough diagnosis and understanding of the patient's disease dynamics.

Table 3.2 Hospital anxiety and depression scale (HADS), Zigmond A. S., Snaith R. P., 1983

Hospital Anxiety and Depression Scale (HADS) *Each statement has four possible replies. Choose the reply that is closest to how you have been feeling, and then add up the scores for each part*	
Part I (Anxiety level)	Part II (Depression level)
1. I feel tense or wound up 3—Most of the time 2—A lot of the time 1—From time to time, occasionally 0—Not at all	**1. I still enjoy the things I used to enjoy** 0—Definitely as much 1—Not quite so much 2—Only a little 3—Hardly at all
2. I get a sort of frightened feeling as if something awful is about to happen 3—Very definitely and quite badly 2—Yes, but not too badly 1—A little, but it doesn't worry me 0—Not at all	**2. I can laugh and see the funny side of things** 0—As much as I always could 1—Not quite so much now 2—Definitely not so much now 3—Not at all
3. Worrying thoughts go through my mind 3—A great deal of the time 2—A lot of the time 1—From time to time, but not too often 0—Only occasionally	**3. I feel cheerful** 3—Not at all 2—Not often 1—Sometimes 0—Most of the time
4. I can sit at ease and feel relaxed 0—Definitely 1—Usually 2—Not often 3—Not at all	**4. I feel as if I am slowed down** 3—Nearly all the time 2—Very often 1—Sometimes 0—Not at all
5. I experience inner tension or trembling 0—Not at all 1—Occasionally 2—Quite often 3—Very often	**5. I have lost interest in my appearance** 3—Definitely 2—I don't take as much care as I should 1—I may not take quite as much care 0—I take just as much care as ever
6. I feel restless as I have to be on the move 3—Very much indeed 2—Quite a lot 1—Not very much 0—Not at all	**6. I look forward with enjoyment to things (activities, hobbies)** 0—As much as I ever did 1—Rather less than I used to 2—Definitely less than I used to 3—Hardly at all
7. I get sudden feelings of panic 3—Very often indeed 2—Quite often 1—Not very often 0—Not at all	7. I can enjoy a good book or radio or TV program 0—Often 1—Sometimes 2—Not often 3—Very seldom

(continued)

Table 3.2 (continued)

Hospital Anxiety and Depression Scale (HADS) *Each statement has four possible replies. Choose the reply that is closest to how you have been feeling, and then add up the scores for each part*	
Part I (Anxiety level)	Part II (Depression level)
Total score:_________ Total score:_________ **0–7 points** **8–10 points** *«subclinical anxiety/depression»* **11 points and higher** *«clinical anxiety/depression»*	

Assessment of the Quality of Life in Hair Disease

Hair disorders, despite relatively minor changes in physical condition, can significantly worsen the emotional and social components of QoL, and are frequently the cause of depression, anxiety, dysmorphophobia, and other disorders. Thus, assessing QoL in patients with this pathology is critical. There are currently few specialized questionnaires designed for patients with hair disease.

The Women's Androgenetic Alopecia Quality of Life Questionnaire (WAA-QOL) was created by hair disease experts and tested in patients at various stages of hair loss using the Ludwig scale. The final version of the questionnaire contains 16 questions, each with 7 possible answers. Patients self-avaluated their condition over the past week. This questionnaire demonstrates content reliability and high reproducibility, and it is useful in studying the effect of AGA on women's QoL as well as assessing therapeutic effects in clinical trials. The WAA-QOL is recommended by international consensus as a tool for measuring QoL in patients with frontal fibrosing alopecia.

The Hair-Specific Skindex-29 questionnaire for assessing QoL in patients with hair diseases was developed on the basis of the Skindex-29 QoL questionnaire for dermatological patients. Skindex-29 was first described in a study that assessed QoL in Korean male AGA patients by replacing the words "skin" with "scalp" and "skin condition" with "AGA." Skindex-29 was later adapted by Spanish researchers and extensively tested for validity and reliability in AGA patients. A rating scale is included in the questionnaire, which is divided into three subscales: physical symptoms (7 items), functioning (12 items), and emotions (10 items). The patient responded to each question by selecting a score ranging from 0 (never bothered) to 5. (always bothered). A high resulting score indicates a low index of quality of life.

The original German Hairdex was a Skindex-29 modification designed for use in women with diffuse alopecia and AGA. The final version includes 48 items divided into 5 subscales: emotions, functioning, symptoms, self-esteem, and stigmatization. The first three subscales are comparable to those found in the Skindex-29 questionnaire. Hairdex takes the majority of patients about 15 min to complete.

A special questionnaire has been developed to assess QoL in alopecia areata patients (AA-QLI). This questionnaire was created by Italian researchers based on prior experiences and clinical evidence: A comparison of AA-QLI and DLQI was performed to investigate the new questionnaire's usability as a more comprehensive tool for assessing patients' QoL. It addressed three aspects of daily life: "Subjective symptoms"; "Relationship"; "Objective signs." AA patients completed both the AA-QLI and the standard DLQI questionnaires. Statistical analysis revealed that the AA-QLI has a higher specificity for assessing QoL in AA.

The AA-QLI is divided into two sections: the first includes questions about gender, age, disease onset, time of last relapse, and percentage of affected skin; the second section includes 21 questions measuring the degree to which the patient was affected by the AA in the previous month, with scores ranging from 1 (not affected at all) to 4 (extremely affected) (highly affected).

Summary

- Thus, QoL as an indicator describing important human functions and allowing for deep multifaceted analysis during the onset of the disease and in the recovery period during treatment has a very important role. QoL assessment is widely used to characterize the severity of the pathological process, its dynamics, and the effectiveness of therapeutic measures. At the same time, it should be remembered that this indicator represents an integral form of the subjective opinion about patient's own health and social opportunities. The QoL assessment should become mandatory in the diagnostic route of patient management.
- Dermatological and hair diseases often lead to significant limitations in the emotional and social aspects and, as a result, decreasing the QoL. To assess QoL in dermatology, general medical scales, special dermatological scales, and dermatological scales for certain diseases are used. To obtain reliable and complete information when assessing QoL, it is necessary to use questionnaires with high validity, reliability, and sensitivity that correspond to the goals and objectives of the study.
- Currently, there are nosology-specific tools for measuring the quality of life of trichological patients, such as WAA-QOL, Hair-Specific Skindex-29, Hairdex, AA-QLI. These dermatological QoL scales at their core are adapted for patients with hair diseases. The use of these instruments in trichological patients is critical in both clinical trials and clinical practice. There is a need for these tools to be optimized and standardized in order to improve their accuracy and validity.

Further Reading

Bjelland I, Dahl A, Haug T, Neckelmann D. The validity of the Hospital Anxiety and Depression Scale; an updated review. J Psychiat Res. 2002;52:69–77.

Capucci S, Vilsboll A, Hahn-Pedersen J, Kragh N. Impact of atopic dermatitis and chronic hand eczema on quality of life comparwith other chronic diseases: a structured review. J Am Acad Dermatol. 2020;83(6):829–34.

Chen SC. Health-related quality of life in dermatology: intrduction and overview. Dermatol Clin. 2012;30(2):205–8.

Chernyshov PV. The evolution of quality of life assessment and use in dermatology. Dermatology. 2019;235:167–74.

Chernyshov PV, Linder MD, Pustišek N, et al. Quimp (quality of life impairment): an addition to the quality of life lexicon. J Eur Acad Dermatol Venereol. 2018;32(5):181–2.

Dolte K, Girman C, Roberts J, et al. Development of a health-related quality of life questionnaire for women with androgenetic alopecia. Clin Exp Dermatol. 2008;25(8):637–42.

Fabbrocini G, Panariello L, De Vita V, et al. Quality of life in alopecia areata: a disease-specific questionnaire. J Eur Acad Dermatol Venereol. 2013;27:276–80.

Finlay AY. Quimp: a word meaning "quality of life impairment". Acta Derm Venereol. 2017;97(4):546–52.

Finlay AY, Khan GK. Dermatology Life Quality Index (DLQI): a simple practical measure for routine clinical use. Clin Exp Dermatol. 1994;19:210–6.

Gerasimchuk PO, Fira DB, Pavlyshyn AV. Assessment of the quality of life associated with health in medicine. J Med Biol Res. 2021;1:112–22.

Guerra-Tapia A, Buendía-Eisman A, Ferrando BJ. Final phase in the validation of the cross-cultural adaptation of the hair-specific Skindex-29 questionnaire into Spanish: sensitivity to change and correlation with the 12-item short-form health survey. Actas Dermosifiliogr. 2019;110(10):819–29.

Mochulska OM. Evaluation of life quality in children with dermatological diseases (literature review). Modern Pediatrics Ukraine. 2021;3(115):61–8.

Olsen EA, Harries M, Tosti A, Bergfeld W, Blume-Peytavi U, Callender V, Chasapi V, Correia O, Cotsarelis G, Dhurat R, Dlova N, Doche I, Enechukwu N, Grimalt R, Itami S, Hordinsky M, Khobzei K, Lee WS, Malakar S, Messenger A, McMichael A, Mirmirani P, Ovcharenko Y, Papanikou S, Pinto GM, Piraccini BM, Pirmez R, Reygagne P, Roberts J, Rudnicka L, Saceda-Corralo D, Shapiro J, Silyuk T, Sinclair R, Soares RO, Souissi A, Vogt A, Washenik K, Zlotogorski A, Canfield D, Vano-Galvan S. Guidelines for clinical trials of frontal fibrosing alopecia: consensus recommendations from the International FFA Cooperative Group (IFFACG). Br J Dermatol. 2021;185:1221. https://doi.org/10.1111/bjd.20567. Epub ahead of print.

Ospanova, editor. Experience in studying the quality of life in a propaedeutic clinic: monograph. Kharkov: KhNMU; 2017. p. 112.

Ring J. Quality of life—an essential parameter for dermatology. J Eur Acad Dermatol Venereol. 2017 Apr;31(4):573–9.

Siafaka V, Zioga A, Evrenoglou T, et al. Illness perceptions and quality of life in families with child with atopic dermatitis. Allergol Immunopathol. 2020;48(6):603–11.

Snyder AM, Brandenberger AU, Taliercio VL, Rich BE, Webber LB, Beshay AP, Biber JE, Hess R, Rhoads JLW, Secrest AM. Quality of life among family of patients with atopic dermatitis and psoriasis. Int J Behav Med. 2022;30:409. https://doi.org/10.1007/s12529-022-10104-7. Epub ahead of print.

Thadanipon K, Suchonwanit P. Measuring patient quality of life following treatment for alopecia. Patient Prefer Adherence. 2021;15:1601–10.

Veenhoven R. Quality of life (QOL), an overview. In: Michalos AC, editor. Encyclopedia of quality of life and Well-being research. Dordrecht: Springer Netherlands; 2014. p. 5265–9.

Ware J, Kosinski M, Turner-Bowker D, et al. User's manual for the SF-12v2 health survey (with a supplement documenting SF-12® health survey). Lincoln, RI: Quality Metric Incorporated; 2007. p. 29–56.

Ware JE, Kosinski M. Interpreting SF-36 summary health measures: a response. Qual Life Res. 2001;10(5):405–13.

Waters A, Sandhu D, Beattie P, et al. Severity stratification of Children's Dermatology Life Quality Index (CDLQI) scores. Br J Dermatol. 2010;163(1):121–7.

Zigmond AS, Snaith RP. The hospital anxiety and depression scale. Acta Psychiatr Scand. 1983;67(6):361–70.

The Art of Consultation

4

Yuliya Ovcharenko, Mohammad Jafferany,
and Ralph Trüeb

Introduction

The professional competence of a physician, their special knowledge, and the art of healing of physical and emotional component of disease are prerequisite conditions in performing clinical activity and alleviating patients' suffering. Medicine is without a doubt the noblest of the arts, and our goal is to master it. Therefore, from psychotrichology standpoint, it is essential for dermatologists to expand their clinical knowledge and therapeutic arsenal to effectively handle the psychodermatological and psychotrichological cases in their practice.

Making the correct diagnosis has crucial implications for successful counseling of patients with any hair disorder. Today, like other branches of medicine, innovative diagnostic methods and tools have been introduced in trichology. However, traditionally, in the management of patients with hair pathology, the correct diagnosis depends on a strictly organized methodical medical thinking. This, in turn, highlights the importance of acquiring appropriate clinical experience.

A general approach to diagnose a patient with psychotrichological disease is through clinical interview. Regardless of a systematic patient history and examination techniques, there remain some subtle mental traps that may lead physicians astray, resulting in misdiagnosis.

Y. Ovcharenko (✉)
V. N. Karazin Kharkiv National University, University Clinic "Trichology Institute", Kharkiv, Ukraine

M. Jafferany
Department of Psychiatry and Behavioral Sciences, Central Michigan University, College of Medicine, Saginaw, MI, USA

R. Trüeb
Center for Dermatology and Hair Diseases, Wallisellen, Zürich, Switzerland

Y. Ovcharenko et al. (eds.), *Psychotrichology*,
https://doi.org/10.1007/978-3-031-64083-4_4

Different physicians have different styles of practice, and different approaches to problems, but all are susceptible to the same types of mistakes in their thinking and diagnosing.

In his book "How Doctors Think," Jerome Groopman focuses on the thinking errors in medicine that account for an estimated 80% of medical errors, while only 20% are due to technical errors. Snap judgment and stereotypical thinking are just two examples of the subtle traps that dangerously narrow the physician's vision.

"If you listen to the patient, he is telling you the diagnosis," said William Osler (1849–1919). The manner in which a physician asks questions and responds to the patient's emotions is critical to patient activation and engagement. However, doctors, like everyone else, are vulnerable to being misled by stereotypes based on an individual's appearance, emotional state, and circumstances. We are all wary of patients who we stereotype as neurotic and anxious. These patients frequently tell their stories in a jumbled manner, making it difficult for the doctor to focus their attention. Medical professionals who dislike their patients frequently interrupt them during their narration of symptoms and complaints, preferring to focus on a diagnosis and treatment that is convenient to the physician. This bias of the physician's thinking potentially leads to inappropriate care. Groopman names this type of mental trap "attribution error." This type of error is frequently made in female patients with a full head of hair who complain of hair loss that clinicians attribute to imaginary hair loss, despite the fact that there is underlying telogen effluvium (TE). Finally, the statement "nothing is wrong with you" is incorrect because it dismisses the possibility of medical error.

Finding some signs or symptoms may be satisfying for the clinician, but despite the natural cognitive tendency to stop searching and thus stop thinking when one makes a significant finding, there is a need to continue thorough evaluation of all possible aspects of the patient's condition.

In modern medicine, the main tools for studying quality of life are standardized professional questionnaires based on psychometric methods. According to World Health Organization (WHO) guidelines, QoL (Quality of Life) questionnaires cover three major areas: physical health, mental/psychological health, and social functions. It is important to note that questionnaires do not assess the degree of health impairment or disease severity, but rather how patients adapt to and endure their illness.

"Search and acceptance of a satisfactory option" is the tendency to stop searching for a diagnosis once you find something [1].

Physicians are taught in medical school and residency training to be focused and be clear in thinking, to apply the law of minimum assumptions, and to seek only one answer to a patient's complaints. This is the correct approach in many cases, but not always. A typical example is limiting the treatment of female patient with hair loss to iron supplementation when iron deficiency is detected, while the patient also suffers from androgenetic alopecia (AGA) and may be on an oral contraceptive treatment with a pro-androgenic action. The question about multiple causes for a given problem should trigger the doctor to initiate a broader search.

We have a tendency to prefer information that suits our expectations and deny that in some cases we accept information selectively and ignore parts of it. A genuine expert in the field, on the other hand, learns about bias and the rule of minimum assumptions, and consciously attempts to keep the mind open to see beyond the preconception and assumptions.

Features of Trichological Consultation

In the authors' experience, it is important to pay special attention to the initial consultation in order to build a working relationship with the patient. In contrast to the classic dermatological visit, along with a detailed history and clinical examination, trichological consultations involve special trichological examinations. When interpreted responsibly, these methods are valuable tools for the diagnosis and management of disease. Diameter, density, and growth phase are the hair growth parameters of greatest importance and interest to physicians. Trichoscopy is recognized as the gold standard for examining a patient with hair and scalp disease. Visualization of a trichological problem or its absence along with the explanation of the visual result, as well as demonstrating the therapeutic effect have a positive impact and involve the patient in the treatment and diagnostic process. The phototrichogram allowing to assess the anagen/telogen ratio remains the ideal choice for quantitative measurements. Nevertheless, clinical practice shows that a prerequisite for testing systems should be safety and simplicity, and from the patient's psychological standpoint, their noninvasive nature. In addition, valid assessment of actual hair loss and monitoring of quantitative parameters for hair growth are simply undeniable and will be evident to both the doctor and the patient. Quantifying, and objectifying the diagnosis has a psychotherapeutic effect. Complementary intelligent TrichoLAB products, created in collaboration with FotoFinder, will help improve the compliance. Their implementation into daily clinical practice, along with a noninvasive assessment of quantitative hair growth (without shaving) parameters, provides an opportunity to support your opinion with an independent second opinion in the same clinic.

Based on the epidemiology of primary and secondary psychopathology, a trichological consultation should include, in addition to trichodiagnosis and effective trichotherapy, identification, proper diagnosis, and treatment of stress-related depressive and anxiety disorders, as well as adjustment disorders, using the framework of psychosomatic psychotherapy.

Some patients lack insight about the recognition of a psychological component associated with their hair disease, and in these situations, the treating physician bears a special responsibility for diagnosis and management. Proper understanding and knowledge of psychopathological factors involved in psychotrichological disorders will help the trichologist to create a specialized management plan. In addition to a comprehensive trichodermatological assessment, patient consultations should include an evaluation of mental status, specifically the identification of underlying stress and psychopathology and the impact of hair disease on the general psychosocial and functional state.

Often patients seek advice from a specialist in hair diseases presenting without abnormalities in hair growth or appearance, or with changes that are age-appropriate and within the normal range. Patients suffering from somatoform disorders who believe their hair is falling out are extremely difficult to treat. The majority of them refuse to participate in psychosomatic diagnostic methods or receive treatment. If diagnostic tests fail to identify a hair disorder that exists in the patient's subjective opinion, it can lead to conflict between the doctor and the patient. Solely referral of the patient to a psychiatrist is rarely helpful. Interdisciplinary consultations such as trichology–psychiatry liaison may be extremely beneficial in these cases. Treatment of patients with chronic TE, as well as patients with hair-related obsessive-compulsive disorder, may be limited to consultations from competent and caring physicians, who is knowledgeable with psychosomatic aspects of the disease.

Despite the availability of innovative diagnostic and therapeutic methods, the communication remains the most powerful tool in the physician's armamentarium. What the doctor says, how it is done, and what the doctor believes have a profound effect on the treatment outcome. A special skill of the doctor is being a master of the spoken word that inspires the patient's faith in healing. The culture of prescribing therapy has the placebo effect. In addition to the brand name, cost, and how the product or procedure is used, the placebo effect depends on how the prescription is made.

We are all aware of the power of words to both hurt and heal. Physicians should be cautious when defining terminology in patient counselling, especially when employing terms like "psychogenic pseudo-effluvium" and others that may be upsetting or challenging for patients. It is recommended to manage and treat challenging patients, who are convinced of their hair loss and often report their symptoms in a categorical and demanding manner, taking into account biopsychosocial aspects.

> Promise less, deliver more.

Identification and monitoring of the patient's expectations is another basic component of the psychotrichological approach. It is necessary to manage both positive and risk expectations at all stages: before, during, and after treatment. The main biological aspects are usually associated with the timing of hair regrowth, the amount of regrowing hair, and the complete cure of the disease. Psychosocial results are recognized as an equally important aspect for monitoring [2]. Thus, the discussion of individual treatment goals and shaping of realistic expectations present important aspects of consultation with patients complaining of changes in their hair and scalp condition [3].

For example, it's necessary to explain the nature of the disease in cases of scarring hair loss, especially at the fibrosing stage, and to emphasize that the major goal of therapy is to halt the inflammatory process that causes additional irreparable hair loss.

When discussing the desired therapy effect with the patient during the initial consultation, it is critical to specify the time frame for this effect to occur. For example, when counseling patients with TE, it is important to emphasize that shedding of "old" hair that completed the growth phase prior to the start of therapy will continue during the first month or two of treatment. Otherwise, by the end of the second month of treatment, or even sooner, the patient may conclude that the treatment is ineffective, be disappointed, and discontinue treatment, or begin unproven self-medication. In the latter case, the patient may notice an improvement but erroneously conclude that it was due to self-medication.

As a result of this common scenario, the patient does not receive appropriate therapy, and, more importantly, it creates conditions for unfounded conclusions, stereotypes, and incorrect beliefs about the ineffectiveness of proven and evidence-based treatments and the efficacy of some nonproven medications.

In a clinical study by Desai [4], it was shown that one in six patients is perceived as "difficult" by clinicians, and patients' expectations are often too high in the case of elective medical procedures such as hair transplantation. The authors note that patient dissatisfaction has to do with multiple factors, both within and outside the control of the surgeon. However, in the present times of development of electronic information and the importance of rankings, managing difficult patients is a critical skill for physicians, as poor patient feedback can undermine the reputation built over years of of meticulous practice.

Despite being one of the most advanced fields of modern medicine, trichology is still riddled with myths that give rise to charlatanism and misinformation. Patients are so concerned about hair loss that they are ready to fall victim to a variety of pseudo-specialists. The Internet and social networks, which are both our friends and foes, have made the situation much worse and complicated.

According to the authors' experience, a physician who is consulting a patient with hair disorder spends a great deal of time, effort, and energy fighting myths, as the poor outcome of "treatment" by charlatans disappoints the patient and casts a shadow on the entire medical community. And this is another characteristic feature of a patient with hair pathology.

In an observational cross-sectional study, Iglesias-Puzas and co-authors concluded that the majority of the contents often shared on social networks are below acceptable quality standards. According to the study, TikTok Patients produced 64.5% (118/183) of videos, while board-certified dermatologists produced 9.8% (18/183). About 54.6% (100/183) of videos were categorized as primarily depicting "personal experiences," followed by 32.8% (60/183) that were considered primarily "educational." Of these "educational" videos, 70.0% (42/60) discussed treatments, 58.3% (35/60) etiology, 15.0% (9/60) diagnosis, and 8.3% (5/60) nutrition.

In order to avoid such incidents, during consultations it is necessary to pay attention to trichopathology and psychological education, providing explanation of the hair cycle dynamics, information about the disease, including its the biopsychosocial aspect, as well as about dermatotrichological "fake-news" [5].

Table 4.1 National associations created for social adaptation and psychological support of alopets and their family members

Country	Organization	Contacts
USA	National Alopecia Areata Foundation	https://www.naaf.org
UK	Alopecia UK	www.alopecia.org.uk
Italy	Associazione areata and friends	www.lopeciaareataandfriends.com
Israel	Heads Up Alopecia areata	headsup.org.il
Germany	Deutschland e.V.	kreisrunderhaarausfall.de
Spain	Spanish Group of Trichology	aedv.es/institucional/grupos-de-trabajo/tricologia
Switzerland	Alopecia Areata Schweiz	/kreisrunderhaarausfall.ch
France	Alopécie areata association	www.Associationalopeciaareata.fr
Lithuania	Nacionalinė alopecijos asociacija	www.alopecia.lt
Ukraine	Alopecia School	https://alopecia.org.ua

Table 4.2 Practical guidelines for counseling patients with psychotrichological diseases

Pay special attention to psychological impact in the initial consultation
Show empathy and build a working relationship with a challenging patient
Perform trichoscopy and give visual presentation of the dermatotrichological problem or its absence along with the explanation of the visual result
Perform a quantitative trichoscopic analysis to objectify the picture and follow up, which will be evident to both the doctor and the patient
Evaluate patient's mental status, including stress levels and the impact of illness on their quality of life
Conduct trichological and psychological education: explain hair cycle dynamics, give information about the disease, including its biopsychosocial aspect
Discuss individual treatment goals and set realistic expectations
Develop a common concept of trichological and biopsychosocial treatment
Explain short-term and long-term goals and compliance measures
Discuss further motivation, indications, use of specific therapies including relaxation techniques, indications for psychotherapy/psychopharmacotherapy
If necessary, refer the patient to a psychological support organization
Get the best management approach through psychiatry and psychology services to provide a holistic approach in the management of psychotrichological patients

For patients with some types of hair loss, the inconsistency between the clinical severity of alopecia and the disease impact on the quality of life (QoL) has been reliably established. These data provide a serious justification for assessing QoL as an integral indicator that describes a deep multifaceted analysis of changes in human functioning, as both a criterion for choosing therapy and a criterion for its efficacy in the process of monitoring patients with hair pathologies (see Chap. 3).

A trichologist in addition to showing concern and professional management, can refer the patient to get psychological help [6–8]. All around the world national associations have been created, and their goals include social adaptation and psychological support for patients and their family members (Table 4.1). Many of these organizations specialize in providing educational materials for patients and their families about the nature and prognosis of their hair disease. These organizations aid in overcoming a feeling of isolation often experienced by these patients. Finally, additional information about various treatment options reduces the risk of premature withdrawal from therapy and come to terms with uncontrolled alopecia. Having hope is essential in maintaining a positive attitude despite chronic or relapsing illness.

The table below contains practical recommendations for counseling patients with psychotrichological diseases (Table 4.2). The intensity of stress experienced by a patient, according to the authors, should be considered when a physician decides how aggressively to treat a hair condition. For example, when there is a significant negative impact on QoL, the degree of stress experienced by a patient due to alopecia may influence the decision to prescribe or not prescribe systemic finasteride in borderline cases of AGA, to recommend or not recommend surgical hair restoration, or to decide about the use of immunosuppressant agent in a patient with limited alopecia areata.

Summary

- The research of the mental components associated with trichological manifestations addresses a modern personalized patient-centered approach. This strategy is aimed not only at managing trichopathology, but also at assessing the most comprehensive picture of the disease, as well as at improving patient's quality of life, which should be considered as the main therapeutic goal.
- The main principle of treating psychotrichological disorders is a multiprofessional approach that combines trichotropic therapy with psychopharmacotherapy (that must be individualized, taking into account the disease's mental manifestations) and is supplemented by psychocorrectional influences

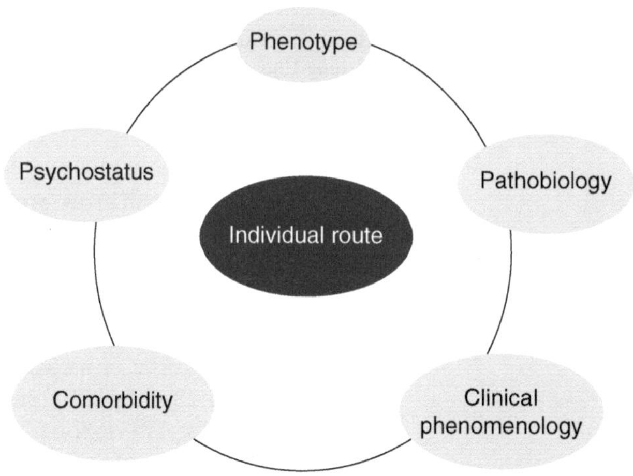

Fig. 4.1 Schematics of an individual therapeutic route based on patient's phenotype, pathobiology, clinical phenomenology, somatic comorbidity, and psychostatus

(cognitive-behavioral psychotherapy with the inclusion of educational methods, elements of indirect suggestions, and relaxation techniques).

- These circumstances define the characteristics of psychotrichological patients' medical management, which entails an interdisciplinary collaboration between dermatotrichologists, psychiatrists, psychologists, and general practitioners.
- In summary, it can be noted that there is a need for a paradigm shift in the treatment of hair diseases from monotargeted to multipurpose therapeutic approaches, and the development of an individual route for each patient should be grounded on phenotype, pathobiology, clinical phenomenology, somatic comorbidity, and psychostatus (Fig. 4.1).

References

1. Groopman J. How doctors think. Boston, New York: Houghton Mifflin Company; 2007.
2. Gorbatenko-Roth K, Wood S, Johnson M, Wallander I, Nugent J, Hordinsky M. Beyond health-related quality of life: initial psychometric validation of a new scale for addressing the gap in assessing the full range of alopecia areata psychosocial burden. Br J Dermatol. 2023;189(1):71–9.
3. Ovcharenko Y. Psychotrichology: new paradigm in management of patients with hair disorders //Abstract book WCHR 2022, Melbourn, Australia, p 140.
4. Desai V. Managing an Unhappy Patient. Indian J Plast Surg. 2021;54(4):495–500. https://doi.org/10.1055/s-0041-1739249.
5. Iglesias-Puzas Á, Conde-Taboada A, Aranegui-Arteaga B, López-Bran E. "Fake news" in dermatology. Results from an observational, cross-sectional study. Int J Dermatol. 2021;60(3):358–62. https://doi.org/10.1111/ijd.15254. Epub 2020 Oct 23. PMID: 33095467.
6. Harth W, Blume-Peytavi U. Psychotrichology: psychosomatic aspects of hair diseases. J Dtsch Dermatol Ges. 2013;11(2):125–35. https://doi.org/10.1111/j.1610-0387.2012.08034.x. Epub 2012 Nov 26
7. Harth W, Gieler U, Kusnir D, Tausk FA. Clinical management of psychodermatology. 1st ed. New York: Springer; 2009.
8. Ovcharenko YS, Serbina IM, editors. Management of patients with alopecia areata: clinical guidelines. Kharkiv: Charisma Plus Publishing House; 2021. p. 96.

Self-Inflicted Pathology of Hair and Scalp

5

Yuliya Ovcharenko, Nino Lortkipanidze, and Lidia Rudnicka

Introduction

Disorders characterized by self-destructive actions toward hair and skin are primary mental disorders that are typically diagnosed by a dermatologist and represent a rather diverse group of conditions.

The literature review on mental disorders with symptoms projected on the skin and its appendages has some terminological difficulties reflecting the dominance of the "dermatological paradigm," and the contradictory interpretation of pathology in official classifications. Pathomimia, for example, is a common dermatology term referring to all skin self-destructive lesions that mask primary mental disorders belonging to various nosological groups (from the Greek "pathos"—disease, pathological process +"mimesis"—imitation). The term is equivalent to the concept of "factitious disorder" in DSM-5 interpretation.

Trichotillomania is the most common pathological destruction of hair caused by self-induced pulling. Other less common forms of obsessive hair damage include shaving and cutting (trichotemnomania), scratching and rubbing (trichoteiromania), and biting (trichodaganomania/trichodacnomania). In some cases, patients eat the extracted hair's roots (trichorizophagy) and/or swallow the extracted hair (trichophagy), which can result in the formation of a trichobezoar (a ball of swallowed indigestible material). The patient's self-destructive behavior may be a combination of different clinical patterns, including self-traumatization of the skin (both within the

Y. Ovcharenko (✉)
V. N. Karazin Kharkiv National University, University Clinic "Trichology Institute", Kharkiv, Ukraine

N. Lortkipanidze
Department of Dermatology and Venereology at D. Tvildiani Medical University, Tbilisi, Georgia

L. Rudnicka
Department of Dermatology, Medical University of Warsaw, Warsaw, Poland

Y. Ovcharenko et al. (eds.), *Psychotrichology*,
https://doi.org/10.1007/978-3-031-64083-4_5

areas of hair damage and in other parts of the body) and nails. Their possible manifestations (neurotic excoriations, onychotillomania, onychophagia, cheilophagy, etc.) will be an additional marker, a psychopathological symptom complex.

In the spectrum of mental disorders characterized by self-induced lesions, including on the scalp, is dermatitis artefacta, although self-damage behavior can also be observed in other psychopathologies, such as delusions of parasitosis. However, it is worth remembering that these clinical consequences, in addition to pathological body sensations of psychiatric origin, which may be the cause of secondary skin lesions, may result from systemic and neurological itching. The management of patients with self-destructive behavior toward hair and scalp is an interdisciplinary task. This chapter proposes a systematic approach on the stages of the diagnostic search for this group of patients and on combination therapy principles using psychopharmacology, psychotherapeutic measures, and dermatologic treatments.

Trichotillomania

Trichotillomania (TTM), among psychiatric pathologies with trichological disorders, is a very interesting nosological unit, insufficiently studied and little known to doctors of many specialties.

TTM is a compulsive habit of consciously or unconsciously pulling one's hair, which results in small or large patches of uneven hair loss without a typical distribution pattern. In this condition eyebrows and eyelashes can also be affected.

TTM is currently classified as a part of the obsessive-compulsive spectrum in DSM-5. TTM can be an episodic psychiatric disorder, but it is more often chronic and difficult to treat. Trichotillomania's comorbidity and phenomenology broaden the concept of obsessive-compulsive disorder to a spectrum of inadequate, excessive manipulation of one's appearance.

The term "trichotillomania" was introduced in 1889 by the French dermatologist François Henri Hallopeau, who presented to the medical community the case of the young man suffering from itching of the scalp. When the itching became unbearable, the patient pulled out his hair. The phenomenon was called trichotillomania. The name comes from three Greek words: "trich"—hair, "tillo"—pulling out, "mania"—pathological attraction.

In 1968 Vaughan, Sawyers, and Scott described the Rapunzel syndrome (named after the protagonist of the Brothers Grimm's fairy tale of the same name about a girl with very long hair)—a type of intestinal obstruction caused by the systematic ingestion of plucked hair (trichophagia), resulting in the formation of a conglomerate consisting of hair (trichobezoar) in the stomach and small intestine [1].

Epidemiology. Previously, it was erroneously believed that TTM was an extremely rare disease. However, epidemiological studies have shown the worldwide prevalence of TTM in the range of 1%–3.5% [2]. There is an opinion that because some respondents denied their behavior and refused to ask for assistance, the true prevalence of TTM is likely underestimated.

TTM is most common in adolescence (between the ages of 11 and 13), has a chronic course, and relapses. Children under the age of five are also prone to hair pulling (baby trich), but this condition usually resolves on its own. TTM is distinguished by a bimodal course (first peak—at preschool age, second—at age of puberty onset). Parents rarely notice their child's behavior, and most do not believe their child is capable of pulling out their own hair. Adult-onset TTM is uncommon, with frequent relapses. The later the disease manifests itself, the more severe its course.

Etiopathogenesis. A dense network of afferent and efferent nerve fibers innervates the skin and its derivatives. This factor is important in the pathogenesis of self-inflicted dermatoses because the skin is frequently the focus of stress reduction and emotionally regulated behavior, particularly during arousal.

TTM most often develops as a syndrome within obsessive-compulsive disorder, depression, post-traumatic stress disorder, schizophrenia, organic brain diseases, congenital developmental anomalies (oligophrenia), but it can also manifest as a separate mental disorder (ICD-1 0 F63.3) [3].

Children raised in strict families with unreasonable demands on the child, which are difficult to meet and may result in the development of a neurotic personality, are especially vulnerable to TTM. Emotional impact, sexual abuse, physical abuse, and emotional deficit at a young age all play a role. In such cases, TTM is a child's reaction to the current situation. The sensation of self-inflicted pain can help to alleviate feelings of isolation and distress.

Another ethological prerequisite for trichotillomanic reactions may include the mechanism of redirected aggression, capable of redirecting repressed anger and irritation toward the offender to uninvolved persons, random objects, and one's own body. Pain from an injury triggers endorphin release giving the patient a short-term sense of satisfaction and further motivating them to repeat similar actions.

In a series of observations, the habit of twisting, pulling, manipulating hair, and other signs of trichomaniac behavior (as a non-pathological or conditionally pathological habit) are noted from infancy and persist for a number of years without the addition of pulling one's own hair. In other cases, this transformation occurs as a result of psycho- or somatogenic harm. Difficulties with adaptation in a child care center, post-influenza asthenia, and other factors may serve as a trigger for such degeneration of an individual habit at the age of 2–3 years. The question arises regarding the criteria for transforming an individual's non-pathological habit into a pathological one, which are currently being researched.

The role of serotonin deficiency in the pathogenesis of TTM is discussed (the theory of neurochemical imbalance). As evidence, they refer to the high efficacy of antidepressants from the group of selective serotonin reuptake inhibitors in the disease treatment. However, according to other authors, antidepressants can increase the severity of TTM.

Investigations into the genetic predisposition of TTM are currently ongoing. Two mutant forms of the SLITKR1 gene, which is responsible for the connections between brain neurons, have been found to occur more frequently in individuals with this pathology, according to research.

A Hoxb8 gene defect is also linked to TTM development. In experiments on mice, it was demonstrated that a pathological urge to pull out one's fur is brought on by a decreased number of glial macrophages brought on by a Hoxb8 gene defect. The majority of mice recovered with the growth of their fur following bone marrow transplantation, but some healthy mice that received mutant bone marrow developed illnesses. Similar research is currently being done on TTM patients to find out if they have Hoxb8 gene mutations.

Clinical Features. The typical clinical picture of TTM is characterized by hair thinning or baldness in the easily accessible frontoparietal region of the scalp, pubis, eyebrows, and eyelashes. There may be a single or multiple patches of baldness, with normal skin and clearly defined follicular ostia [4].

Hair pulling can be classified into three types: automatic (unconscious), conscious (focused), and combined. Patients are overwhelmed by emotional strain prior to the hair pulling action, and after the hair is pulled, they feel relief and satisfaction. Clinical patterns include local (limited and large-scale, up to total damage), diffuse and geometric (Fig. 5.1a–d). Eyebrow and eyelash damage can be both symmetrical and asymmetrical (Fig. 5.1e).

The habit of pulling hair transforms into a complex fixed behavioral ritual at the stage of behavioral automatism. Children are the most commonly affected. The established behavioral habit becomes more automated the longer it exists. Patients are unaware that they are pulling out their hair, and the consequences, in the form of patches of pseudo-alopecia, are only known to others. It is also difficult to obtain information from patients about the duration, frequency, and number of auto-depilations during a single episode of hair-pulling [5].

TTM is an important ritual in conscious pulling. The process is usually carried out in solitude. A person is preparing for the procedure by getting tweezers, making a suitable setting, etc. In most cases, a patient spends 1–3 h per day pulling out their hair. Hundreds of hairs are plucked during this time period. Occasionally, plucking occurs in short bursts where only a few hairs are pulled each time.

Social consequences of the disease are the most common complications of TTM: a patient is avoiding social contacts in fear of being discovered.

Because of the constant irritation of hair growth sites, there are skin and eye infections. There is also a risk of irreversible damage to hair follicles in the damaged area as a result of repeated trauma.

Addictive behavior can be combined with onychophagia (nail biting) and trichophagia, resulting in dental problems such as enamel erosion and other tooth damage. Hair cannot be expelled normally from the stomach and they keep accumulating. As a result, a trichobezoar, which can reach to enormous proportions, forms in the stomach (Fig. 5.2). These trichobezoars necessitate surgical intervention. Cases of 1.5 and even 2 kg hairball removal have been described.

The following variants are described in the clinical phenomenology of obsessive self-traumatization of hair.

Trichotemnomania (from Greek "temnein"—to cut). This condition is characterized by deliberate shortening of the hair with various sharp instruments. Patients usually cut or shave the hair in secret to attract attention. Areas of shaved or cut hair

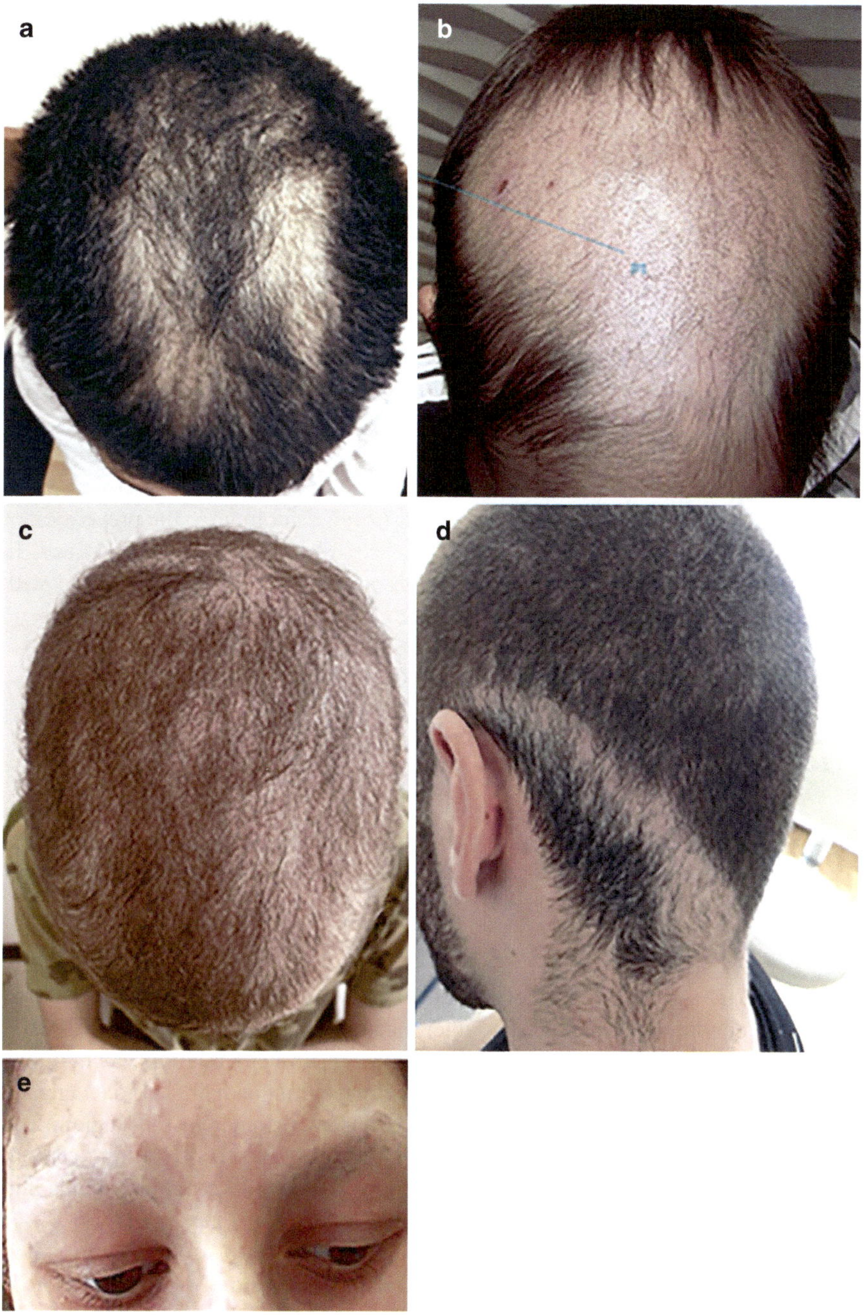

Fig. 5.1 Clinical patterns of trichotillomania: focal limited (**a**); focal large-scale (**b**); diffuse (**c**); and geometrical (**d**); trichotillomania of the eyebrows and eyelashes (**e**)

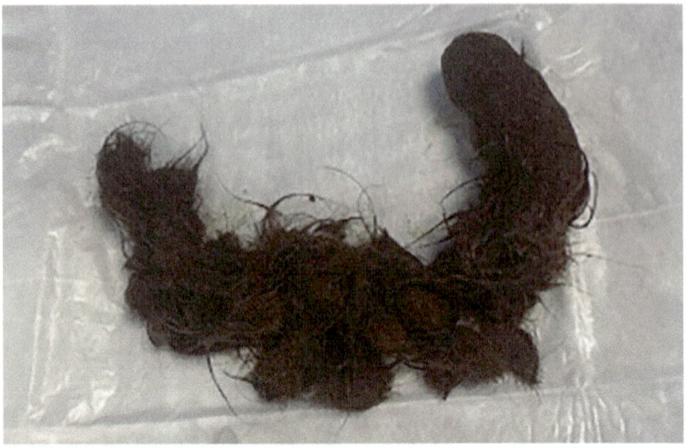

Fig. 5.2 Trichobezoar

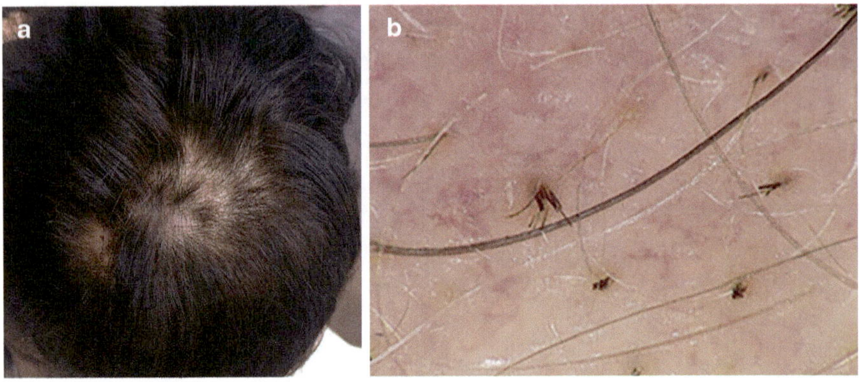

Fig. 5.3 Trichoteiromania: Split ends of the hair shaft in a pseudoalopecia lesion, as well as lichenification of the scalp skin (**a**); trichoscopic image of the trichoteiromania patch shows broom hairs and diffuse congestive erythema (×60) (**b**)

most often are visible on the scalp or other hairy areas of the body. To a greater extent, the condition is a simulation rather than an obsessive-compulsive disorder.

Trichoteiromania (from the Greek "teiro"—to scratch) is a type of fictitious hair loss caused by constant friction of the scalp, resulting in hair shaft damage and pseudo-alopecia. The disease is linked to a sensory disorder in this region. The unaided eye can see the tufted ends of the hair (Fig. 5.3a). Hair splitting (broom hairs) is visible on trichoscopy (Fig. 5.3b) Many patients have mild erythema and broken off hair shafts of varying lengths [6].

Trichodaganomania (from the Greek "dagano"—to bite) is an uncontrollable habit of, an addiction to biting one's hair. **Trichodaknomania**—is an addiction to biting other people's hair. Patients with trichodaganomania/trichodaknomania bite hair on their own or another person's arm. Diagnosis is confirmed by clinical history. Comorbid depression, anxiety, and obsessive-compulsive behaviors are commonly seen [7].

Trichophagy. In rare cases, patients swallow hair that they pull out or otherwise extract. This can lead to trichobezoar formation in the stomach, which sometimes moves to the small intestine. In Rapunzel syndrome, the hair ball can even reach the large intestine. The condition is associated with an increased risk of intestinal obstruction, perforation, or anorexia due to impaired nutrient absorption [1].

Trichorizophagia, an extremely rare type of trichophagia, has been reported in adults. Patients with this condition eat the roots of plucked hair. It is an obsessive-compulsive spectrum disorder with associated psychopathology, like other forms of self-inflicted hair loss. Patients' extracted hair is frequently manipulated, examined, and played with before being eaten. These patients frequently exhibit obsessive behaviors, anxiety, and depression.

Diagnosis of TTM is based on the patient's medical history and findings at clinical examination. Additionally, trichoscopy, biopsy, and hair pull test can confirm the diagnosis of TTM.

According to the American Psychiatric Association's Diagnostic and Statistical Manual of Mental Disorders, fifth edition (DSM-5), the diagnostic criteria for TTM are:

1. The recurrent pulling out of one's own hair, resulting in noticeable hair loss.
2. Repeated attempts by the patient to stop these actions or reduce their frequency.
3. Hair pulling causes clinically significant distress or
4. impairment in social, occupational, or other important areas of functioning.
5. Hair pulling or loss is not due to any other medical condition (e.g., dermatological).
6. Hair pulling is not a symptom of another psychiatric disorder (such as patient's attempts to improve apparent defects in appearance, observed in body dysmorphic disorder).

Psychiatric assessment of TTM is based on the use of questionnaires. Several psychometric scales for assessing the severity of TTM have been developed (see Chap. 2).

On examination, bald or thinning hair areas are visible on the scalp, pubis, brows, and eyelashes. Alopecia patches can be single, multiple, rounded, linear, or irregular in shape. The follicular ostia are clearly visible, and the skin of these patches feels normal or coarse to the touch. The majority of the time, hair shafts are irregular in length, can be split in the middle, or simply appear as small black dots or stubble. In the hair loss areas, excoriations, pustules, erythema, and peeling are frequently seen. It's important to look at the patient's nails because constant friction can make them appear very sharp and shiny [5].

Trichoscopic examination plays a significant role in objectifying the TTM clinical picture and demonstrates the following: decrease in hair density; hair broken at different lengths, black dots (Fig. 5.4a); short hairs with trichoptilosis (split ends); asymmetrically twisted hair, upright regrowing hairs; perifollicular erythema and hyperpigmentation or hemorrhage may be seen (Fig. 5.4b); yellow dots are not typical. In a recent study, new trichoscopic signs of TTM have been identified: residues

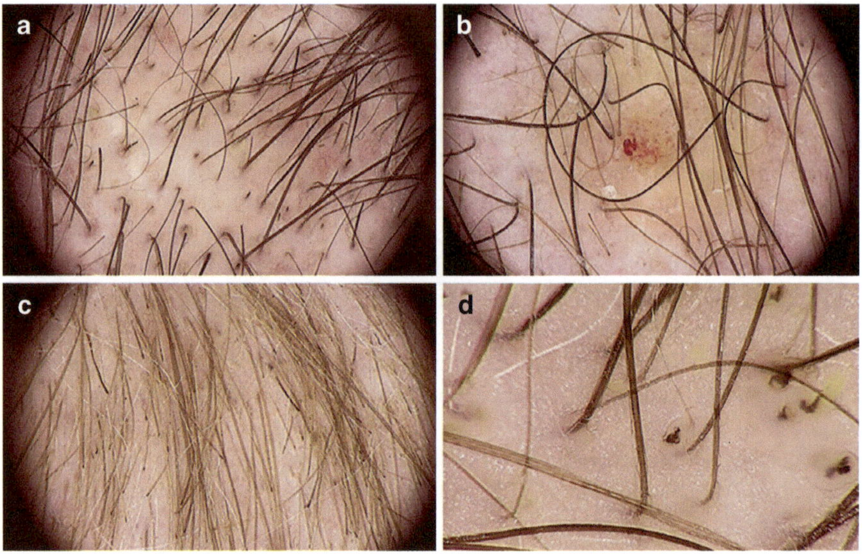

Fig. 5.4 Trichoscopic signs of trichotillomania: irregularly broken hairs, black dots (**a**) (×20); hemorrhage (**b**) (×20); tulip hairs (**c**); flame hairs, trichomalacia (**d**) (×60)

of hair shafts by shape resembling a tulip (tulip hairs) (Fig. 5.4c), flames (flame hairs) (Fig. 5.4d), the letter V as well as shapeless hair residues (trichomalacia) (Fig. 5.4d). Exclamation mark hairs are rare in trichotillomania, but they can become a diagnostic trap and lead to misdiagnosis of alopecia areata (AA), which in rare cases may become a triggering event. These two conditions can coexist, further complicating trichoscopic differential diagnosis. TTM is the most difficult differential diagnosis of AA. In over 50% of cases, the diagnosis of AA is initially established. A negative pull test is another differential criterion for trichotillomania, which will help to distinguish it from AA [8–10].

Histology. Hemorrhages, intrafollicular fissures, and perifollicular fissures are visible in the early stages. Perifollicular fibrosis and sometimes granulomas appear as the illness progresses. Trichomalacia and empty hair channels are distinguishing characteristics. Perifollicular inflammation characteristic of AA is absent [11].

Children with trichophagia should have an iron level tested as part of their screening because iron deficiency has been linked to pica, an unusual craving for nonfood items. Treatment with therapeutic doses of oral iron usually resolves compulsive behavior. Iron deficiency can cause trichophagia or be the result of gastrointestinal bleeding in the case of trichobezoar [12].

Differential diagnosis. Some disorders present with similar or even the same symptoms. Therefore, for clinicians to make an accurate diagnosis, it is necessary to differentiate the following dermatological disorders:

- Alopecia areata
- Loose anagen hair

- Mycosis of the scalp
- Traumatic alopecia due to abuse (battered child syndrome)

and psychiatric disorders

- Telogenomania (obsessive-compulsive fits of fierce hair brushing usually in women)
- Trichophobia (plucking hair due to a delusional conviction in the need to extract something from the hair roots)
- Factitious disorder

Trichotillomania associated with alopecia areata can sometimes cause diagnostic impasse. Trichotillomania can be caused by scratching the AA patch when symptomatic itching occurs, resulting in a habit-forming behavior, or it can be caused by patients with a psychological predisposition deliberately prolonging the disfigurement. These behaviors may be maintained to meet the dependency needs that were previously met during the AA episode [13].

Treatment. TTM therapy should be tailored to the individual. It is necessary to identify and eliminate the psychological cause. Reducing emotional pressure and demands from parents as well as increasing trust are factors that will help to improve the child's condition [14, 15].

Dermatologist's task is to confirm the diagnosis of TTM and convince the patient and their relatives to visit a psychiatrist. Symptomatic treatment is possible: hair growth stimulants, antiseptics and local antibiotics in secondary infection, etc.

Habit Reversal Therapy, a modified type of Cognitive-behavioral psychotherapy is the "gold standard" and evidence-based treatment for TTM treatment. Its multiple components include awareness training, stimulus control, substitution techniques and generalization techniques, and social support. Numerous studies have confirmed the effectiveness of therapy in many patients [16].

Group psychotherapy is based on the patient's active participation in the psychotherapist-directed treatment. Support groups for TTM patients are uncommon. TTM can, however, be treated in groups for patients with obsessive-compulsive disorder. Hypnosis is an effective alternative method that produces quick results without the need for multiple sessions or hard work on self-improvement. It works especially well on children.

With no FDA-approved treatments for TTM, psychopharmacotherapy remains controversial. In some cases, oral N-acetylcysteine has been reported to be effective. It is also possible to use selective serotonin reuptake inhibitors (SSRIs), particularly if concomitant anxiety or depression component is strong [17].

Physicians who use SSRIs to treat obsessive-compulsive disorder or TTM should be aware that the duration of treatment is critical. When drugs are taken for more than 8–12 weeks, noticeable improvement occurs. In most patients, stopping pharmacotherapy results in relapse [18–20].

Prognosis. From a prognosis standpoint, there are two types of trichotillomania: a temporary localized form in infants and children with a good prognosis (tic d'epilation) and severe adult form, usually found in young women and characterized with larger lesions and poorer prognosis.

Neurotic Excoriation of the Scalp

The term "neurotic excoriations" refers to self-inflicted skin damage in the absence of an underlying specific dermatological disease. From the psychiatry point of view, patients with neurotic excoriations are not a homogeneous group, each requires an individual therapeutic approach.

Patients may present with isolated scalp lesions or, in some cases, excoriations of the face, upper torso, and arms. Because patients can only injure easily accessible areas of the body, the clinical distribution of lesions other than the scalp provides a clue to the diagnosis. The initial cause of the excoriations may be a pre-existing skin disease or minor skin surface irregularities (keratin plug, insect bite, acne papule (acne excoriee), or irritation of the hair follicle), but they frequently occur de novo. These patients have a lower itching sensitivity threshold and a proclivity for habitual or neurotic scratching. Scratching can begin inadvertently when the hand comes into contact with irregularities on the skin's surface, or it can occur as a ritual, sometimes accompanied by the use of additional tools such as a knife tip, etc. Itching may be caused by tissue damage, and the itch-scratch cycle takes on a life of its own. Typically, such activity is observed in conjunction with the induction of psychosocial stressors. The condition can manifest itself at any age, from childhood to old age, with the most severe and persistent cases manifesting themselves in the third to fifth decade of life [4].

Etiopathogenesis. Neurotic excoriations are common across the entire psychopathology spectrum. In mild and transient cases, they may be a reaction to stress, particularly in younger patients, such as exam stress (mental itch), and are more common in people with obsessive-compulsive personality traits. These patients have poor impulse control, and the tension caused by the conflict is relieved by skin damage.

In more severe and persistent cases, a generalized anxiety disorder (ICD-10 F41.1), depression (ICD-10 F34.1), or obsessive-compulsive disorder (ICD-10 F42.x) may be diagnosed. From a psychobiological standpoint, obsessive-compulsive disorder is associated with decreased activity in serotonin-mediated neural pathways.

Clinical features. Self-inflicted lesions are nonspecific. Lesions range in size from a few millimeters to several centimeters and can be seen at any stage of development, from small superficial excoriations to deep skin defects (Fig. 5.5), thickened hyperpigmented skin, and finally hypopigmented atrophic scars. Secondary bacterial infection (most commonly caused by *Staphylococcus aureus*) can cause regional lymphadenopathy [4].

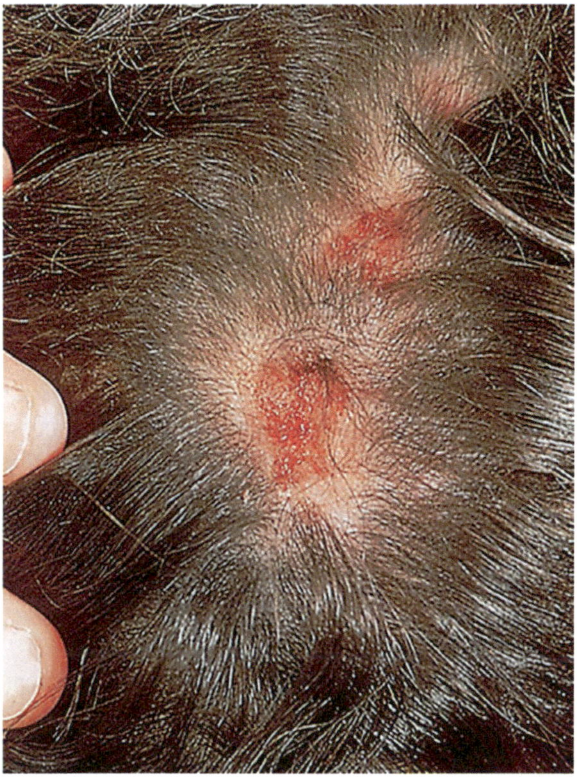

Fig. 5.5 Neurotic excoriations of the scalp. *Clinical observations of Ralph Trüeb*

Histology. The histological picture is typical for excoriation with nonspecific inflammatory changes.

Differential diagnosis. Neurotic excoriations of the scalp are observed in some itchy dermatoses:

- Atopic dermatitis
- Folliculitis necrotica
- Discoid lupus erythematosus
- Pemphigus vulgaris
- Pemphigoid
- Parasitic infection

May cause neurological disorders, drug or substance abuse, and psychiatric disorders:

- Cocaine intoxication
- Delusions of parasitosis
- Factitial dermatitis

The diagnosis is confirmed by the presence of psychopathology based on history and clinical observation.

Topical agents containing glucocorticoids, as well as sedative antihistamines (hydroxyzine or doxepin), are used to treat dermatological condition. Cold soothing and moisturizing compresses are used to relieve itching and facilitate wound cleaning. If there is a secondary bacterial infection, oral antibiotics may be prescribed. Shampoos for sensitive skin are advised for both therapeutic and preventative care.

Many patients who visit a dermatologist, however, are hesitant to accept the psychiatric component of their skin condition and are unaware of the circumstances that cause the urge for excoriations.

Pharmacological and non-pharmacological therapeutic options are both used in psychiatric treatment. The best treatment option or drug will be determined by the underlying mental disorder.

Specific and nonspecific approaches are used in patients suffering from excessive stress. Exercise, biofeedback, yoga, self-hypnosis, progressive relaxation, and other techniques taught in stress management programs are examples of non-pharmacological methods [21].

Pharmacological treatment is available for patients with neurotic excoriations and obsessive-compulsive disorder. Anxiolytics may be an alternative for patients who demonstrate high anxiety and stress. Non-benzodiazepine slow-release anxiolytics (such as buspirone) exhibit a higher level of safety in this drug class. It is important to keep in mind that the buspirone effect typically does not appear for the first 2–4 weeks of treatment. Low-dose doxepin may be considered in patients with chronic anxiety disorder who are not responsive to buspirone. Doxepin is a tricyclic antidepressant, but in low doses, it has an anxiety-relieving effect similar to benzodiazepines. Selective serotonin reuptake inhibitors are safe to use for anxiety. Benzodiazepines should be discouraged at all costs due to addiction potential.

In depressed patients with neurotic excoriations, doxepin is the most effective tricyclic antidepressant. If doxepin's sedative properties are intolerable, the newer selective serotonin reuptake inhibitors such as fluoxetine, sertraline, or paroxetine, may be an option. Due to its potential to lessen compulsive behavior, SSRI is thought to be the most efficient. One of the newer SSRIs (fluoxetine or fluvoxamine maleate), or clomipramine, an older generation antidepressant with extensive published evidence of efficacy in treating obsessive-compulsive disorder, may be prescribed. The patient should be scheduled for regular, brief visits to monitor their dermatological condition and offer emotional support. Individual psychotherapy may be beneficial for patients who need to discuss specific psychological issues, such as workplace frustration, maladaptive behavior in interpersonal relationships, and the presence of maladaptive beliefs about themselves, such as unrealistic expectations or fear of failure [4].

The 1–5 min rule, a behavioral technique that prevents the progression from obsessive thoughts to compulsive behavior, is one of the non-pharmacological approaches to patients who refuse to be referred to a mental health professional. The patient is instructed to wait for some time to pass—ideally 1–5 min—before acting on an obsessive thought or urge to engage in a compulsive behavior. The interval's length is gradually extended to 5, 10, or even 15 min after the patient successfully controls their impulses for 1 min. Finally, such a long interval between compulsive behavior and obsessive thought allows for disruption of the flow from one to the other [21].

Prognosis. In the absence of treatment, the condition persists, and its severity fluctuates in parallel with the level of psychological pressure. Short-term cases are characterized by a more favorable prognosis.

Factitial Dermatitis of the Scalp

Factitial dermatitis (physically manifested simulation disorder) (ICD-10 F68.1) describes a condition in which a patient tries to intentionally harm their skin to satiate an unconscious psychological need, typically to play the role of the sick person [4].

Such patients feign symptoms, but deny their participation in the production of lesions. They tend to play the sick role and may go from one doctor to another to get help. They are typically loners who suffered trauma and deprivation as young children, are unable to form strong interpersonal bonds, and have severe personality disorders. Patients with factitious disorder self-injure themselves for psychological reasons rather than for any benefits, unlike conscious malingerers (ICD-10 Z76.5): they undergo medical procedures and run the risk of developing drug dependence and postoperative complications. A series of hospitalizations turn into a lifelong habit in a more severe form known as Munchausen's syndrome, also known as laparotomophilia. The condition is common in women in all of the series of cases that have been described: from 3:1 to 20:1 female to male ratio, with an average onset age of early adulthood; many patients are employed in the medical field [22].

Etiopathogenesis. Factitious disorder's etiology is not well understood. According to some researchers, patients with factitious disorder as children frequently go through traumatic experiences, particularly abuse and deprivation, endure numerous hospitalizations, and as adults, they lack support from friends and/or family. The majority of patients have borderline personality disorder. Self-inflicted wounds serve several functions: the need for dependence is satisfied by the sick role, while excitement and stimulation reduce feelings of emptiness and isolation, the sensation on the skin establishes boundaries, and the formation of a personal and sexual identity.

Clinical features. Factitious dermatitis may manifest as on any part of the body including scalp. A visit to a dermatologist may be part of a series of appointments with other medical professionals. The patient usually arrives at the appointment with normal laboratory results and a full bag of medications. These patients can be described as having a "blank history," as they are unable to explain how they sustained their injuries. The patient's relatives frequently accuse the medical staff of incompetence.

The injuries themselves are as varied as the methods used to inflict them; ulceration usually occurs on the scalp (Fig. 5.6). These lesions are unusual in shape and distribution and typically appear on normal skin [4, 22].

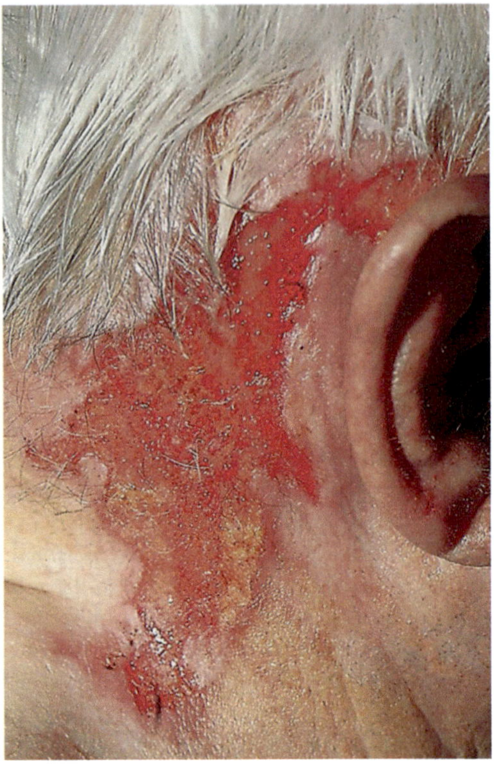

Fig. 5.6 Factitial dermatitis of the scalp. *Clinical observations of Ralph Trueb*

Differential diagnosis. A number of dermatological, neurological, and mental disorders are characterized by similar symptoms. Clinical considerations are determined by morphology and cover the field of clinical dermatology:

- Necrotizing herpes zoster
- Temporal arteritis
- Angiosarcoma
- Neurotrophic ulcers of the scalp
- Neurotic excoriations of the scalp

Treatment. Dermatologic therapy in factitious dermatitis is symptomatic, as it is in other psychotrichological conditions, and its selection is guided by the clinical picture. Wet dressings, emollients, and other soothing topical agents can replace destructive behavior and thus be beneficial, but their effect is only temporary. Occlusive dressings can be used as a diagnostic tool as well as a therapeutic intervention.

The most difficult step is establishing a strong and stable relationship between a patient and a doctor. To achieve this goal, most clinicians advocate a non-conflict strategy that views the symptoms as a "cry for help." The "contractual conference" approach is described. A psychiatrist using this approach emphasizes the need for the patient to express themselves in universal language of complex relationships, feelings, and life problems rather than the disease's fictional language.

Another critical aspect of treatment is identifying and adequately treating commonly associated disorders such as personality disorder, depression, drug and/or alcohol abuse, and dependence. A good response to the antipsychotic drug pimozide has been reported in terms of pharmacological agents. Because of the condition's similarity to obsessive-compulsive disorder, clomipramine or the SSRIs such as fluoxetine, and fluvoxamine maleate were also suggested. [4]

Prognosis. The disease is chronic in the majority of cases, but with the successful establishment of a stable physician–patient relationship, unnecessary hospitalizations and medical procedures can be avoided.

Management of Patient with Self-Inflicted Diseases of Hair and Scalp

Early diagnosis is critical for the effective management of patients with self-inflicted diseases of hair and scalp. It will prevent treatment errors in dermatology, help start appropriate treatment and psychotherapy in timely and adequate manner, preventing the development of complications. In turn, timely psychiatric assessment depending on the range of identified conditions, will reduce the urge to damage one's own skin and increase the effectiveness of interaction between a dermatotrichologist and a psychiatrist in the joint management of this group of patients. Table 5.1 summarizes practical recommendations for early detection of self-inflicted hair and skin diseases.

The type of mental disorders associated with dermatotrichological manifestations should guide psychopharmacotherapy in these patients.

Table 5.1 Clinical, history-based and morphological diagnostics of self-inflicted hair and skin pathologies

Inconsistency between patient history and clinical dermatotrichological picture
Dysfunctional emotional and behavioral patterns
Pathological bodily sensations preceding self-harm, the projection of which reflects the topography of injuries
Clinical observations: unusual, unnatural (chaotic or strictly geometric) configuration of pseudoalopecia or elements of rash
Morphological elements of rash: uniformity with dominant phenomena of linear excoriations and hemorrhagic crusts, erosions, and/or ulcers, in areas with hyper- or hypopigmented spots and scars
Dermatotrichoscopic (chaotic morphology of destroyed hair) and histological (empty hair canals and trichomalacia, hemorrhages, intrafollicular and perifollicular fissures, perifollicular fibrosis and sometimes granulomas) evidence of hair autodestruction
Monitoring: unusual dynamics of hair regrowth/evolution of the skin process in the lesions (sudden appearance of large-scale areas of baldness, rapidly growing hair in areas of pseudoalopecia, long-term nonhealing ulcerative defects and/or relatively rapid resolution of skin lesions without treatment, spontaneously formed scars)

Psychotherapy (cognitive-behavioral with the inclusion of educational approach methods, elements of indirect suggestion, relaxation techniques), in combination with psychotropic drugs, is a valuable method of the treatment.

Topical dermatological treatment should include tissue regeneration stimulators. After skin reepithelization in the pseudoalopecia patch, trichotropic treatment with hair growth stimulants can be prescribed. In patients with somatoform vegetative dysfunction of the skin, topical therapy should include moisturizing agents that, in addition to reducing skin dryness, help to reduce somatoform itching. In patients with impulsive excoriations, limited hypochondria, and delusion of parasitosis, an occlusive protective dressing can be used to reduce skin trauma and accelerate reepithelialization.

Summary

- Disorders characterized by self-destructive actions toward hair and skin are primary mental disorders that are typically diagnosed by a dermatologist and represent a diverse group of conditions.
- Among pathological hair injuries, the most common is trichotillomania, characterized by self-inducted impulsive hair pulling—a mysterious and insufficiently studied disease that motivates further study and identification of key factors in the development of this pathological process. New data will contribute to the understanding of potential disease mechanisms and will be the key to the effective treatment strategies.
- Given the disease's psychotrichological profile, managing patients with pathological hair and scalp destruction necessitates considerable effort, experience, and knowledge, as well as patience and a multidisciplinary diagnostic approach.
- Dermatological treatment in combination with long-term intensive psychotherapy focused on unconscious psychological conflicts can cure patients who meet the criteria for this approach. In other cases, topical agents, emotional support, and psychopharmacological therapy will provide the improvement. Stressful situations frequently lead to exacerbations of existing conditions.

References

1. Vaughan ED Jr, Sawyers JL, Scott HW Jr. The Rapunzel syndrome. An unusual complication of intestinal bezoar. Surgery. 1968;63:339–43.
2. Grzesiak M, Reich A, Szepietowski JC, Hadryś T, Pacan P. Trichotillomania among young adults: prevalence and comorbidity. Acta Derm Venereol. 2017;97(4):509–12.
3. Monzani B, Rijsdijk F, Harris J, Mataix-Cols D. The structure of genetic and environmental risk factors for dimensional representations of DSM-5 obsessive-compulsive spectrum disorders. JAMA Psychiatry. 2014;71(2):182–9.
4. Trüeb RM, Gieler U. Pschychocutaneous disorders of hair and scalp. In: Blume-Peytavi U, Tosti A, Whiting D, Trüeb RM, editors. Hair growth and disorders. New York: Springer; 2008. p. 407–26.

5. Ovcharenko Y. Trichopathies in children. Kharkiv: Maidan; 2017. p. 264.
6. Freyschmidt-Paul P, Hoffmann R, Happle R. Trichoteiromanie. Eur J Dermatol. 2001;11:369–71.
7. Jafferany M, Feng J, Hornung RL. Trichodaganomania: the compulsive habit of biting one's own hair. J Am Acad Dermatol. 2009;60:689–91.
8. Rudnicka L, Olszewska M, Rakowska A. Atlas of trichoscopy. Dermoscopy in hair and scalp disease. London: Springer-Verlag; 2012.
9. Rakowska A, Slovinska M, Olszewska M, Rudnicka L. New trichoscopy findings in trichotillomania: flame hairs, V-sign, hook hairs, hair powder, tulip hairs. Acta Derm Venereol. 2014;94(3):303–6.
10. Abraham L, Torres F, Azulay-Abulafia L. Dermoscopic clues to distinguish trichotillomania from patchy alopecia areata. An Bras Dermatol. 2010;85:723–6.
11. Muller SA. Trichotillomania: a histopathologic study in sixty-six patients. J Am Acad Dermatol. 1990;23:56–62.
12. McGehee FT, Buchanan GR. Trichophagia and trichobezoar: etiologic role of iron deficiency. J Pediatr. 1980;97:946–8.
13. Trüeb RM, Cavegn B. Trichotillomania in connection with alopecia areata. Cutis. 1996;58:67–70.
14. Flessner C, Penzel F, Trichotillomania Learning Center–Scientific Advisory Board, Keuthen NJ. Current treatment practices for children and adults with trichotillomania: consensus among experts. Cogn Behav Pract. 2010;17:290–300.
15. Franklin ME, Zagrabbe K, Benavides KL. Trichotillomania and its treatment: a review and recommendations. Expert Rev Neurother. 2011;11(8):1165–74.
16. Gupta S, Gardi P. Habit reversal training for trichotillomania. Int J Trichol. 2012;4(1):39–41.
17. McGuire JF, Ung J, Selles D, Rahman R, Lewin O, Murphy A, Storch T, et al. Treating trichotillomania: a meta-analysis of treatment effects and moderators for behavior therapy and serotonin reuptake inhibitors. J Psychiatr Res. 2014;58:76–83.
18. Sheikha SH, Wagner KD, Wagner RF. Fluoxetine treatment of trichotillomania and depression in a prepubertal child. Cutis. 1993;51:50–2.
19. Swed SE, Lenane MC, Leonard HL. Long-term treatment of trichotillomania (hair pulling). N Engl J Med. 1993;329:141–2.
20. Johnson J, El-Alfy AT. Review of available studies of the neurobiology and pharmacotherapeutic management of trichotillomania. J Adv Res. 2016;7:169–84.
21. Fruensgaard K. Psychotherapeutic strategy and neurotic excoriations. Int J Dermatol. 1991;30:198–203.
22. Gandy DT. The concept and clinical aspects of factitious dermatitis. South Med J. 1953;46:551–5.

Alopecia Areata

6

Inessa Serbina and Yuliya Ovcharenko

"I have alopecia since I was 9 years old, now I'm 36. First focal, a year ago it progressed to total. I'm hairless practically everywhere: legs, arms, armpits, eyebrows—no hair. I wear a wig. I think about it all the time. Even when I'm sleeping, I worry that the wig would move about. Anyone who hasn't lived through this kind of experience would never understand a living without hair ..."

"When I shaved the rest of the hair on my scalp and saw myself in the mirror ... It was impossible to put into words. Who was that? An alien ... Horror, tears, fear, resentment ... Why me? It was the deepest depression. How to live without hair? ..."

"When people first meet my hairless daughter, they wonder if she has cancer."

"I'm bald. I haven't shaved my head and I'm not going through chemotherapy. This is alopecia, I have had it since I was four. Since five I have been wearing a wig. The more I tried to cover and hide it, the easier it was for people to offend and hurt me. For many years I didn't even think about appearing without a wig ... It was the worst nightmare."

This is a cry from the heart of people who faced reality of living with alopecia areata.

People are cruel, society exists within certain standards, and stereotypes prevail. If you are not like others, you are a "white raven" and people unceremoniously point a finger at you.

I. Serbina (✉)
Department of Infectious Diseases and Clinical Immunology of the V. N. Karazin Kharkiv National University, University Clinic "Trichology Institute", Kharkiv, Ukraine

Y. Ovcharenko
V. N. Karazin Kharkiv National University, University Clinic "Trichology Institute", Kharkiv, Ukraine

Y. Ovcharenko et al. (eds.), *Psychotrichology*,
https://doi.org/10.1007/978-3-031-64083-4_6

Introduction

Alopecia areata (AA) is a chronic relapsing autoimmune inflammatory disease mediated by T-lymphocytes in conditions of impaired immune tolerance of the hair follicle (HF) and activation of the JAK-STAT (Janus Kinases—Signal Transducer and Activator of Transcription) signaling pathway. Manifestations and clinical diversity of AA are conditioned by a complex combination of triggers and genetic factors. The disease has an unpredictable course with non-scarring hair loss, can affect the scalp and/or other hair-bearing body surfaces and manifest as damage to nail plates. It is characterized by various psycho-emotional disorders, social maladaptation with a significant reduction in patients' quality of life (QoL) [1].

> The importance of the problem is confirmed by the efforts to create a international project—Global Registry of Alopecia Areata Disease Severity and Treatment Safety (GRASS) conducted by world renowned experts with the goal of improving the database for future research and development of treatment strategies, as well as improving patient management and outcomes. A community of dermatologists is involved in this initiative, as are patient groups, pharmaco-economists, and pharmaceutical representatives committed to improving patient outcomes and safety [2].

Epidemiology, Genetics, and Immunopathogenesis of Alopecia Areata

According to epidemiological studies conducted in various countries, AA affects between 1.7% and 5% of the population. The disease has a prevalence of 1:1000–3300. The onset of AA can occur at any age, but it is most common before the age of 40. The condition most commonly affects children between the ages of 10 and 25, with 60% of patients falling into this category. According to recent studies, 1%–2% of people with AA are under the age of 2, and 21%–24% are under the age of 16. AA is uncommon in adults over the age of 60.

AA has a 1.7% lifetime risk. Most patients report more than one episode of the disease. The relapse occurs in the form of local small alopecia foci as well as large alopecia patches with complete loss of hair. Severe forms of AA, alopecia totalis (AT) and alopecia universalis (AU), may also develop during the first episode of the disease. Approximately 5%–10% of patients with limited AA progress to complete scalp hair loss (alopecia totalis, (AT)), and 1%–2% progress to complete scalp and trunk hair loss (alopecia universalis, AU). The prevalence of an AA family history in patients with AA was reported to be 10%–20%, compared to 1.7% in controls [3–5].

Information obtained from candidate gene analysis and epidemiological studies have suggested that AA is a disease involving complex interactions between different genes. Among external triggers that could be the basis for the genetic predisposition of AA are environmental factors such as effects of pro-inflammatory substances and, possibly, other modulators, including the most important neurogenic, metabolic, endocrine disorders, allergic conditions, and infectious pathogens [6].

A meta-analysis of genome-wide association studies revealed a strong link between the HLA locus and AA, giving support to the autoimmune origin hypothesis. Individuals with IL-2RA and TNF/LTA loci, as well as the SPATA5 gene on the fourth chromosome, have been shown to be more susceptible to AA. SNPs, STX17, Cxcr3, Cxcl9, Cxcl10, CTLA4, PRDX5, IKZF4/ERBB3, and TNF-308G/A have all been linked to AA development. Polymorphisms in the IL-17A and IL-17RA (IL-17A receptor) genes were discovered in patients with AA. Additional loci for genes involved in the apoptosis activation pathway, regulatory T cells (Treg), and JAK-STAT signaling have been identified, with some of these genes implicated in the development of other autoimmune diseases. The ULBP3 gene (cytomegalovirus-binding protein) on the sixth chromosome (6q25), which encodes activating ligands of the natural killer cell receptor NKG2D and initiating an autoimmune response, was found to be overexpressed in AA. These findings suggest that abnormal antigen presentation and autoimmunity regulation may play a role in the onset of AA [7].

Cytokines are considered as a mediator in the pathophysiological stage of autoimmune reactions in AA, which disrupts the mechanisms maintaining the state of immune tolerance in HF structures. The primary role in the pathogenesis of the disease is given to the T-lymphocytes (of Th-1 and Th-17 types) activation followed by the synthesis of pro-inflammatory cytokines IL-2, IL-15, IL-17, IFN-γ, TNF-α, etc. New facts are emerging about the significance of the JAK-STAT-signaling system in the development of several autoimmune diseases, including AA.

In AA, CD8 + T cells + NKG2D produce IFN-γ, which binds to its receptor on the HF surface and activates the JAK1/2–STAT1 pathway. This, in turn, promotes IL-15 release, which, by binding to its receptor on the surface of T cells, activates JAK1/3–STAT5 and stimulates IFN-γ, supporting immune inflammation. Skin biopsy from AA patients revealed JAK1, JAK2, and, to a lesser extent, JAK3 overexpression [8].

Stress, Neurogenic Inflammation, and Adaptive-Regulatory Mechanisms in Alopecia Areata

The stress response is based on feedback regulation, which modulates the hypothalamic-pituitary-adrenal (HPA) axis and autonomic nervous system activity to protect and adapt the body to stress through a variety of adaptive responses. Failure of adaptive mechanisms can result in structural and functional disorders at all levels, particularly in the neuroendocrine and immune systems, which serve as the pathogenetic basis for disease development [9].

From the standpoint of health risk, AA is known to be a benign condition that is not associated with death. Nonetheless, its psychotraumatic effect outweighs that of other injuries associated with a loss of external attractiveness (for example, obesity or scars on visible areas of the body) and can be comparable to the consequences of life-threatening or disabling diseases. The persistence of immune disorders, the relationship between dermatosis development and recurrence and psychotraumatic factors indirectly indicate the inadequacy of the adaptive potential of the patient's body.

Whether stressful life events can cause the development of AA is a controversial issue. There have been documented cases in which psycho-emotional stress clearly preceded the onset or relapse of AA. However, it is difficult to objectively distinguish stress as a true disease trigger from distress caused by the disease itself, which can be identified retrospectively and incorrectly as the cause of hair loss in AA. Even if stressors play a role in the onset of AA, anxiety and depression caused by various forms of the disease may affect the disease's course via stress mediators [10].

The skin and HF have a local neuroendocrine axis similar to hypothalamic-pituitary-adrenal (HPA) axis. During periods of stress, the axis is activated to release corticotropin-releasing hormone, substance P, nerve growth factor, which leads to degranulation of mast cells, accelerates catagen regression of HF, and may contribute to neurogenic inflammation resulting in the loss of the immune privilege of the HF.

There is evidence of neurohumoral changes in AA. A recent study using a mouse model found that AA is linked to changes in the HPA axis's function. Following the development of AA in mice, there was a significant increase in the tone of the central and peripheral components of the HPA axis when compared to the control. The presence of high activity of the corticotropin-releasing hormone receptor in AA foci, which can cause mast cell differentiation from the HF mesenchyme, was also discovered. It has been observed that the progression of AA alters the expression of substance P. Substance P skin injections in mice with AA cause mast cell degranulation, accelerated hair follicle catagen regression, and an increase in CD8 + T cells [9].

The role of stress and maladaptive disorders in AA was evaluated in the study by Bolotnaya and Serbina [11]. Changes were revealed based on the research of adaptive hormones—cortisol and insulin, as well as the coefficient of stress of adaptive potential "K". Two types of reactions in AA have been identified—an increase or decrease in the level of blood cortisol and insulin, depending on the activity, severity, and duration of AA. Change in the K index in patients with signs of AA progression, high severity, and duration up to 3 years indicated the tension and disruption of adaptive capabilities. Decrease of the coefficient "K" during chronicity and duration of the disease of over 3 years indicates depletion of adaptive mechanisms of organism with possible failure of regulatory processes. An inadequate hormone response to immunoinflammatory stimuli is a factor in the chronicity of the pathological process. Under conditions of inflammation in AA, an acute protective inflammatory reaction is transformed into a chronic uncontrolled pathological process, manifested by a change in the corresponding phases from an increase to a decrease in the level of cortisol and insulin, as well as a similar change in the K index with tension and disruption of adaptive capabilities, which can lead to structural and functional disorders at all levels, and especially in the neuroendocrine and immune systems being the pathogenetic basis for the disease development. Such disruptions justify the use of therapeutic means and methods aimed at breaking pathological pathways—increasing stress resistance and adaptive capabilities in patients with AA.

A high level of psychological comorbidity was found in AA patients (66%). A recent systematic review found that people with AA frequently regard hair loss as a serious problem, which causes stress and has a negative impact on QoL and mental health. The "distorting effect" of AA is thought to be a factor in the development of a wide range of secondary mental disorders. AA frequently causes anxiety and depression, as well as social phobias associated with low self-esteem. Furthermore, patients with severe AA are more prone to stress, making them less effective in dealing with difficult life situations than healthy people. Avoidant behavior is common in this patient group, particularly in those with pathological adjustment disorders [12].

The study by Bolotnaya and Serbina (2017) showed a significant relationship between psychological disorders such as anxiety disorder, depression, and sleep disorders with the clinical form of AA. Seventy-three percent of patients with AA had more severe forms of the disease such as multifocal alopecia, AT and AU. Depressive disorders increase the risk of medical comorbidities, reduce QoL and functional impairment in these patients [11].

Bullying of various types (aggressive harassment including physical and/or verbal harassment, threats, etc.) is experienced by 23% of children with AA of various ages more than once a week. One-eighth of all children were beaten at least once a day. The study emphasized the psychological impact of AA on children and the importance of discussing the emotional and social consequences of this disease with pediatric patients, even those who are very young, as well as their family members. Frequently, the children were concerned about how their illness would affect their family members. According to Sinclair [13], AA is associated with suicidal attempts in adolescents, indicating a clear underestimation of the role of the psychosocial aspect in hair loss.

Diagnosis of Alopecia Areata

The Ukrainian Clinical Guidelines for the Management of Patients with AA [14] offer a diagnostic algorithm taking into account the clinical form, severity, stage of the pathological process, comorbid pathology, QoL, and risk factors for severe disease, which are important criteria for the differentiated therapy (Table 6.1). The unified examination protocol for patients with AA enables more effective disease monitoring, and the outpatient card, developed in accordance with international recommendations, contains data with epidemiological and prognostic significance, as well as key stages in disease progression. This approach to AA patients improves patient management and medical care and serves as the foundation for the All-Ukrainian register of AA patients.

The first step in AA diagnosis is detailed patient history, trigger factor assessment, and clinical examination. When taking a patient history, consider the onset, nature of the disease course, number and duration of episodes and remissions, as well as the role of potential triggers such as stress, endocrine disorders, medication, pregnancy, trauma, comorbidities, and others. Given the genetic predisposition, assessing the AA prevalence in close relatives or family members is essential.

Table 6.1 Diagnostic algorithm for alopecia areata

Patient with hair loss similar to alopecia areata		
History, evaluation of trigger factors, clinical examination		
Differential diagnosis		
Special diagnostic methods: • pull test • trichoscopy	**Additional research methods:** • fungal testing (scraping, plating, Wood's lamp) • antinuclear antibodies, antibodies to native DNA • syphilis serology screening • skin biopsy	
Diagnosis of alopecia areata, determination of the clinical form, stage and affected area		
Clinical form		
• local scalp • local beard • supra- and ciliary • ribbon-like (ophiasis, sisaipho)	• subtotal (multifocal) • totalis • universalis	• diffuse • incognita • canites subita • with nail involvement
Stage (trichoscopy, pull test)		
• **Active** (black dots, broken hairs, exclamation marks, tapered hairs, Pohl Pinkus constrictions (moniletrix-like hairs), coudability hairs); positive pull test • **Chronic** (no signs of activity, yellow dots, vellus); negative pull test • **Hair regrowth stage** (regrowing hair, twisted hair, poliosis); negative pull test		
Affected area (SBN)		
Affected area of the scalp (S) and other parts of the body (B), the degree of nail plate (NP) changes (N):		
• S0—without hair loss • S1—<25% hair loss • S2—from 25% to 49% hair loss • S3—from 25% to 74% hair loss • S4—from 75% to 99% hair loss • S5–100% hair loss	• B0—no body hair loss • B1—some body hair loss • B2–100% body hair loss • N0—no nail involvement • N1—some nail involvement • N1a—20-nail dystrophy	
Definition of severity		
Mild: $S_1B_0N_0$; $S_{\circ}B_1N_0$	**Moderate:** $S_1B_{0\text{-}1}N_{0\text{-}1a}$; $S_2B_0N_0$	**Severe:** $S_2B_{1–2}N_0$—$S_2B_0N_{1\text{-}1a}$—$S_2B_{1–2}N_{1\text{-}1a}$; $S_3B_{0\text{-}2}N_{0\text{-}1a}$—$S_5B_{0\text{-}2}N_{0\text{-}1a}$
• local (scalp) • local (beard) • supra- and ciliary	• local (scalp) (+ NP damage and/or envelopment other parts of the body) • multifocal • ribbon-like (ophiasis, sisaipho) • diffuse • incognita • canites subita	• ribbon-like (ophiasis, sisaipho) • diffuse • incognita • canites subita • multifocal • totalis • universalis (±NP damage and/or involvement of other parts of the body)

(continued)

Table 6.1 (continued)

Patient with hair loss similar to alopecia areata
History, evaluation of trigger factors, clinical examination
Differential diagnosis
Assessment of comorbid pathology
Laboratory and instrumental research methods As per indications (presence of complaints, clinical manifestations) and before treatment: • Clinical and biochemical blood test; • Serological diagnosis of celiac disease, autoimmune diseases (IgA and IgG to tissue transglutaminase, to deaminated peptides (gliadin)); • Acute phase proteins, antinuclear antibodies, antibodies to native DNA and etc. • Deficiencies (iron, ferritin, serum total iron binding capacity, 25 (OH) D, selenium, zinc, etc.); • Cortisol; TSH, free T3 and T4, antibodies to structures of the thyroid; prolactin; • Fluorography; • Interdisciplinary consultations.
Determining patients' quality of life on DLQI scale (0–30 points)
Identifying of risk factors for severe disease course • Early disease onset; • AT, AU or ribbon-like hair loss; • Nail involvement; • Hair loss on the body associated with localized forms on the scalp; • Disease duration more than 5 years (the absence of yellow dots on trichoscopy); • Presence of atopy; • Presence of other autoimmune diseases; • Positive family history.
Development of a treatment plan
Therapy monitoring

Clinical form Clinical examination reveals alopecia foci presented as completely hairless areas on hair bearing skin (scalp, eyebrows, eyelashes, body) with marked boundaries, smooth surface, without signs of scaling, infiltration, and atrophy. The skin of the lesion may be hypotrophic, in severe forms its thinning is detected. The following clinical forms of AA are distinguished depending on the region and area of involvement: Local of scalp and beard, ciliary and supraciliary, ribbon-like (ophiasis and sisaipho), subtotal, AT, AU, diffuse, incognita, canities subita.

The local form is usually presented by several nummular foci on the scalp or beard ("Barbe" type) (Fig. 6.1a, b). In patients with this form, spontaneous hair regrowth within 3 months from the onset or long-term persistence with migration of foci can be observed.

Small foci fusion into larger affected areas are characteristic for multifocal AA as a variant of subtotal form, in which areas with long hair are still preserved on the scalp (Fig. 6.2). Some authors distinguish its subtype—the reticular form, demonstrating many small isolated alopecia foci without fusion.

The supraciliary form (madarosis) is described as the loss of eyebrows, the ciliary form (milfosis)—the loss of eyelashes (Fig. 6.3). These forms can be a manifestation of the disease and its only symptom, creating diagnostic difficulties. Partial, unilateral, complete, combined loss of eyebrows and eyelashes usually correlates with the stage of AA.

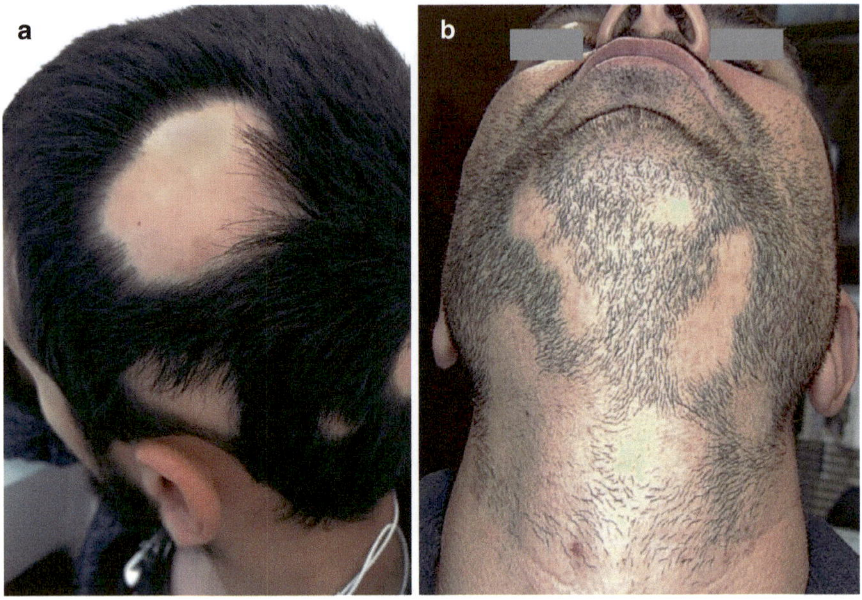

Fig. 6.1 Local form of alopecia areata: scalp (**a**); beard "Barbe" type (**b**)

Fig. 6.2 Subtotal form of alopecia areata

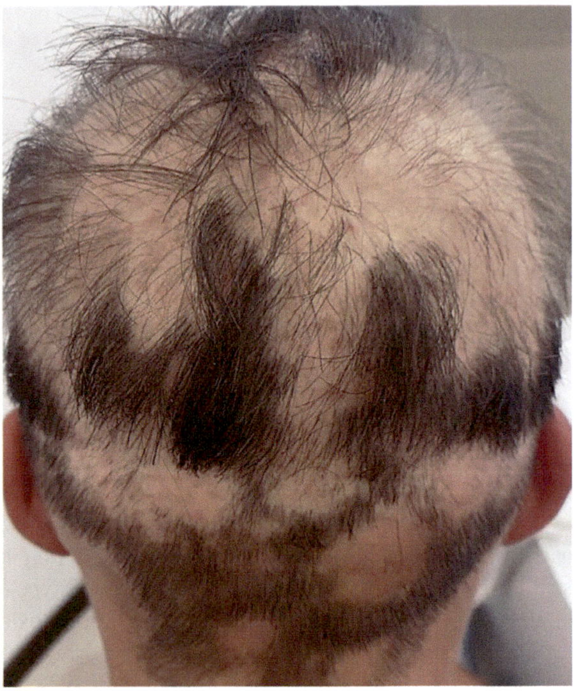

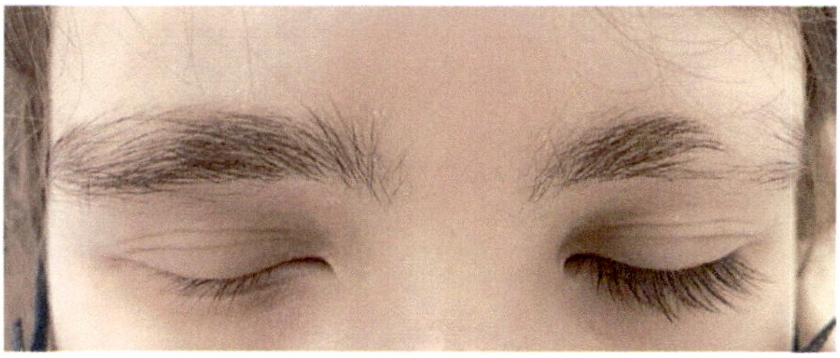

Fig. 6.3 Ciliary and supraciliary form of alopecia areata

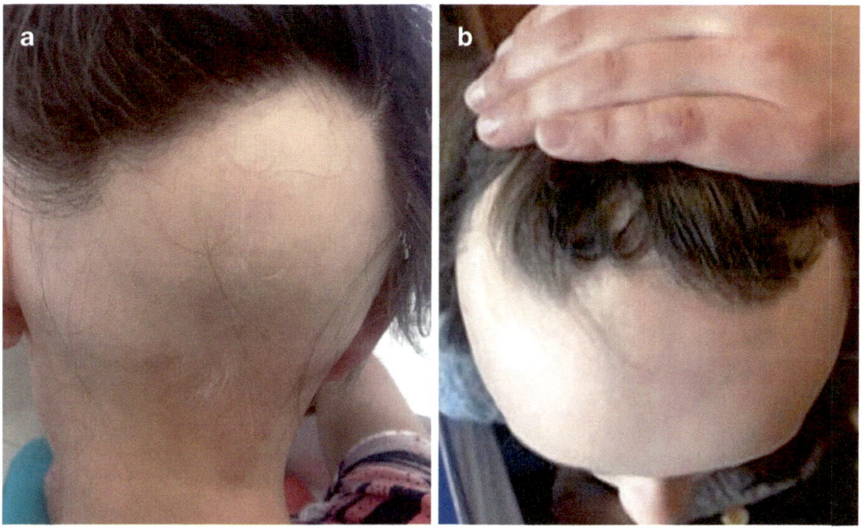

Fig. 6.4 Ribbon-like forms of alopecia areata: ophiasis (**a**); sisaipho (**b**)

The ribbon-like form (ophiasis) is characterized by bald patches in the occipital area, which, merging, spread in the form of a ribbon toward the auricles, reaching the temples.

This clinical subtype is believed to be a poor prognostic factor (Fig. 6.4a). Inverse ophiasis (sisaipho) is a rare type of hair loss in the opposite direction of ophiasis (frontal-temporal-parietal region) (Fig. 6.4b). At present, it is generally accepted that the sisaipho type can be an AA evolutionary model. In AT, hair is absent on the entire scalp, and in men—in the beard area (Fig. 6.5). AU is characterized by the complete loss of hair on the scalp and body. AA onset before puberty poses a risk of AT development at 50%. The chance of a complete recovery in patients with AT and AU is less than 10% [6].

At present, the list of AA patterns has been supplemented with diffuse forms: alopecia areata incognita (AAI), diffuse form of AA (DAA), and canities subita (Fig. 6.6a–c). The absence of smooth lesions of baldness with visible hair loss is characteristic for these subtypes that clinically resemble acute telogen effluvium, since hair loss in these subtypes develops diffusely over the entire scalp without

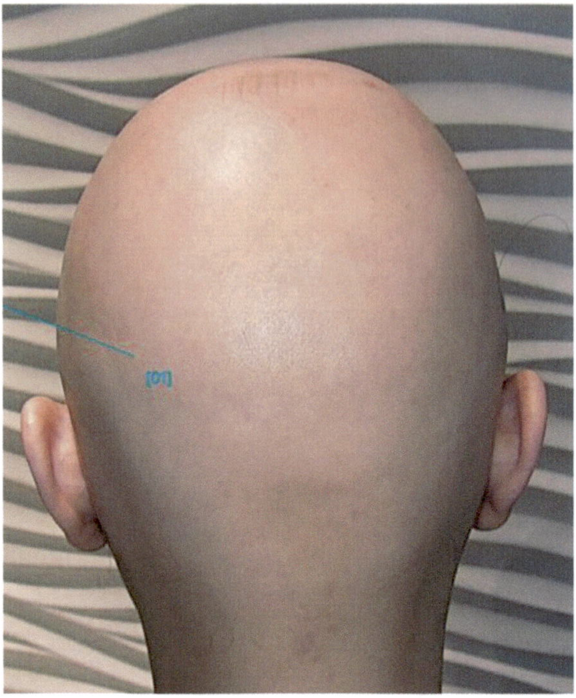

Fig. 6.5 Totalis form of alopecia areata

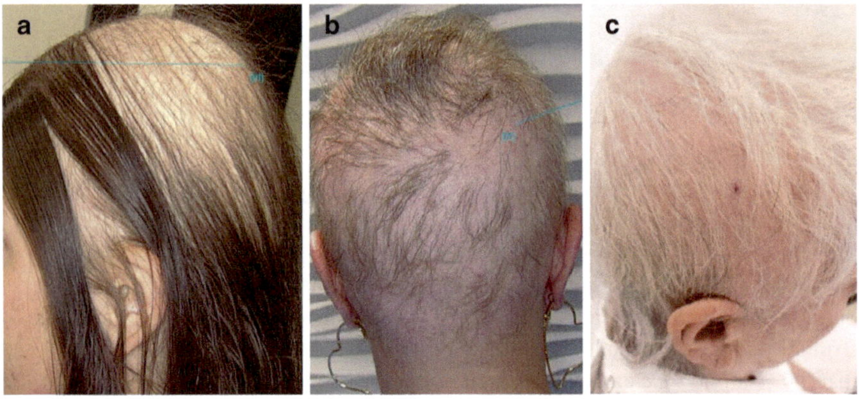

Fig. 6.6 Diffuse forms of alopecia areata: alopecia areata incognita (**a**); diffuse form of alopecia areata (**b**); canities subita or Marie Antoinette syndrome (**c**)

forming patches of alopecia. AAI and DAA are the two most common variants of diffuse forms of AA.

AAI is more common (about 86%) in young women. It has an abrupt onset, severe hair loss, and diffuse thinning that is more noticeable in androgen-dependent areas, as well as involvement of the temporal regions. The pull test is distinctively positive in patients with IAA. A microscopic examination of shed hair reveals telogen roots of varying maturation, with an emphasis on early telogen. At follow-up, some patients develop classic lesions. To confirm the diagnosis, a biopsy is required [15–17]. It is hard to distinguish the condition from DAA. In contrast to AAI, published comparison data of clinical, trichoscopic, and histological characteristics revealed a diffuse pattern of clinical distribution over the entire scalp. Although these AA subtypes are benign and respond to topical steroid therapy, the diffuse form can quickly progress to alopecia totalis [18].

Today canities subita or Marie Antoinette (in women) and Thomas More (in men) syndromes are a rare variant of the diffuse form of AA, in which autoimmunity predominantly targets pigmented hair in naturally graying patients. Acute and selective loss of pigmented hair over several days gives the impression of abrupt graying [19].

Clinical forms can transform into each other, which is especially evident in severe cases. On the one hand, a spontaneous hair regrowth is quite usual in AA, and on the other hand, there are severe torpid forms of hair loss resistant to therapy, or cases where hair growth can be preserved only with continuous treatment, after its cessation hair falls out again within few days.

A physician must evaluate the condition of the nail plates when examining a patient with AA. Nail damage in AA is a nonpermanent symptom. The incidence of nail involvement observed in AA ranges from 7% to 66% (Fig. 6.7).

Stages of the pathological process. In clinical presentation of AA, successive stages are distinguished: active, chronic, and hair regrowth. It is noted that the disease duration often does not correlate with the activity of the pathological process.

The active, or progressive, stage is characterized by increased hair loss along with the expansion of the alopecia patch, as well as several clinical signs such as a positive pull test (especially pronounced along the border of the pathological focus of alopecia), and symptoms of soreness, moderate itching, burning, and a sensation of "swarming" in the alopetic area.

The presence of a formed alopecia patch with unchanged boundaries, a negative pull test, and the absence of hair growth within the lesion characterize the **chronic or stationary stage.** Patients have not complained about altered sensations in the alopetic area. The skin within the alopecia patch is regular in color and appears hypotrophic on clinical examination.

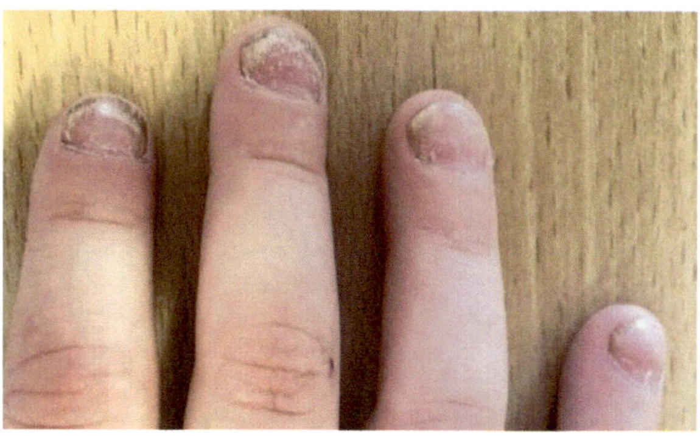

Fig. 6.7 Involvement of all nail plates

Hair regrowth or recovery stage is characterized by hair growth; as a rule, when growth resumes, unpigmented hair shafts grow first, and their repigmentation occurs later, clinically and trichoscopically demonstrating poliosis (Fig. 6.8).

Special diagnostic methods (pull test, trichoscopy, and biopsy when needed) help in the differential diagnosis and are the key to identifying the stage of the pathological process.

Trichoscopy reflects the pathophysiological process in AA, markers are similar for almost all of its clinical subtypes, the main differences are dependent on the disease stage. Observations of the process dynamics within lesions provide additional data regarding the prognosis and the expected therapy efficacy [14].

The dystrophic process in active stage of AA is characterized by black dots, broken hairs, exclamation mark hairs, coudability hair, and monilethrix-like hair (Fig. 6.9).

The absence of the above-mentioned signs of dystrophic activity is the main criterion for the chronic stage. However, yellow dots and vellus hairs are variables, not specific, but characteristic signs of this stage (Fig. 6.10). The number of yellow dots is proportional to patient age and is nearly the only criterion for distinguishing supraciliary and ciliary AA from trichotillomania. Yellow dots are uncommon in prepubertal children and elderly patients.

Yellow dots may be absent in patients with AT and AU who have had the disease for more than 5 years, which is a poor prognostic factor for therapy response. Vellus hair can also indicate the severity of a disease. In the chronic phase, vellus hair growth indicates that the follicle is unable to reproduce terminal hair fiber.

Trichoscopic signs of hair regrowth include vertically growing hairs (Fig. 6.11) and hair that has been symmetrically twisted into rings ("pigtail"), which can be seen alongside signs of activedisease. Pigtail-like hairs twisted into oval or round

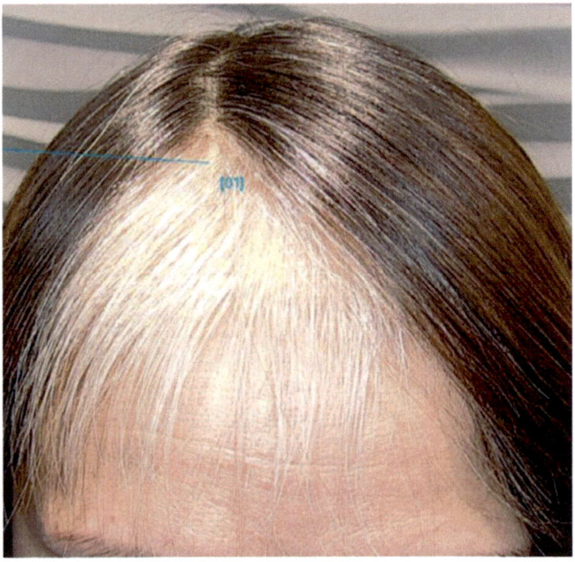

Fig. 6.8 Alopecia areata patient with poliosis in the area of hair regrowth

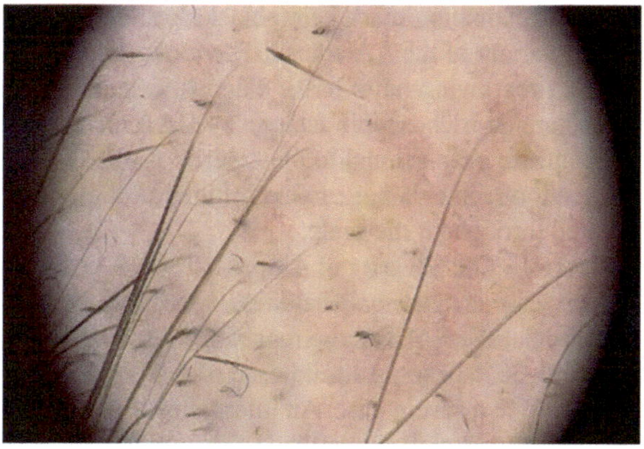

Fig. 6.9 Trichoscopic image demonstrating signs of the alopecia areata active stage—black dots, broken hairs, and exclamation mark hairs on the alopecia patch margin

Fig. 6.10 Trichoscopy showing yellow dots—signs of alopecia areata chronic stage

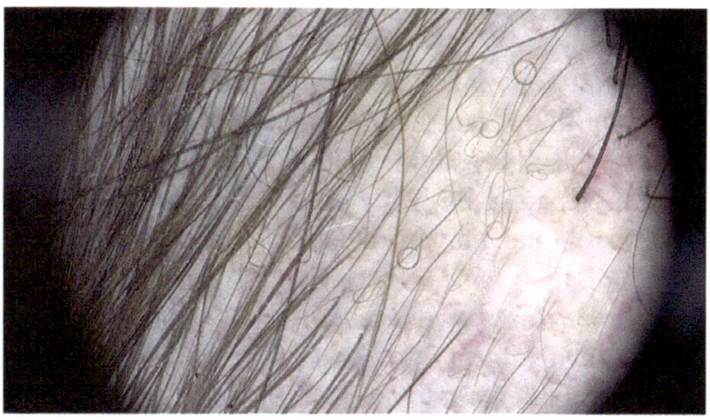

Fig. 6.11 Trichoscopic image demonstrating vertically regrowing hairs and pigtail hairs— signs of alopecia areata hair growth renewal stage

ring with pointed tip indicates the regrowth of terminal hair shaft by partially damaged hair follicles [20].

The trichoscopic picture of AA diffuse forms reflects pathophysiological process features of these patterns and demonstrates the differences from classical forms of the disease described above. The role of trichoscopy in AAI was first described by Tosti et al. [15], who recorded the presence of diffuse yellow dots in 95% of patients. Short regrowing hairs are another typical trichoscopic feature of AA incognita.

- Atopy
- Other autoimmune diseases
- Positive family history

The Level of Psycho-Emotional Stress and Quality of Life in Patients with Alopecia Areata

The Hospital Anxiety and Depression Scale (HADS) is used to diagnose psycho-emotional disorders in patients, allowing for the identification of severity and timely intervention (Table 3.2). For each statement, there are four possible responses. The patient is asked to select the option that best describes their condition, and the results are summarized. A score of 8–10 is considered subclinical anxiety/depression, while a score of 11 or higher is considered clinical anxiety/depression.

A recent study using the HADS questionnaire found depression and anxiety in 38% and 62% of AA patients, respectively, which was significantly higher than in healthy controls ($p = 0.047$ and $p = 0.005$, respectively) [10]. These findings, along with those of other similar studies, confirm the high prevalence of anxiety and depressive symptoms in AA. Dermatologists should be aware of the psychological impact of AA, especially given the limited efficacy of current treatments.

It is important to evaluate QoL in AA as an integral indicator describing the most important functional domains and allowing analysis of changes in these domains during the disease course.

AA causes relatively minor changes in physical condition, but significantly worsens the emotional and social components of QoL, frequently leading to depression, dysmorphophobia, and, in some cases, even suicidal ideation. The severity of AA's negative impact on QoL varies widely and is not well correlated with the objective state of the clinical severity of a patient's disease. Furthermore, there is no direct correlation between patient and physician perceptions of AA. As a result, standard clinical measures used to assess disease severity, such as the percentage of affected skin, cannot accurately describe the psychological status of AA patients.

There are currently several dermatology-specific questionnaires tailored to trichology patients. Because of its high degree of objectivity and reliability, the DLQI (Dermatology Quality of Life Index) is the most cited tool for assessing quality of life. DLQI is intended for use in adults (Table 3.1). Completing the questionnaire is easy and does not require additional detailed explanations by the physician. Questions are classified under the following six subscales: symptoms and feelings (questions 1–2), daily activities (questions 3–4), leisure (questions 5–6) and personal relationships (questions 8–9) with a maximum score of 6 points for each item, work (question 7), and treatment (question 10) with a maximum score of 3 points for each item.

Bolotnaya, Serbina [11] investigated the quality of life in AA patients. The questionnaires were divided into two sections. The first, completed by the doctor, included questions about gender, age, AA family history, AA history, disease duration, stress in the previous 6 months, employment status (currently working or not), education level, and other diseases. The second section consisted of DLQI questions. The authors proposed a system for clinical DLQI interpretation. The higher the score (number of points), the lower the quality of life. A score of 0–1 is interpreted as having no effect on the patient's life, a score of 2–5 as having a minor effect, a score of 6–10 as having a moderate effect, a score of 11–20 as having a very strong effect, and a score of 21–30 as having an extremely strong effect on life.

The DLQI was administered to 120 AA patients. The indicator score ranged from 1 to 30, with a mean of 9.85 ± 7.22. At the same time, the impact of the following factors was assessed: gender, age (under 30 years and over 30 years), level of education, disease duration (up to 12 months and more than 12 months), family history of AA, history of AA (primary episode or relapse), stress in the previous 6 months, AA severity, and other concomitant diseases (thyroid disease, diabetes mellitus, atopy, etc.).

Mean DLQI scores for various severity degrees were 4.8 ± 2.5; 7.8 ± 5.2 and 17.4 ± 6,5, corresponding to mild, moderate, and severe, and statistically significant ($p < 0.001$). Correlation analysis revealed a positive correlation between the DLQI score and AA patient age (under 30 years); severe course (AT and AU); acute stress in the last 6 months; hair loss for more than 12 months—$r = 0.51$, $r = 0.58$, $r = 0.52$, and $r = 0.64$, $p < 0.01$ respectively.

AA-QLI (Alopecia Areata Quality of Life Index), a special questionnaire to assess the quality of life in patients with AA, has been developed (Table 6.2). Developers of the questionnaire conducted a study to introduce and to validate a

Table 6.2 AA-QLI questionnaire/ From: Fabbrocini G., Panariello L., De Vita V. et al. Quality of Life in Alopecia Areata: A Disease-Specific Questionnaire, 2013

Subjective symptoms
• I feel uncomfortable using a wig • I tend to hide my scalp with hats or bandanas • I am sad about the appearance of my hair/eyebrows/eyelashes • I worry about having this hair problem for the rest of my life • I cannot forget that I have this hair problem I worry that it might spread • I do not take my wig/hat/bandana off in front of my partner/relatives/friends • It costs me a lot of money to look after my hair • I am afraid my children may have alopecia areata
Relationships
• I feel that people find it unpleasant to look at me • I think that other people notice my hair/eyebrows/eyelashes problem • I am afraid that other people think my hair looks badly cared for • I am embarrassed when going out to a party • I have to explain to others what is wrong with my hair/eyebrows/eyelashes • I feel that others are afraid of catching diseases from me • I feel I have sexual difficulties because of alopecia areata • I feel I have difficulties in establishing relationships with friends and/or relatives • My work/studying has deteriorated because of alopecia areata
Objective signs
• My scalp is visible • I lose tufts of hair when I comb or shampoo • I feel itchy on my scalp

new disease-specific questionnaire for AA, and to compare the Quality of Life Index (QLI) using DLQI [25].

The AA-QLI is divided into two sections: the first includes questions about gender, age, age of disease onset, time of last relapse, and percentage of affected skin, and the second section includes 21 questions measuring the degree to which the patient was affected by the AA in the previous month, scored from 1 (not affected at all) to 4 (extremely affected) (highly affected). Patients with AA were asked about the impact of their disease and treatment on their lives, and their responses were used to guide the development of the AA-QLI. Thus, three aspects of daily life are addressed: "subjective symptoms," "relationships," and "objective signs."

The comparison of these results with the DQLI questionnaire results confirmed the validity of this new system scale. This demonstrates the significance of the AA-QLI as a specific statistical tool that allows the QLI to be decomposed into main components, as opposed to the DLQI, which aggregates the results using arithmetic or weighted means.

The authors conclude that, statistically, AA-QLI is a valid and suitable specific alternative to DLQI; the modeling approach allows for the estimation of individual and average AA-QLI scores, highlighting that "Relationship" affects patients' QoL more than "Objective signs." Statistical analysis revealed that the AA-QLI has a higher specificity for assessing QoL in AA.

Therapeutic Strategies

Treatment of AA patients presents a challenge to treating physicians. The lack of consensus for AA development mechanisms, causes of the onset and patterns of the disease course hinders the emergence of effective methods of therapy. Despite the availability of various treatments, it is not always easy to manage the disease in an effective and safe manner. The review of international treatment protocols for AA shows that currently there is no universal method of therapy that guarantees the relapse-free course in future. Of particular difficulty is the treatment of AA patients with comorbid pathology, which can require close interdisciplinary collaboration.

The Ukrainian clinical guidelines for management of patients with AA [14] define the principles and algorithm of therapy. The treatment criteria selection for AA is the following: age; degree of severity; stage of the process activity; and QoL score. It is critical to weigh the risk of adverse events against the expected therapeutic effect of the drugs prescribed.

Consider the following when administering treatment for AA:

1. The disease does not directly endanger general health
2. In localized forms, hair can regrow spontaneously within a year of the disease's onset even without treatment

(continued)

3. The disease's impact on physical and emotional state (including aspects like self-confidence, relationships in society, and assessment of quality of life
4. The level of anxiety, disappointment, helplessness, and guilt in family members of AA patients, and
5. Comorbid pathology

It is critical to focus on the dynamics of the QLI when evaluating the efficacy of various AA treatment methods (the results are determined after 6 months of treatment initiation).

Leaving AA without treatment ("waiting tactics") is an acceptable and, in some cases, the most correct option, as evidenced by the following facts:

- Spontaneous remission occurs in 80% of patients with limited focal alopecia within a short period (<1 year)
- Patients with severe forms of AA may be unresponsive to various types of therapy for a long period of time without any improvement
- The long-term prognosis for severe AA forms is poor, and the best option may be the use of a wig (prosthesis) rather than continued therapy, which is unlikely to be effective

The modern arsenal of AA therapy includes both potent pathogenetic pharmacological drugs and various adjuvant agents. According to the antigenic concept of the AA pathogenesis, the main group of medication for pathogenetic therapy includes glucocorticosteroids (GCS) and other drugs with immunosuppressive effect.

Topical GCS, due to ease of administration, are the first-line therapy for both adults and children with mild to moderate AA when used as monotherapy or in combination with other treatments. In adults with severe AA, topical GCS are regarded as an adjunct to systemic treatments. The most commonly used is a highly potent clobetasol propionate 0.05% available as an ointment, lotion, foam, or shampoo.

In AA, topical application of minoxidil solution or foam during the period of hair regrowth promotes faster pigmentation and density renewal. It is not recommended to use minoxidil in the active stage of the disease, as this can provoke its spread and increase the area of hair loss. The experience of using a 5% minoxidil solution showed its higher efficacy in combination with topical GCS in patients after managing the signs of disease activity. According to the results of various studies, topical 5% minoxidil reduces the rate of post-steroid relapse in AA.

The most common treatment in patients with AA with up to 50% affected area are injections of long-acting GCS (betamethasone dipropionate and betamethasone sodium phosphate suspension, triamcinolone acetonide suspension) into deep dermis on the lesion allowing to achieve optimal tissue concentrations with minimal systemic absorption. A retrospective analysis of the observations in patients with more than 50% affected area of the scalp receiving intralesional injections of GCS showed a better response at young age, with shorter duration of AA. This therapy was more effective in patients with signs of activity.

Intralesional GCS as monotherapy is ineffective in advanced forms of AA, but it can be used as an adjunct to systemic treatment to accelerate the action of oral GCS and JAK inhibitors.

Cyclosporine and methotrexate have been shown to be effective as monotherapy in severe forms of AA, as well as in combination therapy with oral GCS or after discontinuation of GCS as steroid-sparing treatment. Potential side effects of long-term use as well as the risk of relapse after dose reduction or treatment discontinuation are factors that limit the use of systemic therapies for AA. In severe AA, the systemic GCS regimen involves a gradual reduction in dosages. Steroid-sparing agents are frequently used to reduce the risk of adverse effects associated with long-term use of high-dose systemic GCS. According to the International Consensus Expert Group, in adults JAK inhibitors, methotrexate or cyclosporine in combination with systemic corticosteroids are effective.

JAK inhibitors are currently the most promising targeted agents in the treatment of AA. In patients with refractory AA, pharmacological inhibition of JAK promotes hair regrowth and reverses dystrophic mail changes. The first systemic medicine, baricitinib (Olumiant), a selective inhibitor of JAK1 and JAK2, was approved by the FDA in June 2022 as a systemic treatment for severe AA in adults at a dose of 4 mg once daily. The decision was made based on the results of two phase three randomized clinical trials (BRAVE-AA1 and BRAVE-AA2) with the participation of patients with severe forms of AA with SALT score >50. About 40% of patients receiving baricitinib in 4 mg tablets had at least 80% scalp hair regrowth, compared to only 6% of the placebo group after 36 weeks of therapy. Adverse effects include upper respiratory and urinary tract infections, acne, increased levels of low-density cholesterol and creatine kinase, and herpesvirus infections [26].

Ritlecitinib, a highly selective JAK3/TEC inhibitor, suppresses the action of signaling molecules and immune cells responsible for hair loss in AA (CD8+ T-cells, CD4+ T-cells, B-cells, Treg and NK-cells). The advantages of using ritlecitinib compared to other JAK inhibitors include the prevention of clinical side effects of JAK1/JAK2 inhibition, in which such pharmacodynamic effects as an increase in cholesterol and liver enzymes as well as thrombocytopenia, anemia, are observed.

On June 23, 2023, the FDA approved 50 mg ritlecitinib (Litfulo) orally once daily for severe AA in adolescents and adults. This is the first and only drug approved by the FDA for the treatment of children suffering from this disease from the age of 12. The approval was based on the results of the ALLEGRO Phase 2b/3 clinical study, in which 718 patients with scalp hair loss with ≥50% SALT score took part, evaluating the efficacy and safety of Litfulo in 18 countries. In this key study, a statistically significantly greater proportion of patients experienced regrowth (SALT score ≤20) with ritlecitinib compared with placebo. The efficacy and safety of the medicine were the same in adolescents (from 12 to 17 years) and adults (from 18 years and older). The most frequent adverse events, reported in at least 4% of patients, included headache (10.8%), diarrhea (10%), acne (6.2%), rash (5.4%), and urticaria (4.6%) [27].

Tofacitinib is a JAK inhibitor that primarily blocks JAK1 and JAK3, and to a lesser extent JAK2. The drug is FDA approved for the treatment of psoriatic and rheumatoid arthritis in adults. "Off label" is used in AA therapy. Oral tofacitinib at a dose of 10 mg/day is an efficacious treatment for severe cases of AA that have not undergone other treatment methods. It is possible to increase the dose to 20 mg/day in torpid forms according to the results of some studies. We should take into account the possibility of developing side effects, which include hematological disorders; increase in the level of liver enzymes and cholesterol; infections, including herpes zoster and reactivation of tuberculosis; venous thromboembolism; and acne rash [28].

Currently, scientists are working on the integration of JAK inhibitors into international and national guidelines for management of patients with AA. Further clinical trials of this group of drugs will allow us to learn more about their efficacy, safety, determine the optimal dosage and duration of treatment, as well as the need for supportive therapy.

Improving Self-Esteem, Overcoming Depression and Anxiety in Alopecia Areata

A treatment strategy in AA should include psychotherapy as well as pharmacological treatment of psychological disorders, as well as advice on aesthetic methods of correction, in addition to the primary treatment of AA.

The evaluation of antidepressant efficacy in AA is worth considering because AA is associated with a high level of anxiety, depression, and sleep disorders. Several studies on small groups of patients with AA who received antidepressants (selective serotonin reuptake inhibitors) found that treatment in the antidepressant group was significantly more effective. Large sample-size randomized controlled trial studies are needed to confirm these findings [29].

A significant decrease in depression and anxiety was observed in the group receiving hypnotherapy in a non-randomized trial comparing 20 patients (most of whom had severe AA) receiving hypnotherapy to 21 patients in the control group who received no treatment. There were no differences in the rates of hair regrowth between the groups. This study supports the significance of treating secondary mental disorders in AA patients, despite the unproven impact on hair growth [30].

The impact of hair prostheses on patients with AA's quality of life has been assessed in a number of studies [31]. The findings showed that aesthetic correction significantly increased QoL, so it should be incorporated into AA therapy algorithms (Fig. 6.12). The degree of an individual's psychological impact from AA depends on both their capacity to accept their altered appearance and their

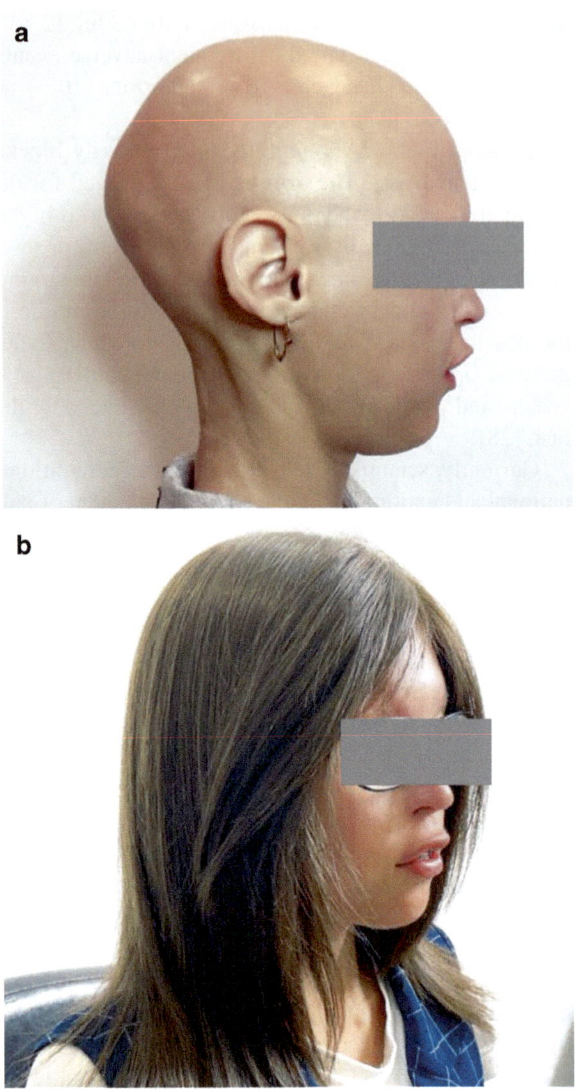

Fig. 6.12 Cesare Ragazzi CNC Hair System in a girl with alopecia areata (pre-manufacturing parameterization step and final result)

subjective perception. The cosmetic correction of hairless areas, which helps them look natural, is crucial for maintaining psychological comfort. The alopetic areas can be covered up with integrated hair replacement systems, wigs, hairpieces, head scarves, false eyelashes, and trichopigmentation.

Psychological Support and Social Adaptation of Patients with Alopecia Areata

Although AA is a relatively benign disease with no life-threatening consequences, its psychotraumatic impact is devastating. The stages of disease perception have been described in patients with severe AA. Fear and loneliness come first, followed by hope and, finally, acceptance of oneself without hair. Not everyone can reach this stage.

The psychological support of AA patients' family members and friends is critical. Another difficult and important task is the adaptation of individuals with AA in society and the adaptation of society to people with alopecia. Support groups that meet on a regular basis for AA patients and their families can be a valuable resource for this population. Patients receive emotional support and information to aid in the development of positive coping strategies, as well as the improvement of QoL and treatment outcomes.

Without a doubt, evidence-based medicine is the foundation of modern medicine. However, we must not overlook another critical component of successful therapy: the patient's trust in the doctor. Even Hippocrates stated that disease treatment necessitates not only "the art of the doctor and medicine, but also a great deal of care and attention in relation to the patient."

The example and inspiring experience of the National Alopecia Areata Foundation (www.naaaf.org), an organization that has been supporting patients and holding seminars and conferences on alopecia areata since 1981, prompted the Ukrainian Hair Research Society (UHRS) (http://uhrs.org.ua) collegium to establish "The School of Alopecia" to support people with AA and their families. Since 2017, the organization has been actively working to achieve its goals.

Here is one of the stories that we go through with our patients. Two girls, both red-haired, almost of the same age. They are just getting to know each other. Their meeting is not accidental; it is very exciting and touching to tears, to goosebumps.

Emilia is a little girl with gorgeous red hair. She was astonished to learn that we were treating alopecia, which can cause children to go completely hairless for an extended period of time. After all, the nearby kids have hair, just like her. We explained to Emilia how painful it is to be hairless and how challenging it is to live a different life from everyone else. Emilia made a decision quickly, saying, "I'd like to share my hair with these kids" (Fig. 6.13). And it became possible.

Ira has been suffering from AT since the age of 6, now she is 13, without hair yet. She is a very kind and modest child with a conscious attitude of an adult. Today Ira is wearing a hair replacement system, custom made of Emilia's hair. "This is exactly what I dreamed of," said the girl with tears of happiness in her eyes when she saw herself in the mirror.

The Cesare Ragazzi Hair Replacement System is a medical product made individually for each patient. The system provides the opportunity to live a full active

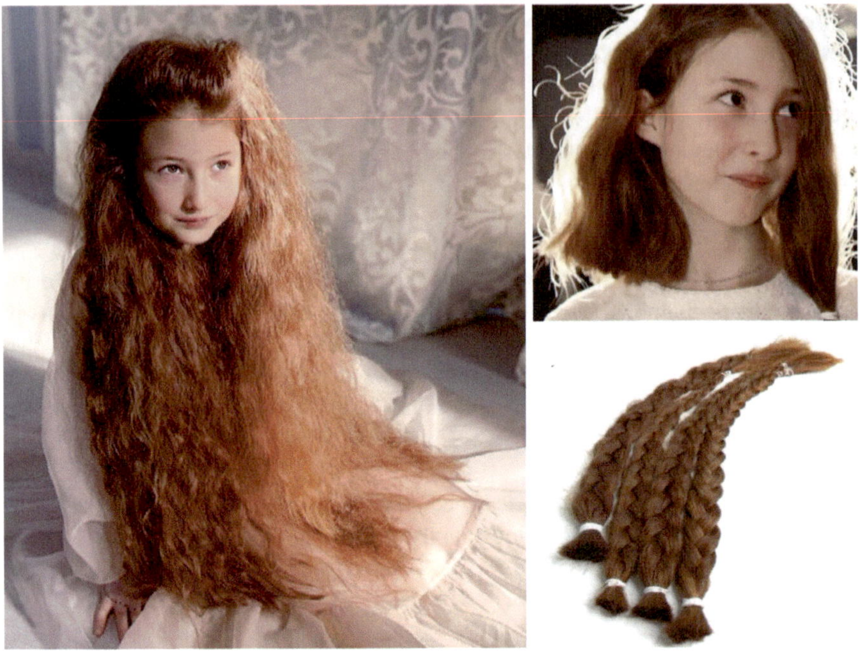

Fig. 6.13 Emilia and her hair

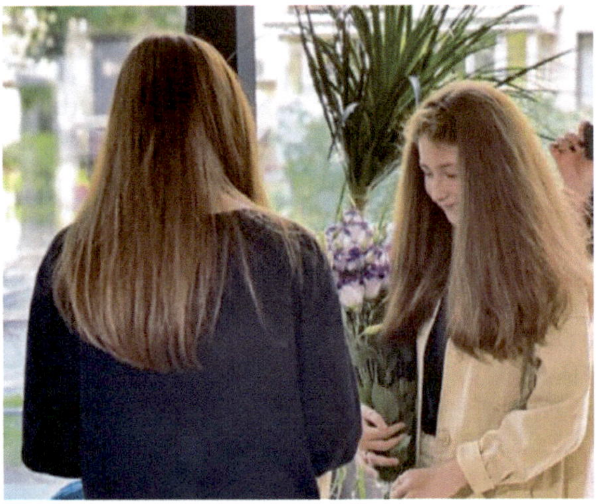

Fig. 6.14 Girls meeting after hair replacement system was placed

life. Helping children and adults with alopecia areata was made possible thanks to the work of a large team of professionals from Italy and Ukraine, doctors from the Institute of Trichology, and the School of Alopecia Charitable Foundation (Fig. 6.14).

Summary

- AA is an immune-mediated disease caused by the interaction of genetic factors and exogenous triggers, which results in autoimmune inflammation and HF immune tolerance impairment. AA's progression is unpredictable. On the one hand, there is spontaneous hair regrowth, and on the other, there are severe torpid forms of hair loss that are resistant to therapy. There are many cases where hair growth can only be maintained with continuous treatment, whereas when it is stopped, hair falls out within a few days.
- Studies presented data on the role of stress, neurogenic inflammation in the HF zone, and adjustment disorders in patients with AA. Although the role of anxiety and depression in triggering AA is still discussed, stressful life events commonly precede the onset and/or exacerbation of the disease. AA leading to relatively minor changes in physical condition significantly worsens the emotional and social components of the QoL, often being the cause of depression, dysmorphophobia, and suicidal attempts. Its psychotraumatic effect is comparable to the consequences of life-threatening or disabling diseases. The "distorting effect" of dermatosis is regarded as a factor provoking a whole range of secondary mental disorders, creating a vicious circle: stress—AA—psycho-emotional status of the patient—AA—stress.
- The degree of AA negative impact on QoL may not correlate with the objective severity of the patient's condition, which is often not taken into account in the diagnosis and treatment of the disease. QoL assessment using special questionnaires is a necessary step in the diagnostic route. The proposed tools for QoL assessment (DLQI, AA-QLI) may offer very useful supports to physicians in order to develop the best strategies for improving QoL of their patients with AA. This will help doctors to comprehend the impact of AA on patient's feelings and daily life, guiding them in the choice of an appropriate therapy and psychological support; it can also help patients by showing them that their pain is understood by others, in particular by their doctor, thereby improving in this way the doctor–patient relationship, which underlies the therapeutic success.

References

1. Aghaei S, Saki N, Daneshmand E, Kardeh B. Prevalence of psychological disorders in patients with alopecia areata in comparison with normal subjects. ISRN Dermatol. 2014;2014(1–4):304370. https://doi.org/10.1155/2014/304370.
2. Wall D, Meah N, York K, et al. A global eDelphi exercise to identify core domains and domain items for the development of a global registry of alopecia areata disease severity and treatment safety (GRASS). JAMA Dermatol. 2021;157(4):439–48. https://doi.org/10.1001/jamadermatol.2020.5839.
3. Pratt CH, King LE Jr, Messenger AG, Christiano AM, Sundberg JP. Alopecia areata. Nat Rev Dis Primers. 2017;3:17011. https://doi.org/10.1038/nrdp.2017.11.

4. Fricke ACV, Miteva M. Epidemiology and burden of alopecia areata: a systematic review. Clin Cosmet Investig Dermatol. 2015;8:397–403. https://doi.org/10.2147/CCID.S53985.
5. Blaumeiser B, van der Goot I, Fimmers R, Hanneken S, Ritzmann S, Seymons K, et al. Familial aggregation of alopecia areata. J Am Acad Dermatol. 2006;54(4):627–32. https://doi.org/10.1016/j.jaad.2005.12.007.
6. Darwin E, Hirt PA, Fertig R, et al. Alopecia areata: review of epidemiology, clinical features, pathogenesis, and new treatment options. Int J Trichol. 2018;10(2):51–60.
7. Biran R, Zlotogorski A, Ramot Y. The genetics of alopecia areata: new approaches, new findings, new treatments. J Dermatol Sci. 2015;78(1):11–20. https://doi.org/10.1016/j.jdermsci.2015.01.004.
8. Ramot Y, Zlotogorski A. Jak inhibitors for the treatment of alopecia areata. Harefuah. 2020;159(1):38–42. Available from: https://www.researchgate.net/publication/338582544_JAK_INHIBITORS_FOR_THE_TREATMENT_OF_ALOPECIA_AREATA
9. Zhang W, Yu M, Yu W, et al. Development of alopecia areata is associated with higher central and peripheral hypothalamic- pituitary-adrenal tone in the skin graft induced C3H/HeJ mouse model. J Invest Dermatol. 2009;129:1527–38.
10. Peters E, Liotiri S, Bodo E, et al. Probing the effects of stress mediators on the human hair follicle: substance P holds central position. Am J Pathol. 2007;171:1872–86.
11. Bolotnaya LA, Serbina IM. Adaptation-regulatory mechanisms in alopecia areata. Georgian Med News. 2017;11(272):75–80.
12. Sellami R, Masmoudi J, Ouali U, et al. The relationship between alopecia areata and alexithymia, anxiety and depression: a case-control study. Indian J Dermatol. 2014;59(4):421.
13. Sinclair R. Alopecia areata and suicide of children. Med J Aust. 2014;200(3):145–8.
14. Serbina I, Andrashko Y, Galnykina S, Kadigrob I, Khobzei K, Liadova T, Litus O, Sviatenko T, Svistunov I, Syzon O, Vozianova S, Ovcharenko Y. Clinical guidelines of the Ukraine Hair Research Society. Diagnosis and treatment of alopecia areata. Actual problems of modern medicine. 2023;12:45–67. https://doi.org/10.26565/2617-409X-2023-12-06.
15. Tosti A, Whiting D, Iorizzo M, et al. The role of scalp dermoscopy in the diagnosis of alopecia areata incognita. J Am Acad Dermatol. 2008;59(1):64–7. https://doi.org/10.1016/j.jaad.2008.03.031.
16. Rebora A. Alopecia areata incognita: a hypothesis. Dermatologica. 1987;174(5):214–8. https://doi.org/10.1159/000249182.
17. Miteva M, Misciali C, Fanti PA, et al. Histopathologic features of alopecia areata incognito: a review of 46 cases. J Cutan Pathol. 2012;39(6):596–602. https://doi.org/10.1111/j.1600-0560.2012.01896.x.
18. Alessandrini A, Starace M, Bruni F, Brandi N, Baraldi C, Misciali C, Fanti PA, Piraccini BM. Alopecia areata incognita and diffuse alopecia areata: clinical, trichoscopic, histopathological, and therapeutic features of a 5-year study. Dermatol Pract Concept. 2019;9(4):272–7. https://doi.org/10.5826/dpc.0904a05. Erratum in: Dermatol Pract Concept. 2019;10(1):e2020027. doi: https://doi.org/10.5826/dpc.1001a27. PMID: 31723460; PMCID: PMC6830548
19. Navarini AA, Trüeb RM. Why Henry III of Navarre's hair probably did not turn white overnight. Int J Trichology. 2010;2:2–4.
20. Rudnicka L, Olszewska M, Rakowska A. Atlas of trichoscopy. Dermoscopy in hair and scalp disease. London: Springer; 2012.
21. Olsen E, Hordinsky MK, Price V, et al. Alopecia areata investigational assessment guidelines. Part II. J Am Acad Dermatol. 2004;51:440–7.
22. Ovcharenko Y. Trichopathies in children. Kharkiv: Maidan; 2017. p. 264.
23. Conic RZ, Miller R, Piliang M, et al. Comorbidities in patients with alopecia areata. J Am Acad Dermatol. 2017;76(4):755–7.
24. Ikeda T. A new classication of alopecia areata. Dermatologica. 1965;131(6):421–45.
25. Fabbrocini G, Panariello L, De Vita V, et al. Quality of life in alopecia areata: a disease-specificquestionnaire. J Eur Acad Dermatol Venereol. 2013;27:276–80.

26. King B, Ohyama M, Kwon O, Zlotogorski A, Ko J, Mesinkovska NA, Hordinsky M, Dutronc Y, Wu WS, McCollam J, Chiasserini C, Yu G, Stanley S, Holzwarth K, DeLozier AM, Sinclair R, Investigators BRAVE-AA. Two phase 3 trials of baricitinib for alopecia areata. N Engl JMed. 2022;386(18):1687–99. https://doi.org/10.1056/NEJMoa2110343. Epub 2022 Mar 26
27. King B, Zhang X, Harcha WG, Szepietowski JC, Shapiro J, Lynde C, Mesinkovska NA, Zwillich SH, Napatalung L, Wajsbrot D, Fayyad R, Freyman A, Mitra D, Purohit V, Sinclair R, Wolk R. Efficacy and safety of ritlecitinib in adults and adolescents with alopecia areata: a randomised, double-blind, multicentre, phase 2b-3 trial. Lancet. 2023;401(10387):1518–29. https://doi.org/10.1016/S0140-6736(23)00222-2. Epub 2023 Apr 14. Erratum in: Lancet. 2023
28. Sanchez-Diaz M, Diaz-Calvillo P, Rodriguez-Pozo JA, Tercedor-Sánchez J, Cantudo-Cuenca MR, Molina-Leyva A, Arias-Santiago S. Tofacitinib for treatment of alopecia areata: real-world evidence and factors associated with therapeutic response. Acta Derm Venereol. 2022;102:adv00736. https://doi.org/10.2340/actadv.v102.2036.
29. Abedini H, Farshi S, Mirabzadeh A, Keshavarz S. Antidepressant effects of citalopram on treatment of alopecia areata in patients with major depressive disorder. J Dermatolog Treat. 2014;25(2):153–5.
30. Willemsen R, Haentjens P, Roseeuw D, et al. Hypnosis in refractory alopecia areata sigificantly improves depression, anxiety, and life quality but not hair regrowth. J Am Acad Dermatol. 2010;62(3):517–8.
31. Park J, Kim DW, Park SK, Yun SK, Kim HU. Role of hair prostheses (wigs) in patients with severe alopecia areata. Ann Dermatol. 2018;30(4):505–7. https://doi.org/10.5021/ad.2018.30.4.505. Epub 2018 Jun 28. PMID: 30065604; PMCID: PMC6029960

Telogen Effluvium

7

Ralph Trüeb, Kuzma Khobzei, Anna Lyakhovitsky, and Yuliya Ovcharenko

Introduction

Few dermatologic problems carry as much emotional burden as the complaint of hair loss, specifically in women with telogen effluvium (TE). Some patients' anxiety may be exacerbated by previous frustrating experiences with physicians, who tend to downplay or dismiss complaints of hair loss. This attitude on the part of physicians can be attributed to either a lack of understanding of the impact of hair loss on the quality of life or a lack of confidence in the treatment of alopecia. Indeed, the most effective way to alleviate the emotional distress associated with hair loss is to treat it effectively. Today's treatment options are limited, both in terms of indications and efficacy. Success depends not only on comprehension of the underlying pathology, but also on proper level of empathy on the part of the physician.

A detailed patient history focusing on chronology of events, examination of the pattern of hair loss and the scalp, a few standard diagnostic tests, trichoscopy, appropriate blood screening, and, in selected cases, a scalp biopsy will usually establish the diagnosis. Once the diagnosis has been confirmed, the appropriate treatment is likely to control the problem of hair loss [1–3].

R. Trüeb (✉)
Center for Dermatology and Hair Diseases, Wallisellen, Zürich, Switzerland
e-mail: r.trueeb@derma-haarcenter.ch

K. Khobzei
Department of Infectious Diseases and Clinical Immunology of the V. N. Karazin Kharkiv National University, Khobzei Clinic, Kyiv, Ukraine

A. Lyakhovitsky
Department of Dermatology, Sheba Medical Center, Tel Hashomer, Affiliated with the Faculty of Medicine and Health Sciences, Tel Aviv University, Tel Aviv, Israel

Y. Ovcharenko
V. N. Karazin Kharkiv National University, University Clinic "Trichology Institute", Kharkiv, Ukraine

Y. Ovcharenko et al. (eds.), *Psychotrichology*,
https://doi.org/10.1007/978-3-031-64083-4_7

Many factors can lead to a pathologically increased hair loss. Whatever the cause, the follicle tends to behave in a similar way. To properly understand this concept requires understanding the varied derangements of the hair cycle leading to hair loss. The hair follicle (HF) is subject to a constant turnover during perpetual cycles through phases of proliferation, involution, and resting, with regeneration in the successive hair cycle. Cyclic hair growth activity occurs in a random mosaic pattern with each follicle possessing its own individual control mechanism over the evolution and triggering of the successive phases, while a number of systemic and environmental factors may have an influence, such as hormones, cytokines, growth factors, toxins, deficiencies of nutrients, vitamins, and calories (Fig. 7.1).

Telogen effluvium is by far the commonest cause of hair loss, and results from increased shedding of hairs from the telogen phase of the hair cycle. This can either be due to synchronization phenomena of hair cycling (Fig. 7.2), with hair thinning usually seen at the temples and shedding of hairs in the hundreds in telogen effluvium or to a decrease of anagen phase duration in androgenetic alopecia (AGA) with its sex-typical patterns of alopecia (male and female pattern hair loss), variable shedding of hair, and increasing diversity of hair shaft diameters. The increase in the percentage of follicles in telogen (>20%) leads to increased shedding of hairs in telogen (Fig. 7.3).

It can be challenging to distinguish between chronic telogen effluvium (TE) and AGA in females due to the overlap of both conditions. To differentiate between

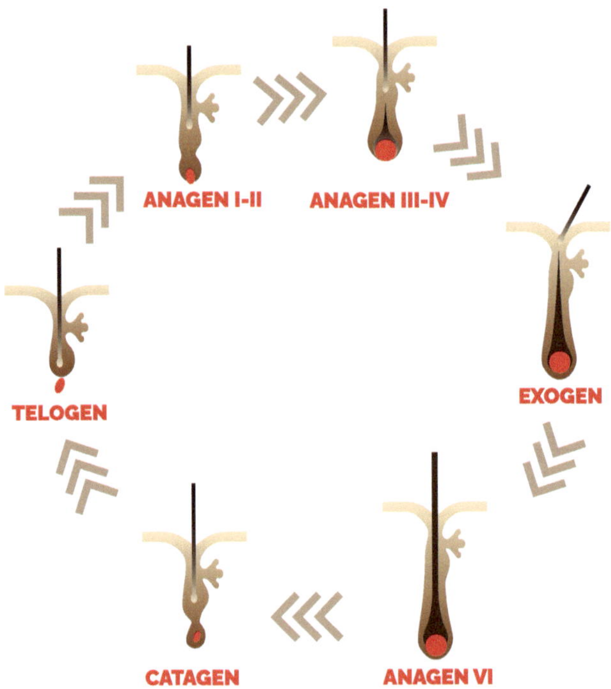

Fig. 7.1 Hair cycle

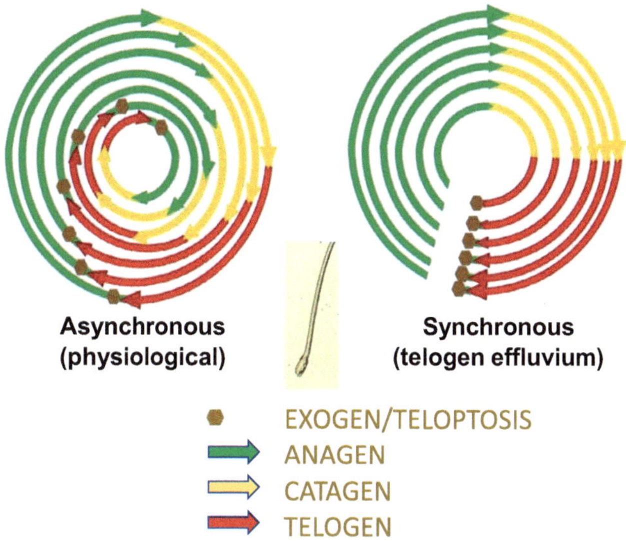

Fig. 7.2 Physiological asynchronous versus synchronous shedding of telogen hairs (teloptosis) in telogen effluvium

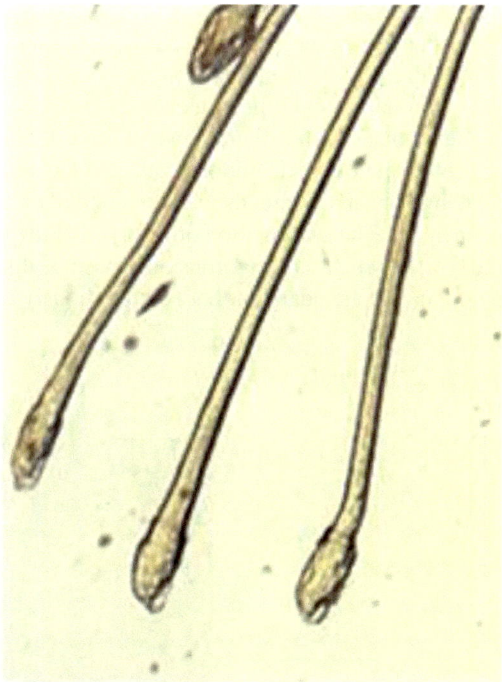

Fig. 7.3 Hair pluck in telogen effluvium: telogen bulbs

AGA and TE and determine the severity of the disease, Guarrera et al. proposed a wash test to measure the quantity of shed hair as well as terminal and vellus hair. Five days after their last shampoo wash, the patient is asked to wash their hair in the sink with the drain gauze-covered. Afterward, the hairs that are tangled in the gauze are counted and divided into lengths of ≤3 and ≥5 cm. According to the research, there are significantly more vellus hairs in AGA than in chronic TE (58.9% vs. 3.5%) [4].

History

Defluvium capillorum was the original term used in 1932 to describe diffuse hair loss. Other researchers used the term to refer to all forms of alopecia, while Sabouraud restricted it to a sudden diffuse loss of hair following a severe emotional shock.

Chronic diffuse alopecia in women was first distinguished from acute and reversible diffuse alopecia due to a clearly identifiable cause in the 1950s. Sulzberger et al. reported an unexplained significant increase in the incidence of diffuse alopecia in women in 1960. This report, however, does not permit discrimination between women with diffuse TE and female AGA [5].

Moreover, female AGA with its more diffuse thinning of the crown area and an intact frontal hairline (Fig. 7.4), as opposed to male-pattern AGA with its characteristic bitemporal recession of the hair and balding vertex, was originally described by Ludwig only in 1977 [6].

Ultimately, in the 1990s, Rushton et al. and Rushton and Ramsay characterized many affected women biochemically and trichologically as having a diffuse androgen-dependent type of alopecia [7].

Nevertheless, a peculiar type of chronic TE does seem to exist that preferentially affects women in their middle ages, and has probably originally been described in 1959 by Guy and Edmundson, who reported on a diffuse cyclic (type of) hair loss in women [8]. The presentation of this type of diffuse hair loss tends to be distinctive: the typical patient is a vigorous otherwise healthy woman with a full, thick head of hair. Patients are adamant that they previously had more hair and are distressed by

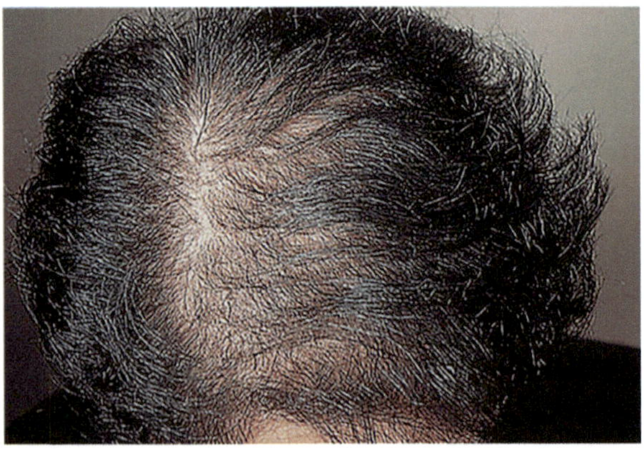

Fig. 7.4 Female pattern hair loss

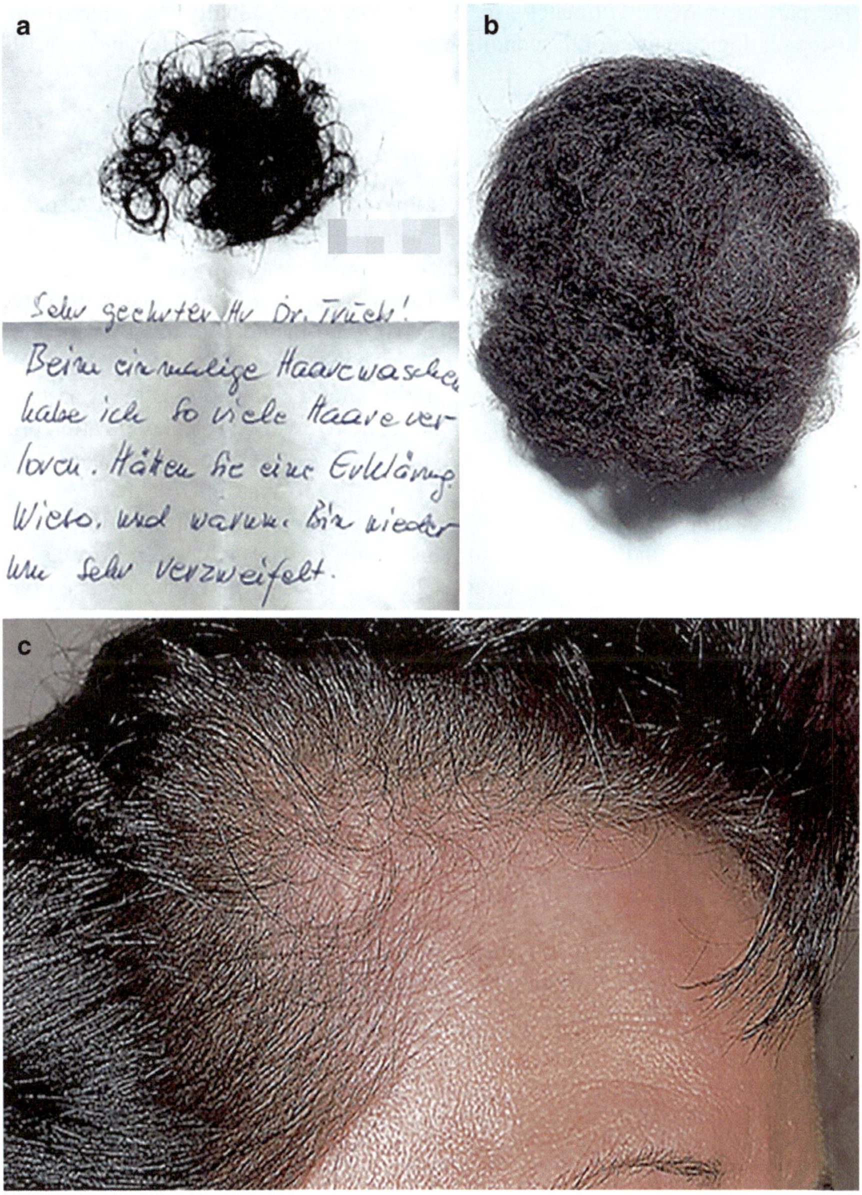

Fig. 7.5 Telogen effluvium: (**a**) letter of patient concern with hair loss, (**b**) ball of shed hairs, (**c**) temporal thinning of hair

the prospect of going bald (Fig. 7.5a), and many bring large balls of hair for inspection (Fig. 7.5b), but despite this do not show any obvious balding.

On examination, there is some bitemporal thinning (Fig. 7.5c), and a positive hair pull test equally over the vertex and occiput. There is no widening of the central hair part as in AGA. Ultimately, in 1996, Whiting additionally characterized the histopathologic features of the condition finally delineating it from female AGA [9].

Classification

Kligman in 1961 revealed the pathophysiology of one common pattern of response of hair follicles to a variety of insults and named it TE [10]. While several attempts have been made with respect to the underlying pathophysiology of TE and its classification, the original classification by Headington from 1993 remains unabated and most comprehensive. Five functional types are included in this classification based on changes in various hair cycle phases (Table 7.1).

While TE represents a monomorphic reaction of the hair follicle to a variety of causes, the underlying pathologic dynamics is more diverse. The classification proposed by Headington covers all clinical types of TE: post-febrile, posttraumatic, and postinterventional (immediate anagen release), postpartum (delayed anagen release), shedding phase upon initiation of topical minoxidil treatment (immediate telogen release), and seasonal hair shedding (delayed telogen release) [11]. Headington's innovative classification predicted the existence of a short anagen syndrome, which was only later confirmed by the original report of the condition as congenital hypotrichosis due to short anagen by Barraud-Klenovsek and Trüeb in 2000 [12]. The condition was later renamed as short anagen syndrome (Fig. 7.6a, b).

Table 7.1 Functional types of telogen effluvium. From: Headington J. T. Telogen effluvium. New concepts and review. Arch Dermatol, 1993

Immediate anagen release
Hair Follicles (HFs) that would normally complete a longer cycle by remaining in anagen, prematurely enter into telogen. It is a very common form of telogen effluvium (TE), typically occurring after periods of physiologic stress including episodes of high fever. Hair loss occurs 3–4 months after the inciting event and is dependent on the transition from anagen to catagen and telogen, with subsequent release of telogen hairs
Delayed anagen release
HFs remain in prolonged anagen rather than cycling into telogen. When finally released from anagen, the clinical sign of increased shedding of telogen hair will be found. This type of TE underlies postpartum hair loss
Delayed telogen release
HFs remain in prolonged telogen rather than being shed and recycled into anagen. The clinical sign of increased shedding of club hairs is observed again after the onset of teloptosis. This process underlies molting (ecdysis) in mammals and probably also seasonal shedding of hairs in humans or mild TE following travel from low-daylight to high-daylight region
Short anagen
A shortened anagen phase duration causes a mild but persistent TE associated with decreased hair length. AGA is a common cause of acquired progressive shortening of anagen. Shortened anagen can also be seen in hereditary hypotrichosis, ectodermal dysplasia (tricho-dental syndrome), and as an isolated disorder in otherwise healthy children, described by Barraud-Klenosvek and Trüeb

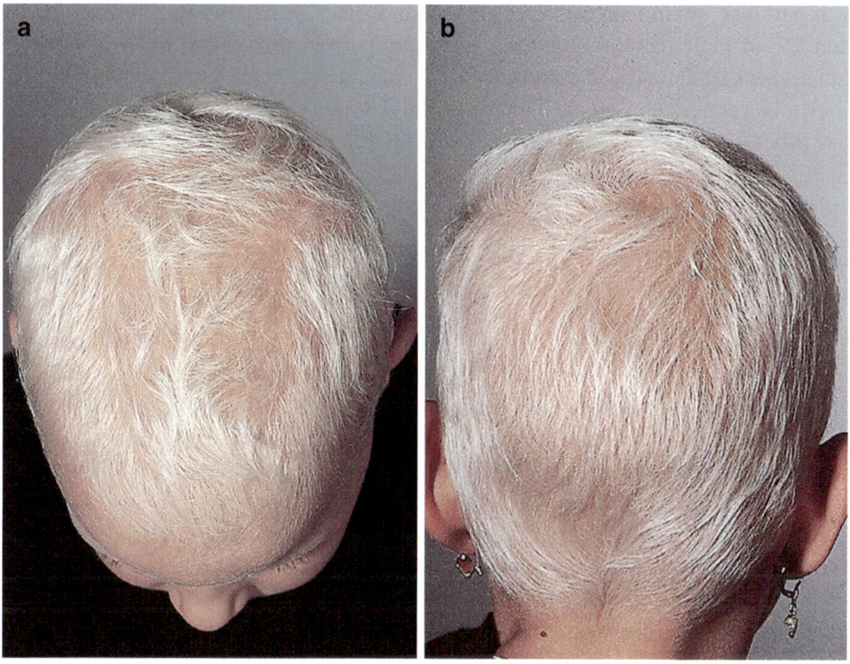

Fig. 7.6 Short anagen syndrome (**a**, **b**)

Chronic Telogen Effluvium and Trichodynia

In the original description of Kligman, TE is an acute diffuse hair loss brought about by a variety of triggers, such as fever, hemorrhagic shock, crash diet, parturition, usually within 3 months of the inciting event. Clinical experience, however, proves that chronic TE also exists. It has arbitrarily been defined as diffuse telogen hair loss that persists longer than 6 months, and either represents a primary disorder and is then a diagnosis of exclusion, or it is secondary to a variety of identifiable systemic disorders, such as iron deficiency, thyroid disease, systemic lupus erythematosus, syphilis, HIV infection, dietary habits, and drugs. These represent frequent culprits and must therefore be systematically investigated. In cases of multifactorial chronic TE, the cause is often difficult to establish.

Rebora [13] proposed an inflammatory or autoimmune type of TE based on the observation of a high frequency of associated scalp dysesthesia (trichodynia), associated autoimmune phenomena (Hashimoto thyroiditis), and a response to topical corticosteroid treatment.

Rebora et al. [14] also originally proposed the term trichodynia for discomfort, pain, or paresthesia of the scalp related to the complaint of hair loss, and found a frequency of 34.2% of female patients who had their hair consultation because of hair loss. In a study on 403 patients (311 females, 92 males) whose main complaint was hair loss, Willimann and Trüeb [15] found that 17% of patients, (20% of female and 9% of male patients) reported hair pain, pain or discomfort of the scalp, not otherwise explained by the presence of a specific dermatologic disease or neurologic disorder, while statistical analysis failed to demonstrate any significant correlation between the scalp discomfort, the extent of hair thinning, and hair loss activity.

It is worth noting that trichodynia typically increases the anxiety related to the patient's preoccupation with hair loss or fear of hair loss.

Contrary to Rebora and colleagues' prediction's that trichodynia would be common in chronic TE, it was found in other hair disorders also, particularly AGA. The exact cause of trichodynia is unknown; however Perifollicular microinflammation was proposed as a possible cause by Rebora et al. However, clear histopathologic evidence for this suggestion is currently lacking.

Acute diffuse and total alopecia of the female scalp, described by Sato-Kawamura et al. [16] as a specific type of inflammatory non-cicatricial alopecia with marked female predominance and a uniquely short clinical course with hair regrowth, is one of the differential diagnoses for TE. This condition is most likely a subtype of alopecia areata with diffuse hair loss, as first described by Braun-Falco and Zaun [17]. The condition typically affects women over the age of 40 who have diffused alopecia and were misdiagnosed with TE. Some authors consider alopecia areata incognita, described by Rebora in 1987, as a similar condition, but the issue remains debatable [18]. Trichoscopic diagnosis (see Chap. 6) and histopathology usually confirm the diagnosis.

Until proven otherwise, the designation "inflammatory telogen effluvium" should be reserved exclusively for TE resulting from inflammatory conditions of the scalp, such as severe seborrheic dermatitis, acute allergic contact dermatitis (usually to para-phenylenediamine in hair coloring agents), erythroderma (of psoriasis or lymphoma), or interface dermatitis from lupus erythematosus or dermatomyositis.

Hoss and Segal [19] interpreted scalp dysesthesia as a cutaneous dysesthesia syndrome related to underlying psychiatric disorders, with affected individuals either suffering from depressive, generalized anxiety, or somatoform disorder.

Ericson et al. [20] found localization of the neuropeptide substance P in the scalp skin of patients with painful scalp suggesting a causal relationship between the presence of substance P and trichodynia. Substance P represents a neuropeptide involved in nociception and neurogenic inflammation. Willimann and Trüeb [15] reported that only a small number of patients with trichodynia showed telangiectasia of the scalp, and this finding strongly correlated with the presence of trichodynia. it is interesting to note that substance P not only represents an important mediator of nociception and neurogenic inflammation, but also exerts a potent vasodilatory effect. The role of substance P and related substances (neuropeptides) in the pathogenesis of trichodynia, and especially its relation to the nervous system and emotional stress, needs further elucidation. By the virtue of their bidirectional effects on the neuroendocrine and immune systems, substance P and other neuropeptides may well represent key players in the interaction between the central nervous system and the skin immune and microvascular system.

Such mechanisms would explain the noxious effects not only of external stimuli (mechanical, thermal, and chemical), but also of emotional distress on cutaneous nociception through the release of neuropeptides, such as substance P.

Arck et al. [21] demonstrated that stress-induced immune changes of the hair follicles in mice could be mimicked by injection of substance P in non-stressed animals and were abrogated by selective substance P receptor antagonism in stressed animals.

More recently, a possible association of trichodynia with cervical spine disease has been reported [22].

> It is noteworthy that trichodynia probably represents a polyetiological symptom with a significant psychosomatic component.

It is still unknown what causes primary chronic TE. Shortening of the anagen phase, premature teloptosis, or persistent or intermittent pathologic synchronization phenomena of the hair cycle have all been proposed as potential causes of the disorder.

There is currently insufficient evidence that TE has an inflammatory or autoimmune origin. In trichodynia-related cases, substance P might be involved. Chronic TE remains a diagnosis of exclusion (disease, medications, deficiencies), requiring consideration of several underlying cause-relationships, including notable seasonal variations in hair growth and shedding, notable overlap with AGA, and widespread psychological overlay [23].

Seasonal Hair Shedding

Several women complain of recurrent hair loss. The condition tends to run a fluctuating course, presumably reflecting seasonal periodicity in the growth and shedding of hair.

Orentreich [24] originally reported three women in New York who experienced maximum hair loss in November. By studying a group of 14 men for 18 months, Randall and Ebling [25] subsequently showed that the proportion of telogen hair and of hair shedding were maximal in September.

Courtois et al. [26] observed ten men, with or without alopecia, for a period of between 8 and 14 years, and demonstrated a maximal proportion of telogen hairs at the end of summer. Some subjects also exhibited a periodicity approximately corresponding to two annual peaks.

To test the hypothesis that periodicity in shedding of hairs in women complaining of hair loss may reflect seasonal changes in human hair growth, Kunz et al. [27] eventually performed a study over a period of 6 years of telogen rates as assessed by the trichogram technique in 832 otherwise healthy women complaining of hair loss with or without clinically apparent alopecia in relation to the season.

The study demonstrated the existence of overall annual periodicity in the growth and shedding of hair, manifested by a maximal proportion of telogen hairs in July. Taking a telogen phase duration of approximately 100 days into account, one would expect shedding of these hairs by autumn. A second peak seems to exist, although less pronounced, in April. The telogen rate was lowest at the beginning of February.

The cyclical activity of the HF is the mechanism by which mammals change their coat of hair to meet the needs of growth, seasonal changes in the ambient environment and, perhaps, normal wear and tear. The fact that human HFs, just as those of other mammals, undergo cyclical activity and are influenced by hormones, implies that human hair is not unaffected by these phenomena. From an evolutionary point of view, the maintenance of the low winter level of hair shedding and the postponement of hair fall until the end of summer might, perhaps, be postulated as having a selective advantage with respect to isolation of the head against the cold in winter, and protection of the scalp against the midday sun in summer, respectively.

More importantly, the existence of seasonal fluctuations in hair growth and shedding complicates the assessment of pharmacological effects. Awareness of these fluctuations is prerequisite to providing the correct cause and prognosis to the patient, ensuring patient compliance with therapy, but also has potentially serious implications for investigations with hair growth-promoting agents. Depending upon the stage of periodicity in growth and shedding of hair for a particular subject, the heterogenicity of included subjects may be enough to distort the clinical efficacy results and the perceived benefit of an investigational agent. In the active stage of seasonal TE, the involved hair follicles would probably fail to respond to the therapeutic agent, which may cause a false-negative result. In the recovery stage, the increase amounts of spontaneously regrowing hair might be interpreted falsely as a positive result.

Psychogenic Effluvium

Published materials about the cause-relationship of emotional distress and hair loss were more controversial than helpful. The emotional stress is not an indisputable proof of its having incited the patient's hair loss. The relationship may also be the inverse. Nevertheless, case-control studies suggest that women who experience high stress are more likely to experience hair loss [23], moreover the distress caused by the alopecia itself may eventually contribute to its chronic course.

Adjustment Disorders

Even though most patients with hair disorders experience significant psychological impact, it is usually not of an intensity to qualify as a mental illness. Nevertheless, the impact that hair disorders have on body image significantly contributes to the overall impact on the patient's quality of life. If one appreciates the psychosocial impact of hair disease, there is no doubt that appropriate treatment frequently has a huge bearing on the patients' quality of life.

The clinician should keep in mind that the distress the patient feels from having a hair disease can be handled both dermatologically and psychologically.

Some patients have difficulties adjusting to hair loss. As a result, the individual may have difficulty with his or her mood and behavior. From a psychopathological point of view, adjustment disorders may result from the stressful event of hair loss, depending on its acuity, extent, and prognosis. An adjustment disorder is a debilitating reaction to a stressful event or situation. These symptoms or behaviors are clinically significant as evidenced by either of the following: distress that is in excess of what would be expected, or significant impairment in social, occupational, or educational functioning.

Adjustment disorder subtypes include:

- Adjustment disorder with depressed mood
- Adjustment disorder with anxiety
- Adjustment disorder with mixed anxiety and depressed mood
- Adjustment disorder with disturbance of conduct
- Adjustment disorder with mixed disturbance of emotions and conduct

Associated features may include somatic and/or sexual dysfunction, feelings of guilt and/or obsession. The most effective way to alleviate the emotional distress caused by hair disease is to eliminate the hair disease that is causing the problem.

Psychogenic Pseudoeffluvium

Patients with imaginary hair loss or psychogenic pseudoeffluvium are frightened of the possibility of going bald or are convinced they are going bald without any objective findings of hair loss. Basically, they suffer from what Cotterill [28] has termed dermatologic nondisease. Although dermatologists are used to seeing patients with minor skin and hair problems in several body areas that cause disproportionate anxiety and cosmetic distress, with dermatologic nondisease there is no dermatologic pathology.

It is important to realize that imaginary hair loss only makes up for a minority of patients complaining of hair loss, and that patients with psychogenic pseudoeffluvium have varied underlying mental disorders that have to be recognized and treated as such, ideally in a combined liaison clinic with an interdisciplinary approach. Nevertheless, the dermatologist is often the physician designated by the patients to handle their chief complaint, even if the main disorder is a psychological one.

> It is essential for dermatologists dealing with such patients to expand their clinical acumen and therapeutic armamentarium to effectively handle the psychodermatologic cases in their practice.

The most common psychiatric problems underlying psychogenic pseudoeffluvium present are depressive disorder and body dysmorphic disorder. The clinical spectrum is wide, and many patients are at the neurotic end of the spectrum and merely have overvalued ideas about their hair, whereas a minority of patients are truly deluded and suffer from delusional disorder. These patients lie at the psychotic end of the psychiatric spectrum. Those parts of the body that are important in body image are the focus of the preoccupation and concern.

True TE resulting from AGA, TE, or from involutional alopecia must carefully be excluded. Differential diagnosis is particularly challenging since there is a considerable overlap between hair loss and psychological problems. Patients with hair loss have lower self-confidence, higher depression scores, greater introversion, as well as higher neuroticism and feelings of being unattractive.

> It is important to recognize that patients with psychogenic pseudoeffluvium are expecting the clinician to treat them with respect as a trichologic patient, and not as a psychiatric case. The most effective approach to pychogenic pseudoeffluvium is to take the chief complaint seriously and offer the patient a complete trichologic examination.

A careful medical history, including medications, hormones, and crash diets, clinical examination of the hair and scalp (no alopecia, normal scalp), hair calendar (normal counts of hairs shed), trichogram (normal anagen and telogen rates), and laboratory workup should be performed to exclude real effluvium, and if necessary repeated.

In addition to the relentless complaint of hair loss, patients suffering from body dysmorphic disorder adopt obsessional, repetitive ritualistic behavior, and may come to spend much of the day in front of a mirror, repeatedly checking their hair. Another aspect of this behavior is a constant need for reassurance about the hair, not only from the immediate family but also from the medical profession and from dermatologists. These patients may become the most demanding and challenging to treat. The first step in the treatment is to establish a good rapport with the patient.

Telogen Mania

Telogen mania refers to the obsessive-compulsive fits of fierce hair brushing usually in women [10].

Individuals with an obsessive-compulsive personality are rigid, perfectionistic, and indecisive for fear of making a mistake; they lack self-confidence, are sensitive to criticism, and are socially reserved. Most importantly they have a profound difficulty in handling anger and aggression, which sometimes is explosive and at other times is displaced into self-manipulation rather than being expressed directly in a modulated fashion. Other conditions of the obsessive-compulsive spectrum are neurotic excoriations of the scalp, tic depilation, nail biting, skin picking, and acne excoriée.

The psychological effects of hair loss may be hard to differentiate clinically from preexisting psychopathology. Nevertheless, patients with personality disorders tend to experience more distress from hair loss than patients with healthy psyche, since these individuals lack a secure sense of self and effective coping skills, and therefore may be especially vulnerable to the adverse effects of hair loss.

Ultimately, patients with personality disorders tend to have difficulties to cope with stress. The physician should be careful not to be judgmental or scolding because this may rapidly close down communication. Sometimes the patient gains therapeutic benefit just from venting concerns in a safe environment with a caring physician.

Management

A comprehensive medical and drug history, physical examination of the hair and scalp, and appropriate laboratory evaluation are all required for a patient complaining of hair loss, just as they are for any other medical problem. A variety of diagnostic techniques are also available to the clinician to determine whether the patient's disorder is a true hair shedding disorder or merely perceived pathology.

Understanding the underlying dynamics of hair loss and the potential multitude of cause relationships is required for providing appropriate patient care. It is important to remember that hair loss is frequently the result of a combination of factors that must be addressed. An individualized treatment plan can be designed by approaching the hair loss patient methodically and beginning with objects ascending step by step from the simplest and easiest to recognize to the more complex ones. It is prudent to divide each problem into as many parts as possible that may be required for its adequate solution, and finally to make enumerations and reviews as complete and general as possible, so that nothing is omitted.

It is important for a trichologist to inform the patient about the nature and mechanism of hair loss since a misunderstanding of these aspects lead to delusions and further aggravation of the emotional and psychological status. A typical example of this situation can be a state for which the authors proposed the term **accumulated effluvium** (AE). This condition occurs in patients who develop a fear of washing, combing, or even touching their hair, because they are convinced that these actions will lead to hair shedding (Ovcharenko and Khobzei 2025) [29].

Because it is no secret that most hair falls out precisely during any physical impact on them, this "careful" handling allows for a slight reduction in shedding. However, this has no effect on the amount of hair that has completed the telogen phase and is preparing to fall out. Hair that hasn't fallen out in time accumulates on the scalp, and even the slightest impact from outside factors, whether it's an attempt to fix the hairdo or a gust of wind, causes a large amount of hair loss. This gives the impression that "the hair are not attached at all" or "the hair roots are very weak," further traumatizing the patient and encouraging them to wash or touch their hair less frequently, entrapping them in the vicious circle of delusion. According to studies conducted by Ovcharenko and Khobzey on 58 female patients with similar symptoms, 74% had previously experienced acute TE. Trichoscopic observations of this condition have shown resemblance to common TE, with some increase in new growing hairs, but this picture is discordant with a markedly positive hair tension test that does not correlate with a relatively small number of growing hairs. In addition, the accumulation of sebum and keratin scales on the scalp due to hygiene problems is characteristic (Fig. 7.7).

The management of these patients includes providing trichological care in a trichology clinic environment. Patients usually are more comfortable if a professional washes their hair because they don't see the whole amount of hair falling out. Additionally, the hair will stop shedding excessively at the smallest impact after complete washing, combing, and hair drying.

The psychosocial study in female patients with AE showed a negative relationship between the hair condition and quality of life, often secondary to primary psychological problems. It is established that the probability of psychological problems development/worsening in female patients with hair diseases are determined by their primary psychopathologies. In 68% of patients in the study cohort, the phobia to touch their hair developed in the context of preexisting psychiatric disorders, including depression and anxiety disorders.

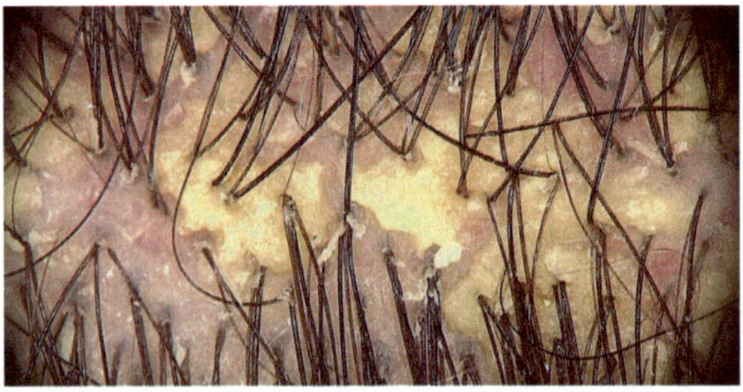

Fig. 7.7 Trichoscopy in a patient diagnosed with accumulated effluvium reveals few growing hairs, a significant amount of sebum and keratin scales due to personal hygiene problems (×60)

In this regard, it is critical for a trichologist to distinguish between the patient's objective fear of baldness and the paradoxical, irrational fear of touching one's hair. Since in the latter case, without psychological treatment, it can be extremely difficult to help the patient.

> Reliably assessing the actual shedding of hair is a crucial diagnostic point in trichology practice. This evaluation should be simple, noninvasive, and quick.

Many methods have been proposed, but there is still no standard test for assessing hair shedding. The simple hair pull test is insensitive, and the trichogram used to determine telogen percentage does not directly correlate with the clinical severity of hair loss. The patient can perform daily hair counts at home. The patient is instructed to collect all hairs that fall out during morning grooming, including hairs on the pillow, sink, comb, brush, and shoulders, as well as all hairs that come out with the morning shampoo, for this purpose. A piece of nylon netting or gauze draped over the drain will help secure hairs that would otherwise be lost during washing. All collected hair is placed in a clear plastic bag with the date and written information on whether or not the hair has been shampooed. In addition, the patient is asked to count each hair in the bag and record the total count on the label.

Typically, the patient is recommended to collect the hair for 14 consecutive days, and then bring 14 bags to the doctor's office. Normal hair shed can range from 35 to 180 hairs per day, depending on the total amount of scalp hair and seasonal factors. The number is usually higher on the day of shampoo, especially when the hair is not shampooed daily. The number of hairs shed daily in TE is in the hundreds, whereas in AGA it may be less than 100.

While the daily hair count is a cumbersome procedure, to find a simple method to evaluate reliably the diagnosis and activity of androgenetic alopecia and telogen effluvium, Guarrera et al. [4] adopted the modified wash test (MWT). The test accomplishes such a task through assessing the number of shed hair and the vellus percentage. Seven days after the last shampoo, the patient washes her hair in the sink with the drain covered by gauze. The number of hairs caught on the gauze is then counted. It is simple, noninvasive, and not expensive and helps to distinguish TE from AGA, to identify cases of association TE+AGA, to assess the severity of these conditions, and to point to the correct treatment tactics.

Trichoscopic Diagnostics

Trichoscopy and quantitative analyses of hair growth indicators allow not only to objectify the patient's condition, but also build synergistic patient–doctor relationships leading to more effective management of trichopathologies. Practical experience shows that patients subjectively perceive a consultation using trichoscopy as more trustworthy than in the case of examination with the naked eye only. Digital trichoscopy and demonstration of changes characteristic for a particular condition allows additionally involving the patient in the process and, probably, improving compliance [30].

An increased number of new regrowing hairs is a common trichoscopic sign in both acute and chronic TE (Fig. 7.8a) [31]. In severe acute TE, for example, following a COVID-19 infection, which is a classic example, the volume of hair loss and, consequently, the amount of newly regrowing hairs will be greater than in chronic TE (Fig. 7.8b). Acute TE can cause panic symptoms even in mentally stable people due to the large volume of shedding and abrupt thinning.

In these cases, a doctor can assure the patient by showing them an abundance of growing hair and explaining that new shafts are growing in place of shed hairs. In most cases, patients respond positively to this information.

Trichoscopy can also be used to see telogen hair roots extracted during a pull test, as well as to determine the duration and mechanism of hair loss. A telogen bulb at one end (Fig. 7.9a) and a pointed tip at the other (Fig. 7.9b) will indicate that the hair has not been broken or trimmed. Hair age can be determined by measuring its length every month at a rate of 1–1.2 cm. Loss of new (less than 2 years old) short (less than 25 cm) hair may indicate anagen phase premature completion, which is one of the mechanisms of TE.

In pseudo-alopecia, the analysis of hair quantitative parameters to objectify the diagnosis and determine the true level of hair loss can be a very powerful tool. It is well-known that in some patients with complaints of excessive hair loss, this loss is not actually excessive. Patients can sometimes interpret hair loss due to the physiological phase change in the hair follicle cycle as increased and seek medical attention.

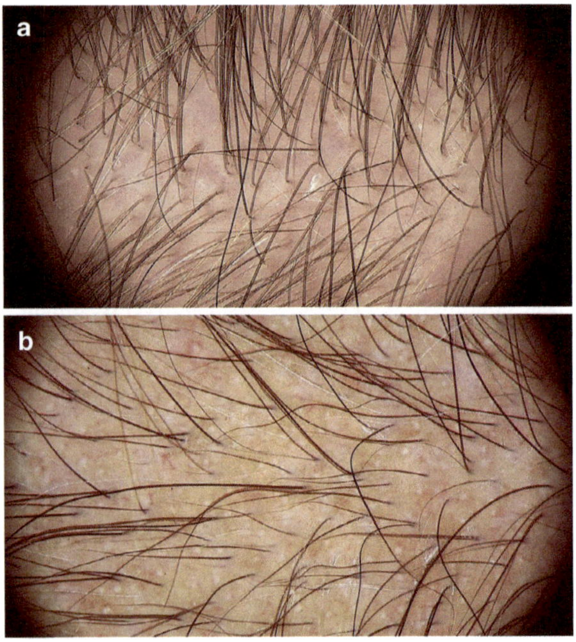

Fig. 7.8 (**a**) Trichoscopic picture of acute telogen effluvium showing an increase of new growing hairs (×20). (**b**). Trichoscopic picture of acute post-COVID telogen effluvium. Multiple new regrowing hairs (×20)

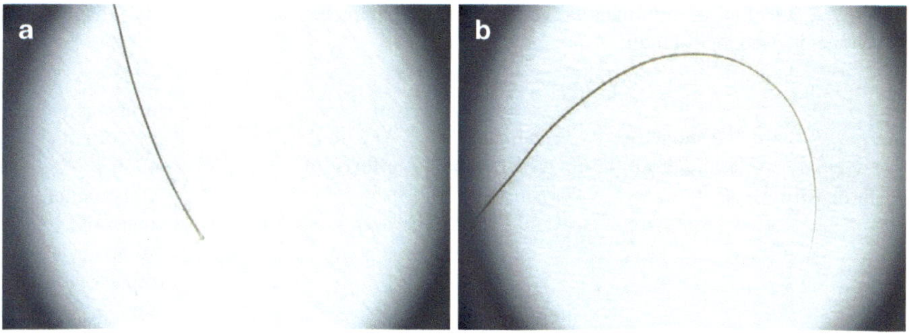

Fig. 7.9 (**a**) Telogen root; (**b**) pointed free tip of an extracted hair (×20)

Often these patients use phrases "I used to have less hair loss," "My tail was twice as thick," etc. Undoubtedly, these statements need to be critically analyzed, since they are based on the patient's subjective perception of the hair loss process.

The diagnosis of TE can be further objectified by a two-stage phototrichogram (PTG). Among the criteria that is being examined are the hair density per 1 cm^2, the average hair diameter, the ratio of vellus and terminal hairs, and the anagen/telogen percentage, which has the most significant clinical value in the diagnosis of TE [32, 33].

That said, trichologists are aware that "persuading" a patient to do an FTG with shaving is sometimes not possible, but the results of the quantitative hair examination in the differential diagnosis of pseudoeflvium, accumulated efluvium, TE and AGA can be crucial (Table 7.2) [30].

TrichoLAB service, available to users of Fotofinder digital dermatoscopy systems, can be considered an effective alternative to classical FTG. The advantage of TrichoScale AI method is obtaining quantitative parameters of hair growth without shaving. The solution is based on images taken with a help of a precise algorithm, and the measurements themselves are performed according to the images produced at 50x magnification (Fig. 7.10). Due to the larger scale, the accuracy of the measurements will be noticeably higher, and the measurements of hair diameter, as well as the parameters dependent on it, will be more accurate than in the case of the 20x magnification used in classical FTG. The documented results of the trichoscopic report allow, among other things, to involve the patient in the therapeutic and diagnostic process and, in case of psychogenic pseudoeffluvium, to assure that patient does not lose hair in the dynamics of subsequent quantitative observations.

The TrichoLAB trichoscopic report includes such parameters as hair density, mean hair diameter, number of thin hairs (diameter less than 30 μm), medium hairs (30-50 μm) and thick hairs (more than 50 μm), hair distribution in follicular units (percentage of follicular units with one, two, three or more hairs), cumulative hair thickness, and Trichoscopy Derived Sinclair Scale assessment of pattern hair loss in women. An increase in the number of thin hairs and a decrease in mean hair diameter in the frontal area are in favour of AGA. Normal characteristics of hair growth density, mean hair diameter and distribution of hair in follicular units combined with an increase in the number of short growing hair are in favour of TE (Table 7.2).

Table 7.2 Qualitative and quantitative trichoscopic parameters in the differential diagnosis of psychogenic pseudoeffluvium

Criteria	Psychogenic pseudoeffluvium	Telogen effluvium	Accumulated effluvium	AGA (androgen-dependent zone)
Hair density	N	N	N	At the initial stage—N, At the progressive stage—decreased
Anisotrichosis	Absent	Absent	Absent	20% and more
Thin hair count	N	Increased due to new growing hair	N or increased due to new regrowing hairs if the condition developed secondary to clinical TE	Increased
Anagen hair count	N	Decreased (85% and less) in different zones	N or decreased, if the condition developed secondary to clinical TE	Decreased (85% and less) In androgen-independent zone—N
Telogen hair count	N	Increased (15% and more) in different zones	N or increased, if the condition developed secondary to clinical TE	Increased (15% and more) In androgen-independent zone—N
Yellow dots	Absent	Absent or single	Absent or single, if the condition has developed secondary to clinical TE	At the initial stage may be absent In progressive stage—from single to dozens per 1 cm^2

Trichological patients frequently inquire, "Am I losing too much hair?" "Am I going bald?" "Is the prescribed treatment working?" and so on. These questions may be difficult for a doctor to answer, but the ability to answer in an empathetic manner would serve as the foundation for a constructive trusting relationship with the patient and, eventually, more effective patient care. This can be accomplished by incorporating modern quantitative hair growth analysis methods into routine clinical practice.

Quantitative trichoscopic methods provides an opportunity to translate subjective complaints into an objective plan.

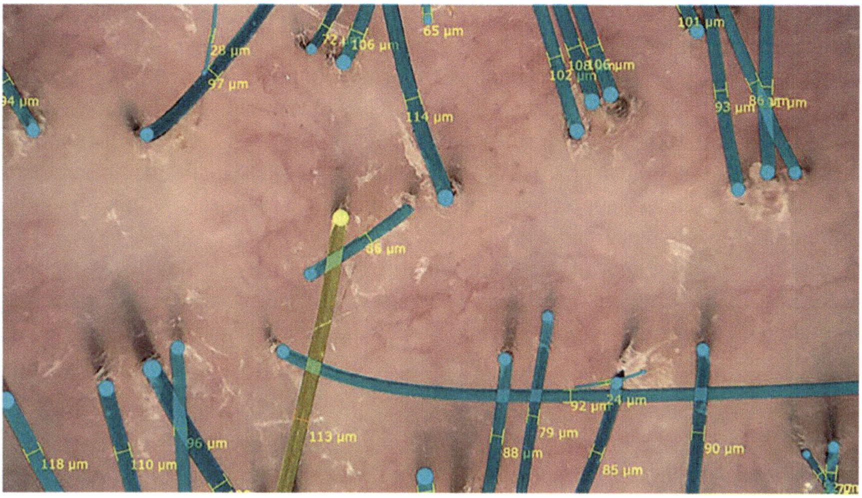

Fig. 7.10 Trichoscale AI—hair thickness measurement with an accuracy of 1 μm (×50)

Treatment

The cause and pathophysiology of TE in relation to the hair growth cycle influence treatment and prognosis. Most acute TE, particularly those caused by acute-onset physiologic events such as post-febrile, postpartum, and seasonal TE, are self-limiting and will resolve completely. If the patient does not recover completely, another diagnosis or a combination of TE and AGA should be considered. Ikeda and Yamada discovered that the presence of AGA increases the risk of developing TE.

Meanwhile, the cause of chronic TE may be multifactorial and difficult to establish. It is critical to rule out or treat many conditions that have been linked to TE, including thyroid dysfunction, systemic lupus erythematosus, and iron deficiency. Medications known to cause hair loss, such as colchicine, antimetabolites (including methotrexate, azathioprine, cyclophosphamide, and others), retinoids, interferon, and pro-androgen hormones (norethisterone, levonorgestrel, and tibolon), should all be discontinued unless the patient absolutely requires them. Finally, in young women, dietary habits should be addressed.

If anorexia nervosa/bulimia is suspected, the aid of a psychiatrist should be sought, in other cases the informed patient will be happy to abandon any dietary culprit.

Differential diagnosis may be complicated through considerable overlap, especially with androgenetic alopecia in women, for instance, in postpartum effluvium that does not necessarily return to the same antepartum texture and length of hair.

In these cases, the addition of topical minoxidil to the treatment regimen is usually helpful. Ultimately, synchronization phenomena of hair cycling, also on a seasonal basis, tend to be more pronounced in patients with AGA, since with a shorter anagen phase a greater proportion of HFs synchronize.

Recommendations for pharmacological treatment of primary chronic TE include corticosteroids, minoxidil, and dietary supplements primarily based on L-cystine, vitamin B1, pantothenic acid (vitamin B5), biotin, vitamin D, zinc, and omega-3 fatty acids [34]. Trüeb RM., Lengg et al. conducted a double-blind, placebo-controlled study in 30 otherwise healthy women suffering of TE and demonstrated by means of the TrichoScan that a L-cystine, medicinal yeast, pantothenic acid and thiamine-based dietary supplement increased the anagen hair rate within 6 months of treatment, while placebo did not [35].

The therapeutic effect of a nutrient-based treatment may be delayed, generally becoming evident not before 3 months. This delayed effect distinguishes active from the placebo effect, which typically is seen early and decays over time.

The placebo effect is about more than just the pill. It is about the cultural meaning of the treatment. The effect of color, packaging, brand name, cost, and route of administration are all of significance. The more elaborate the ritual, the more effective is placebo [36].

An injection is a much more dramatic intervention than just taking a pill. For example, intravenous vitamin B5 and biotin for treatment of TE in women has been reported to be more effective than the respective oral or intramuscular way of administration.

Treatment outcomes are influenced by what the doctor says, how it is done, and what the doctor believes. Even if the doctor remains silent, what he knows or assumes leaks out in his body language, affect, eyebrows, and nervous smiles.

Finally, the issue of psychogenic effluvium and of overvalued ideas in relation to the hair condition is not always easy to resolve, however it is important to control stress as a complication of hair loss or fear of hair loss. For this purpose, strong psychological support is essential to help limit patient anxiety, and patients need to be educated about the basics of the hair cycle. Information about the hair cycle can be useful to explain how hair loss is not related to cycle shortening, as in AGA, which generally precedes new regrowth, and why considerable patience is required for effective cosmetic recovery.

Most importantly, women with primary chronic TE need to be reassured that the condition represents exaggerated shedding rather than actual hair loss and that the shed hair is mostly being replaced, therefore the risk of total baldness is remote. Over time this can be demonstrated by means of regular standardized global photographic assessments and quantitative trichoscopy.

Summary

- Many factors can lead to pathologically increased hair shedding. The pathophysiology of hair shedding can be directly related to disorders of hair cycling.
- TE results from increased shedding of hairs from the telogen phase of the hair cycle. Based on changes in different phases of the hair cycle, TE has been classified into five functional types.
- TE presents either as an acute diffuse hair loss brought about by a variety of identifiable triggers, or as chronic TE, which is defined as telogen effluvium that persists >6 months with multiple, or unknown etiologies.
- Management depends on the cause and underlying pathophysiology in its relation to the hair growth cycle. Once the diagnosis is certain, treatment appropriate for that diagnosis is likely to control the problem.
- Chronic TE of unknown origin can be successfully treated with empathetic approach and a firm explanation of the dynamics of hair growth and has a generally favorable prognosis.
- Overvalued ideas in relation to hair condition and psychogenic pseudoeffluvium are not always easy to resolve and may necessitate interdisciplinary management.

References

1. Trüeb RM. Female alopecia. Guide to successful management. Berlin/Heidelberg: Springer; 2013.
2. Trüeb RM. The difficult hair loss patient. Guide to successful management of hair loss and related conditions. Cham, Switzerland: Springer International Publishing; 2015.
3. Trüeb RM, Lee W-S. Male alopecia. Guide to successful management. Cham, Switzerland: Springer International Publishing; 2014.
4. Guarrera M, Cardo PP, Rebora A. Assessing the reliability of the modified Wash Test. G Ital Dermatol Venereol. 2011;146:289–94.
5. Sulzberger MB, Witten VH, Kopf AW. Diffuse alopecia in women. Its unexplained apparent increase in incidence. Arch Dermatol. 1960;81:556–60.
6. Ludwig E. Classification of the types of androgenetic alopecia (common baldness) occurring in the female sex. Br J Dermatol. 1977;97:247–54.
7. Rushton DH, Ramsay ID, James KC, et al. Biochemical and trichological characterization of diffuse alopecia in women. Br J Dermatol. 1990;123:187–97.
8. Guy WB, Edmundson WF. Diffuse cyclic hair loss in women. Arch Dermatol. 1960;81:205–27.
9. Whiting DA. Chronic telogen effluvium: increased scalp hair shedding in middle-aged women. J Am Acad Dermatol. 1996;35:899–906.
10. Kligman AM. Pathologic dynamics of human hair loss. 1. Telogen effluvium. Arch Dermatol. 1961;83:175–98.
11. Headington JT. Telogen effluvium. New concepts and review. Arch Dermatol. 1993;129:356–63.
12. Barraud-Klenovsek MM, Trüeb RM. Congenital hypotrichosis due to short anagen. Br J Dermatol. 2000;143:612–7.
13. Rebora A. Proposing a simpler classification of telogen effluvium. Skin Appendage Disord. 2016;2(1–2):35–8.
14. Rebora A, Semino MT, Guarrera M. Trichodynia (letter). Dermatology. 1996;192:292–3.

15. Willimann B, Trüeb RM. Hair pain (trichodynia): frequency and relationship to hair loss and patient gender. Dermatology. 2002;205:374–7.
16. Sato-Kawamura M, Aiba S, Tagami H. Acute diffuse and total alopecia of the female scalp. A new subtype of diffuse alopecia areata that has a favorable prognosis. Dermatology. 2002;205:367–73.
17. Braun-Falco ZO. Über die Beteiligung des gesamten Capillitiums bei Alopecia areata. Hautarzt. 1962;13:342–8.
18. Rebora A. Alopecia areata incognita: a hypothesis. Dermatologica. 1987;174:214–8.
19. Hoss D, Segal S. Scalp dysesthesia. Arch Dermatol. 1998;134:327–30.
20. Ericson M, Gabrielson A, Worel S, Lee WS, Hordinsky MK. Substance P (SP) in innervated and non-innervated blood vessels in the skin of patients with symptomatic scalp. Exp Dermatol. 1999;8:344–5.
21. Arck PC, Handjiski B, Peters EM, Peter AS, Hagen E, Fischer A, Klapp BF, Paus R. Stress inhibits hair growth in mice by induction of premature catagen development and deleterious perifollicular inflammatory events via neuropeptide substance P-dependent pathways. Am J Pathol. 2003;162:803–14.
22. Thornsberry LA, English JC 3rd. Scalp dysesthesia related to cervical spine disease. JAMA Dermatol. 2013;149:200–3.
23. York J, Nicholson T, Minors P, Duncan DF. Stressful life events and loss of hair among adult women, a case-control study. Psychol Rep. 1998;82:1044–6.
24. Orentreich N. Scalp replacement in man. In: Montagna W, Bobson RL, editors. Advances in biology of skin. Hair growth, vol. IX. Oxford: Pewrgamon; 1969. p. 99–108.
25. Randall VA, Ebling FJG. Seasonal changes in human hair growth. Br J Dermatol. 1991;124:146–51.
26. Courtois M, Loussouarn G, Hourseau S, Grollier JF. Periodicity in the growth and shedding of hair. Br J Dermatol. 1996;134:47–54.
27. Kunz M, Seifert B, Trüeb RM. Seasonality of hair shedding in healthy women complaining of hair loss. Dermatology. 2009;219:105–10.
28. Cotterill JA. Dermatologic nondisease. Dermatol Clin. 1996;14:439–45.
29. Ovcharenko Y., Khobzei K. Accumulation Effluvium: clinical trichoscopic characteristics of the new psychotrichological disorder, 2025. (in press).
30. Ovcharenko Y. Trichology. In: Ovcharenko Y, Serbina IA, Khobzei K, editors. Practical guide. Kharkov: Publishing house "Charisma plus"; 2025. p. 380.
31. Rudnicka L, Olszewska M, Rakowska A. Atlas of trichoscopy. Dermoscopy in hair and scalp disease. London: Springer-Verlag; 2012.
32. Hoffmann R. TrichoScan: a novel tool for the analysis of hair growth in vivo. J Investig Dermatol Symp Proc. 2003;8(1):109–15.
33. Van Neste MD. Assessment of hair loss: clinical relevance of hair growth evaluation methods. Clin Exp Dermatol. 2002;27(5):358–65.
34. Ovcharenko Y. Use of a nutraceutical agent in women with telogen effluvium: results of a prospective clinical observation. Ukr J Dermatol Venerol Cosmetol. 2024;4(95):51–9.
35. Lengg N, Heidecker B, Seifert B, Trüeb RM. Dietary supplement increases anagen hair rate in women with telogen effluvium: results of a double-blind placebo-controlled trial. Therapy. 2007;4:59–6.
36. Wolf S. The pharmacology of placebos. Pharmacol Rev. 1959;11:689–704.

Anagen Effluvium

8

Ralph Trüeb

Introduction

Novalis (Georg Philipp Friedrich von Hardenberg, poet, author, and philosopher of early German Romanticism, 1772–1801) wrote: *"When we dream that we are dreaming, the moment of awaking is at hand."* I personally realized the extent of psychological trauma resulting from the loss of hair in clumps from a respective dream, in which I pulled out my hair in clumps in front of the mirror while attempting to groom them. In that moment I realized that I was dealing with dystrophic anagen effluvium of whatever cause, but almost simultaneously also that I was dreaming. Since hair is a power symbol, as exemplified by the Biblical Samson in *Judges 16*, it is customary that hair falling out in dreams is interpreted as loss of power and control. The same type of helpless feeling is experienced in everyday life when hair is lost. The hair loss dream is typically a manifestation of a stressful situation. Ultimately, hair dreams represent a situation that is beyond one's control, exactly as when losing hair in true life.

Dystrophic Anagen Effluvium

Dystrophic anagen effluvium (DAE) is hair loss that results from the shedding of large numbers of hairs from the anagen phase of growth. It is a major characteristic of anagen that the epithelial hair follicle (HF) compartment undergoes proliferation, with the hair matrix keratinocytes showing the highest proliferative activity in building up the hair shaft. The common pathogenesis, which unites the different etiologies of DAE, is a direct insult to the rapidly dividing bulb matrix cells. The abrupt cessation of mitotic activity leads to the weakening of the partially keratinized

R. Trüeb (✉)
Center for Dermatology and Hair Diseases, Wallisellen, Zürich, Switzerland
e-mail: r.trueeb@derma-haarcenter.ch

Y. Ovcharenko et al. (eds.), *Psychotrichology*,
https://doi.org/10.1007/978-3-031-64083-4_8

proximal portion of the hair shaft, its narrowing, and subsequent breakage within the hair canal and shedding. The morphological consequence is the dystrophic anagen hair with a tapered proximal end and lack of root sheath. Hair loss is usually dramatic, involving 90% of affected hair that are shed within days to few weeks of the inciting event.

Causes of dystrophic anagen effluvium are antineoplastic drugs (chemotherapy-induced alopecia), X-ray exposure (radiation-induced alopecia), environmental or occupational exposure to toxins (toxic alopecia), or immunologic injury due to alopecia areata.

Dystrophic anagen effluvium may present in an either diffuse, patterned, or focal manner depending on the cause. Whatever the cause, the experience of hair loss is usually dramatic and traumatizing for patients, irrespective of the extent, due to its acuity, particularly if unexpected. Ultimately, an important question that arises for the patient is the reversibility of the condition.

Chemotherapy-Induced Alopecia

Chemotherapy-induced alopecia is the hair loss that is induced by cancer chemotherapy. It manifests as hair shedding that usually begins at 1–3 weeks after initiation of chemotherapy. Due to its long anagen phase, the scalp is the most common location for hair loss, while other terminal hairs are variably affected depending on the percentage of hairs in anagen. Since, normally up to 90% of scalp hair is in the anagen phase, hair loss is usually copious, and the resulting alopecia is quite obvious (Fig. 8.1). Nevertheless, chemotherapy given at high doses for a sufficiently

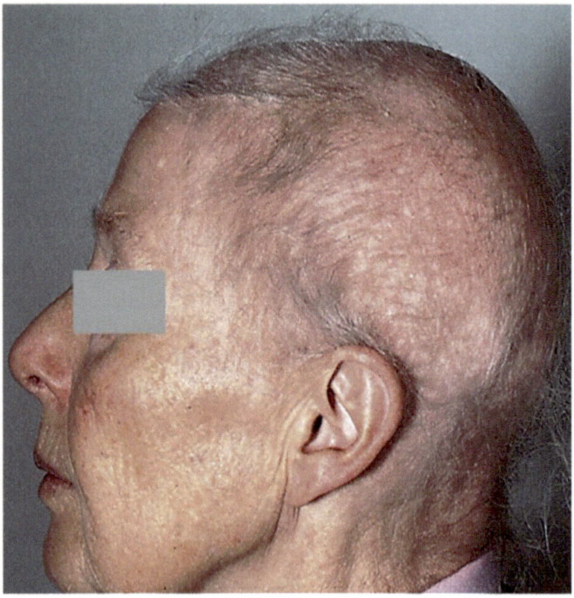

Fig. 8.1 Alopecia from dystrophic anagen effluvium (chemotherapy)

long time and with multiple exposures may also affect the beard, eyebrows, eyelashes, axillary, and pubic hairs.

Chemotherapy-induced alopecia occurs with an estimated overall incidence of 65%. The incidence and severity of the hair loss are variable and related to the particular chemotherapeutic agent and protocol. Multiple classes of anticancer drugs induce alopecia (Table 8.1), with frequencies of chemotherapy-induced alopecia differing for the four major drug classes. More than 80% for anti-microtubule agents (for example, paclitaxel), 60–100% for topoisomerase inhibitors (for example, doxorubicin), more than 60% for alkylators (for example, cyclophosphamide), and 10–50% for antimetabolites (for example, 5-fluorouracil plus leucovorin). Combination therapy consisting of two or more agents usually produces greater incidene of more severe hair loss compared with single-agent therapy.

While chemotherapy-induced alopecia has traditionally been categorized as acute diffuse hair loss due to a DAE, more recently it has been pointed out that, in fact, chemotherapy-induced alopecia may present with different pathophysiologic mechanisms and clinical patterns [1–4]. Evidence exists that the hair follicle may respond to the same insult capable of stopping mitosis with both shedding patterns, DAE, and telogen effluvium (TE). Accordingly, the hair may fall out very quickly in clumps, or gradually. When mitotic activity is arrested, numerous and interacting factors may influence the shedding pattern. One of these factors is the mitotic activity of the hair follicle at the time of the insult.

When the hair is in its late anagen phase, in which the mitotic rate is slowing down spontaneously, it simply accelerates its normal path to telogen, while mitotically inactive phases (catagen and telogen) are not affected. Since anagen duration is diminished in androgenetic alopecia (AGA), the probability is increased that the

Table 8.1 Cytotoxic agents causing hair loss

Cytostatic agents that usually do cause hair loss:	
Adriamycin	Docetaxel
Daunorubicin	Paclitaxel
Etoposide	Ifosfamide
Irinotecan	Vindesine
Cyclophosphamide	Vinorelbine
Epirubicin	Topotecan
Cytotoxic agents that sometimes cause hair loss:	
Amsacrine	Vincristine
Cytarabine	Vinblastine
Bleomycin	Lomustine
Busulfan	Thiotepa
5-Fluorouracil Melphalan	Gemcitabine
Cytotoxic agents that unusually cause hair loss:	
Methotrexate	Procarbazine
Carmustine	6-Mercaptopurine
Mitoxantrone	Streptozotocin
Mitomycin C	Fludarabine
Carboplatin	Raltitrexate
Cisplatin	Capecitabine

antimitotic insult strikes the hair close to the resting phase resulting in TE. While synchronization of hair cycles also plays a role, and again in androgenetic alopecia, the hair cycles tend to synchronize due to the diminished duration of anagen, even a minor antimitotic insult may produce marked hair loss that may be patterned.

The hair loss generally is usually reversible, with hair regrowth typically occurring after a delay of 3–6 months. In some patients, the regrown hair shows changes in color and/or texture. It might be curlier than it was before, or it could be gray until the follicular melanocytes begin functioning again. But the difference is usually temporary. However, there is an increasing number of reports of permanent chemotherapy-induced alopecia. Originally reported in children treated with busulfan and cyclophosphamide after bone marrow transplantation for leukemia [5], it has been associated with certain risk factors, including chronic graft versus host reaction, previous exposure to X-ray, and patient age [6]. More recently, reports have accumulated, related specifically to breast cancer chemotherapy by sequential fluorouracil/epirubicin/cyclophosphamide (FEC) and docetaxel. Miteva et al. [7] studied scalp biopsies from the affected scalp areas of permanent alopecia after systemic chemotherapy. The histology was characterized by a non-scarring pattern with a preserved number of follicular units and lack of fibrosis. The hair count revealed fewer terminal hairs, an increased number of telogen, and miniaturized vellus-like hairs. There was an increased number of fibrous streamers (stelae) in both the reticular dermis and the subcutis, with Arao-Perkins bodies found in the subcutaneous portions of the streamers. The histological findings of permanent alopecia after chemotherapy are like those in AGA. It may be speculated that exposure to chemotherapy may lead to an accumulation of DNA damage with defective renewal of HF stem cells.

Chemotherapy-induced hair loss is considered one of the most traumatic factors in cancer patient care, since hair loss negatively affects a patient's perception of appearance, body image, sexuality, and self-esteem, and patients feel deprived of their privacy because the hair loss is readily interpreted by the lay public as associated with having cancer.

According to McGarvey et al. [8] and Rosman [9], 47% of female cancer patients consider chemotherapy-induced hair loss the most traumatic aspect of their therapy, and 8% would even decline chemotherapy because of this fear of hair loss.

Finally, hair loss induced by cancer chemotherapy has been reported to cause changes in self-concept and body image that do not return to the previous state after regrowth of hair for many patients. In such cases, patients have difficulties expressing their feelings (alexithymia) and may be more prone to avoiding family conflicts. Family therapy can help families to cope with these psychological problems if they arise [10].

Of the preventive measures so far investigated, scalp cooling (hypothermia) has been the most widely used and studied [11]. Fifty-three studies were published between 1973 and 2003 on the results of scalp cooling for the prevention of chemotherapy-induced hair loss. Out of these, seven trials were randomized. In six of the seven randomized studies, a significant advantage was observed with scalp cooling. The positive results were most evident when anthracyclines or taxanes were the chemotherapeutic agents. In the most recent open-label, prospective, non-randomized clinical trial, patients with solid tumors receiving docetaxel in a palliative setting were allocated according to patients' preference to short-term cooling (over 45 min postinfusion) with a Paxman® PSC-2 machine (PAX), with cold cap (CC) or no cooling. The combined endpoint was alopecia World Health Organization (WHO) III or IV, or the necessity to wear a wig. Two hundred thirty-eight patients were included in the trial (128 patients PAX, 71 CC, and 39 no cooling). The number of cycles (median 4) and median docetaxel doses were similar across the three groups (55–60 mg/day on weekly therapy, 135–140 mg/day on 3-weekly therapy). Alopecia occurred with PAX, CC, and no cooling under 3-weekly docetaxel in 23%, 27%, and 74%, and under weekly docetaxel in 7%, 8%, and 17%, respectively. Overall, cooling (PAX and CC combined) reduced risk of alopecia by 78% (hazard ratio 0.22; 95% confidence interval 0.12–0.41). CC and PAX prophylaxis led to the same degree of prevention of alopecia. In this first comparison study published to date, both PAX and CC offered efficacious protection against hair loss, in particular when docetaxel was administered in a 3-weekly interval [12].

Patients undergoing scalp cooling commonly report feeling uncomfortably cold and complain of headaches. In several studies, authors have expressed concerns about the risk of scalp skin metastases after cooling. Therefore, scalp cooling has remained contraindicated for those with hematological malignancies, and its use remains controversial in patients who undergo curative chemotherapy for non-hematological malignancies with propensity to scalp metastasis.

So far, no approved pharmacologic treatment exists for chemotherapy-induced alopecia. Among the agents that so far have been evaluated, the topical hair growth promoting agent minoxidil was able to shorten the duration, albeit did not prevent chemotherapy-induced hair loss.

Among the agents that so far have been evaluated in cancer patients, the topical hair growth-promoting agent minoxidil was able to shorten the duration, though did not prevent chemotherapy-induced hair loss [13]. Minoxidil also fails to induce significant regrowth of hair in busulfan- and cyclophosphamide-induced permanent alopecia [14]. Nevertheless, topical minoxidil has proven to be effective in the management of endocrine therapy-induced alopecia in patients with breast cancer (Fig. 8.2a,b).

Freites-Martinez et al. [15] reported patients with endocrine therapy-induced alopecia (n = 112) with information on the drug-related frequencies, clinical features, impact on quality of life, and response to dermatologic therapy. Alopecia was attributed to aromatase inhibitors in 67% and tamoxifen in 33% of patients, the presentation was androgenetic alopecia-like, both clinically and on trichoscopic examination, negative impact on quality of life was significant, and topical minoxidil improved alopecia in 80% of treated patients. Patients who had previously received cytotoxic therapy were excluded from the study. However, patients with breast cancer often receive a combination of chemotherapy and endocrine therapy. While in many instances chemotherapy-induced alopecia is reversible, permanent

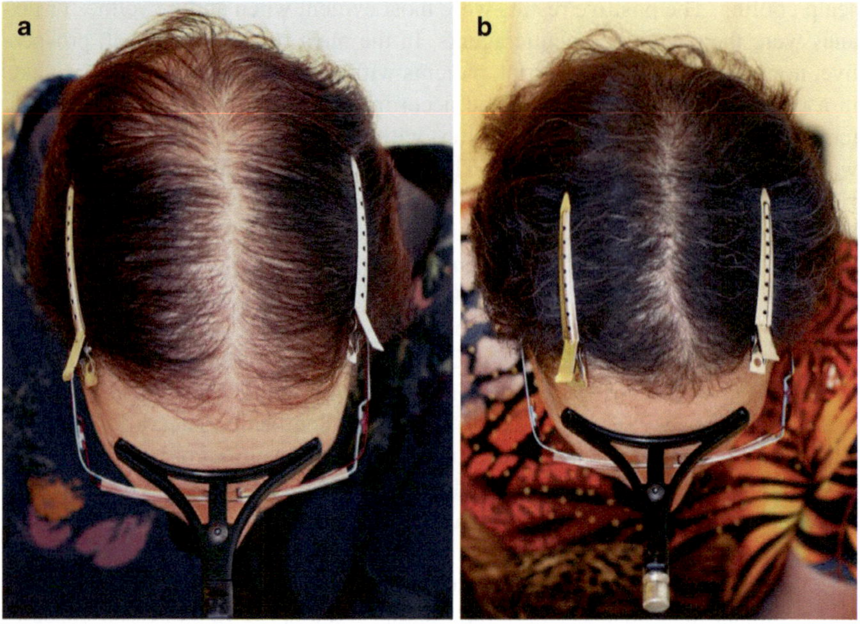

Fig. 8.2 Endocrine therapy-induced alopecia in patient with breast cancer: (**a**) before, and (**b**) after 6 months topical 5% minoxidil treatment b.i.d

chemotherapy-induced alopecia has been reported in women treated for breast cancer [16]. While permanent chemotherapy-induced alopecia is irreversible, endocrine therapy-induced alopecia is amenable to treatment with minoxidil in the same way androgenetic alopecia (AGA) is, if treated timely. At the time-point of the clinical consultation, the pattern of hair loss is not always reliable to distinguish the two conditions, since chemotherapy-induced alopecia is not always diffuse, but can also be patterned [1]. Rather, the chronology of events will help determine prognosis, since a history of recovery from chemotherapy-induced alopecia with worsening following initiation of endocrine therapy will point to endocrine therapy-induced alopecia and potential improvement with topical minoxidil. The mean time to development of alopecia from endocrine therapy initiation has been16.8 months (range 1–91 months) with 58% reporting alopecia within the first 12 months of endocrine therapy. Minoxidil should be used for the whole duration of endocrine therapy to preserve the hair that are at risk of gradually being permanently lost during endocrine therapy-induced alopecia, just as in AGA. Furthermore, after cessation of endocrine therapy, there is the potential for further and sustained recovery of hair, irrespective of duration (usually from 5–10 years) of endocrine therapy [17].

Since chemotherapy-induced hair loss cannot be reliably prevented, the best way to deal with it is to plan ahead with a focus on making the patient as comfortable as possible with his appearance before, during, and after cancer treatment.

The major approach to prevent or minimize chemotherapy-induced hair loss remains scalp cooling, while topical minoxidil may speed up hair regrowth and is effective for treatment of endocrine therapy-induced alopecia.

Even if chemotherapy-induced hair loss cannot be prevented, it can be managed. Anticipating hair loss, coming to terms with the inevitability of hair loss, and taking control are the key steps in coping with chemotherapy-induced hair loss. Recommendations for hair care are summarized in Table 8.2.

Finally, nutritional supplements are widely used among patients with cancer who perceive them to have anticancer and/or antitoxic properties [18]. A significant proportion of people with cancer have been found to supplement their diets with antioxidants and immune system stabilizing micronutrients, depending on the type of malignancy and the gender of the patient [19] often without consulting their attending physician. However, from the oncological viewpoint, there have been concerns that dietary supplements may decrease the effectiveness of chemotherapy and radiotherapy, specifically the antioxidants may reduce toxicity of chemotherapy and radiotherapy at the cost of reduced treatment efficacy since radiotherapy and many chemotherapy agents exert their anticancer effects by production of reactive oxidative species and apoptosis [20].

Recent studies, however, have provided evidence of improved patient compliance, fewer adverse effects and, subsequently, a lower rate of treatment discontinuations, when selected micronutrients, such as selenium and vitamin D, were added to an adequate supply of energy substrates (proteins, fats, and carbohydrates) [21]. Moreover, a majority of cytostatics used in treatment today, specifically the antimetabolites (methotrexate), nitrogen mustard derivatives (cyclophosphamide), platinum complexes (cisplatin), vinca alkaloids (vinorelbine), taxanes (paclitaxel), and anthracyclines (epirubicin) do not primarily act through oxidative stress. Therefore, the often uncritical blanket renunciation of dietary supplements with antioxidant and immunomodulating micronutrients during chemotherapy does not seem justified [22]. In fact, the success of treatment and the healing process in cancer patients

Table 8.2 Chemotherapy-induced hair loss. Recommendations for hair care

- **Avoidance of physical or chemical trauma**, such as bleaching, coloring, or perming of hair, curling irons, and hot rollers.
- **Gentle hair strategies** should be continued throughout chemotherapy, using a satin pillowcase, which is less likely to attract and catch fragile hair, using a soft brush, washing hair only as often as necessary and using a gentle shampoo.
- **Cutting hair short or shaving hair**. Short hair tends to look fuller than long hair, and when the hair is shed, it won't be as noticeable when it is short. Moreover, cut hair might help to make a better transition to total alopecia. Also, a shaved head may be easier for securing a wig or hairpiece.
- **Appropriate head covering should be planned**. Head covering as the hair falls out is a very personal decision. For women in particular, chemotherapy-induced hair loss involves a confrontation with the nature of their disease, while for men it is a normal and inevitable consequence of treatment. Depending on individual preference, temporarily wearing a wig or another head covering until the hair regrows may be the most effective way of dealing with this condition, while protecting the scalp from sun and cold exposure at the same time.

are significantly influenced by the nutritional status of patients [23], and possibly also the condition of the hair.

Radiation-Induced Alopecia

The anagen hair follicle is highly susceptible to the genotoxic effect of X-ray exposure. Again, a DAE results from acute damage to the actively dividing matrix cells of anagen follicles. This is followed by a telogen shedding due to premature catagen entry of follicles in late anagen at the time of the insult. Hair loss occurs within the exposure area, and most patients notice hair loss 2–3 weeks following radiation exposure.

Radiation-induced alopecia may either be temporary or permanent, depending on the amount of radiation and other treatments received, such as concomitant chemotherapy.

Hair loss occurs on hair-bearing skin with doses above 300–400 cGy, and is permanent with a single dose above 1200 cGy. If the dose is fractionated, permanent hair loss my not occur until the dose exceeds 4500 cGy. If the hair loss is temporary, complete hair regrowth occurs 2–4 months after X-ray exposure.

Endovascular procedures have become a widely used treatment of cerebral vascular malformation. Krasovec and Trüeb [24] originally reported temporary radiation-induced epilation following a neuroradiologically guided embolization procedure in the dermatologic literature (Fig. 8.3). Transient alopecia following therapeutic embolization is probably underreported, since it seems not to be an uncommon event. It has been misinterpreted to be due to arterial occlusion; moreover, excluding the differential diagnosis of alopecia areata may be difficult, since the bald patch is devoid of inflammatory signs, and hair loss is characterized by dystrophic hair. The patient history, chronology of events, the localization and the geometry of the bald patch usually allow correct diagnosis.

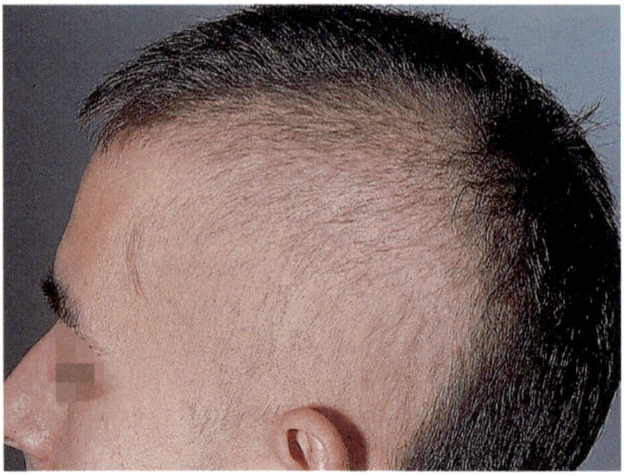

Fig. 8.3 Temporary radiation-induced epilation following a neuroradiologically guided embolization of an intracranial vascular malformation

Knowledge of the condition is important to prevent any myths and misinformation about the etiology and prognosis of the hair loss in patients. It is helpful to inform the patient about the possibility of temporary hair loss following neuroradiological interventions and its reversibility, to avoid anxiety related to the condition. Neuroradiologists usually are aware of the condition but underestimate the impact on the patient's psychological well-being and often fail to provide their patients the necessary information.

The scalp skin is sensitive to radiation, and more so after hair loss. The skin may become erythematous, tender, or inflamed, much like a sunburn. After 2 or 3 weeks of radiation exposure the scalp may become dry and itchy. If necessary, treatment can be prescribed to relieve discomfort and itching. Protection from UV radiation is mandatory. Recommendations for hair and scalp care are summarized in Table 8.3.

Hair loss from high dosages of X-rays, usually for treatment of brain tumors, is permanent (Fig. 8.4). In this case, hair loss can be psychologically devastating. In such cases, a psychological approach with an empathic consideration of the patient's concerns as well as the provision of practical medical-aesthetic and styling tips are important.

Table 8.3 Suggestions for patients to minimize scalp reaction to radiation treatment

- Avoid frequent shampooing. Use a mild shampoo without any perfumes.
- Wash scalp with warm water only. Avoid rubbing or scratching. Pat dry with a soft towel.
- Avoid excessively combing or brushing hair.
- Avoid using hair spray, oils, or creams.
- Avoid using heat sources, including hair dryers, rollers, or curling irons.
- Do not perm or color hair until about 4 weeks after radiation treatment is complete.
- Protect head from sun, cold, and wind by wearing a head covering.

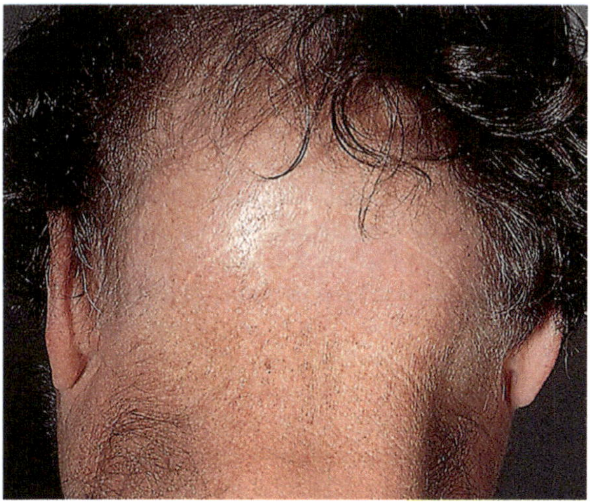

Fig. 8.4 Permanent radiation-induced alopecia from treatment of brain tumor

Toxic Alopecia

Toxic alopecia from occupational exposure to hazardous chemicals has decreased over the years due to more stringent government regulations. More recently, interest has focused on the effects from toxic metals of the environment.

Many heavy metals can disrupt the formation of the hair shaft through covalent binding with the sulfhydryl groups in keratin: thallium, mercury, arsenic, copper, cadmium, and bismuth.

A study conducted in 1979 by Piérard [25] in Belgium reported diffuse alopecia related to ingestion of toxic metals in 36 of 78 patients with diffuse alopecia. Toxic metals in abnormal amount in blood and urine were observed only when >10% of hair bulbs were dystrophic. Copper was involved in 17 alopecia cases, arsenic in 12, mercury in 5, and cadmium in 2 cases. Copper intoxication was found to be related to ingestion of tap water containing a high concentration of copper salts, presumably from low pH, presence of chelating agents, or connection of electrical ground wires to copper water pipes, which caused sufficient flow of electrical current to ionize the metal.

Adverse effects related to dental amalgam, including hair loss, have also been the subject of recent attention. In one study, mercury levels in blood and urine correlated with the number of amalgam surfaces, indicating the release of mercury from dental amalgam restorations [26]. Since the mercury levels were far below those where negative health effects would be expected and were similar in patients with complaints self-related to dental amalgam restorations and healthy control individuals, mercury was not found to be a likely cause of the impaired health reported by the patients [27]. In another study, assays of mercury in urine samples of patients with amalgam illness indicated that the exposure was far below the levels at which symptoms could be indicated by psychometric tests [28]. Psychologic investigation indicated that the symptoms were psychosomatic [29–31]. All patients had experienced important psychic traumata in close correlation with the first appearance of symptoms [32].

The diagnosis of heavy metal toxicity requires clinical suspicion, observation of presenting symptoms, including acute alopecia [33], obtaining a thorough history of potential exposure (occupational, environmental, accidental), and the results of laboratory tests. These include measuring urine, blood, or hair levels of the suspected heavy metals. Chemical hair analysis may prove useful for retrospective purposes when blood and urine are no longer expected to contain a particular contaminant, and are primarily used for forensic purposes [34]. The results of such forensic studies on hair have also been of historical interest when performed on hair clippings of famous personalities, such as Beethoven (1770–1827) [35] and Napoleon (1769–1821) [36], where high levels of lead and of arsenic, respectively, were detected.

Hair analysis refers to the chemical analysis of a hair sample. Its most widely accepted use is in the fields of forensic and environmental toxicology. Hair analysis is also used for the detection of recreational drugs, including cocaine, heroin, benzodiazepines, and amphetamines. Chemical hair analysis may prove particularly useful for retrospective purposes when blood and urine are no longer expected to contain a particular contaminant, typically a year or less. On the other hand, an increasing number of commercial laboratories are committed to providing multielement hair analyses in which a single test is used to determine values for many minerals simultaneously. This type of analysis used by several alternative medicine fields with the claim that hair analyses can help diagnose a wide variety of health problems and can be used as the basis for prescribing natural chelation therapy, mineral, trace elements, and/or vitamin supplements. However, these uses remain controversial for several reasons:

Most commercial hair analysis laboratories have not validated their analytical techniques by checking them against standard reference materials.

Hair mineral content can be affected by exposure to various substances such as shampoos, bleaches, and hair dyes. No analytic technique enables reliable determination of the source of specific levels of elements in hair as bodily or environmental.

The level of certain minerals can be affected by the color, diameter, and rate of growth of an individual's hair, the season of the year, the geographic location, and the age and gender of the individual.

Normal ranges of hair minerals have not been defined.

For most elements, no correlation has been established between hair level and other.

known indicators of nutrition status. It is possible for hair concentration of an element to be high even though deficiency exists in the body, and vice versa.

Alopecia Areata

Alopecia areata (AA) is a common hair loss condition involving a dystrophic anagen effluvium, either localized or diffuse, occurring in the otherwise healthy child or adult. It is characterized by an acute onset of non-scarring hair loss in usually sharply defined areas. Any hair-bearing area can be affected, but the most noticeable are the scalp, the beard area, and the eyebrows. The characteristic patch of AA is usually round or oval, and is completely bald and smooth. Trichoscopic markers of classical forms of alopecia areata are similar and depend on the stage of the disease. The activity of the process is characterized by signs of dystrophy, such as black dots, broken hairs, exclamation mark hairs. The absence of the signs of dystrophic activity is the main criterion for the chronic stage, which also includes yellow dots and vellus hairs (See Chap. 6).

The condition is of autoimmune origin with an organ-specific, T-cell-mediated assault on the hair follicle at the level of the bulb, though a psychosomatic origin has also been implicated and triggered much controversy [37].

The hair bulb is an immune protected site with deficient MHC expression. There is circumstantial evidence suggesting that alopecia areata results from loss of immune privilege with presentation of autoantigens. A peribulbar lymphocytic infiltrate induces hair follicle keratinocytes to undergo apoptosis resulting in inhibition of cell division in the hair matrix [38].

The progress of AA in an individual patient is unpredictable, though a large surface area, a long disease duration, and associated nail abnormalities have related to a poorer prognosis, and psychological factors may also play a role. Some patients lose hair in only a small patch, while others may have more extensive or less frequently diffuse involvement. Alopecia totalis is the loss of all scalp hair, alopecia universalis is the loss of all scalp and body hair.

Depending on the patient age, disease severity, activity, adverse prognostic factors, and impact on quality of life, a treatment algorithm can be designed [39] (see Chap. 6).

> Trüeb and Cavegn [40] reported trichotillomania in connection with alopecia areata, and suggested that patients with a mental predisposition may artificially prolong the disfigurement as the hair on the bald patches of AA regrows, with the aim to maintain gratification of dependency needs, which were being met during alopecia areata.

Some experts therefore advocate combination treatment with antidepressant agents in alopecia areata with comorbid depression. Antidepressants that have been used with success include imipramine, paroxetine [41, 42], and citalopram [43]. Others suggest that hypnotherapy may enhance the mental well-being of patients with AA, though no effect on hair regrowth could be shown [44].

As there is no definite cure for AA, and conventional therapy has its clear limitations; several AA patients resort to complementary and alternative medical remedies and therapies (CAM). Hay et al. [45] reported a randomized, double-blind, controlled trial of 7 months' duration aromatherapy with follow-up at 3 and 7 months to investigate the efficacy in the treatment of AA. Eighty-six patients were randomized into two groups. The active group massaged essential oils (thyme, rosemary, lavender, and cedarwood) in a mixture of carrier oils (jojoba and grapeseed) into their scalp daily. The control group used only daily carrier oils for their massage. Treatment success was evaluated on sequential photographs. The degree of improvement was measured by two methods: a 6-point scale and computerized analysis of traced areas of alopecia. Nineteen (44%) of 43 patients in the active group showed improvement compared with 6 (15%) of 41 patients in the control group ($p = 0.008$). The authors concluded that aromatherapy is a safe and effective treatment for AA.

A more recent review of CAM addressed two pertinent aspects, an overview of the published medical literature on CAM used in alopecia areata and second, a thorough assessment of the considerations and limitations of the use of CAM for treatment of alopecia areata. A systematic MEDLINE search yielded 13 studies of the clinical use of CAM in the management of alopecia areata, all belonging to one of the five main categories of CAM. Methodological quality was analyzed using objective assessment scores (Wilson and Lawrence scores). No study was of sufficient internal validity to provide robust evidence of the benefit of CAM for treatment of alopecia areata [46].

Ultimately, the options available for adapting to the disease rather than treating to cure are to be taken into consideration in selected long-standing widespread cases or recurrent small spot disease. In one study, 46% of participants reported that wearing a wig had a positive impact on their everyday life with negative experiences related to fears of the wig being noticed. Psychological interventions alongside wig provision would be beneficial for people living with alopecia [47].

Normal Anagen Effluvium

In contrast to DAE, Delmonte et al. [48] originally coined the term normal anagen effluvium for an anagen hair loss due to a disruption of the anchoring of the normal anagen hair shaft in the follicle. This phenomenon may be observed in the loose anagen hair syndrome and in anagen effluvium in pemphigus vulgaris.

Loose Anagen Hair

Loose anagen hair or loose anagen hair syndrome is a condition characterized by easily pluckable anagen hairs and a disorder predominantly observed in children [49]. The cause is unknown, but a keratinization disorder of the internal hair root

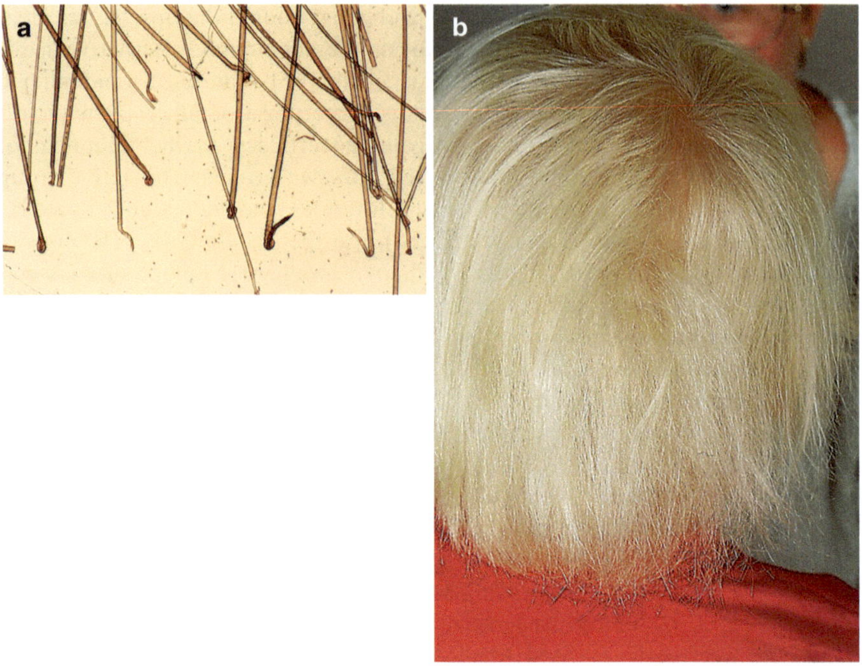

Fig. 8.5 Loose anagen hair: dry and lusterless hair (**a**), anagen hairs devoid of root sheaths (**b**)

sheath with a disruption of the anchoring of the hair shaft has been postulated. The condition often recedes with age.

The diagnosis of loose anagen hair is based on the criteria including painless extraction of >10 anagen hairs (devoid of hair root sheaths) on Pull test; trichogram showing >80% of plucked hairs are anagen hairs devoid of sheaths (Fig. 8.5a) [50]. Clinically, the hair may show uneven ends. Additionally, there may be variations in hair texture, and the hair is often dry and lusterless (Fig. 8.5b).

Histological studies of scalp biopsies have demonstrated abnormal clefts between the internal root sheath and the hair shaft, premature keratinization, poor cohesion of the cells of the outer sheath, and degeneration of the inner sheath. Ultrastructural studies show longitudinal grooves of the hair shaft. The presence of these alterations supports the hypothesis of some abnormality of the root sheath adversely affecting anchoring of the anagen hair in the follicle.

There is no specific treatment for loose anagen hair, except for careful grooming of the hair to avoid extracting the loose anagen hairs.

The proportion of children under the age of 10 years among patients complaining of hair loss in a dermatologic clinic is 5%. Pediatric alopecia is caused by several conditions, and patterns are different from those seen in adults.

Alopecia in childhood is a source of high concern, frustration, and anxiety. Young children usually lack self-awareness, and it may be the parents who, projecting their own concerns onto the child, most acutely feel any associated anxiety.

A thorough understanding of normal hair development enables accurate assessment of the child with hair loss. Knowledge of the normal range and variation observed in children's hair additionally enhances this assessment. The differential diagnosis of alopecia in the pediatric age group is simplified by the fact that 90%–95% of cases are caused by four major entities including alopecia areata, tinea capitis, telogen effluvium, and trichotillomania, and in some cases trichotillomania-by-proxy and battered child syndrome [51]. Sometimes, clinically, more elusive conditions such as congenital triangular alopecia, or premature androgenetic alopecia, may be responsible for hair loss. Finally, conditions peculiar to the pediatric population are the short anagen syndrome and the loose anagen hair syndrome.

Eventually, hair loss for the older child can lead to low self-esteem, depression, bullying, and humiliation. Ultimately, hair loss in children can have psychologic effects that interfere with a child's normal development. Therefore, delineating types of alopecia and those that are chronic or potentially related to underlying medical problems and psychological counseling of parents and support of both parents and child are important.

Anagen Effluvium in Pemphigus Vulgaris

Delmonte et al. [48] originally reported on normal anagen effluvium in pemphigus effluvium due to autoimmune-mediated acantholysis within the outer hair root sheath. Subsequently, Schaerer and Trüeb [52] were the first to propose direct immunofluorescence studies on plucked hairs for diagnosis of autoimmune pemphigus. Hair is plucked in the same manner as for the trichogram, snap frozen, and processed much the same way as scalp biopsies for direct immunofluorescence (DIF) studies. The observation of positive immunofluorescence within the outer hair root sheath of plucked anagen hairs (Fig. 8.6) in patients with pemphigus vulgaris and foliaceus has stimulated subsequent authors to further elaborate on the method. Positive DIF findings are seen in scalp hair, irrespective of the presence of skin lesions. All pemphigus variants (pemphigus vulgaris, foliaceus, erythematosus, and vegetans) have early positive DIF findings in the outer hair root sheaths. Regarding the high sensitivity of DIF on plucked hair in autoimmune pemphigus patients, it seems that hair plucking is a suitable alternative to the more invasive techniques of skin biopsy for obtaining specimens for DIF for an early diagnosis in patients with scalp erosions as initial manifestation of pemphigus that may otherwise be misinterpreted as neurotic scalp excoriations or factitial dermatitis.

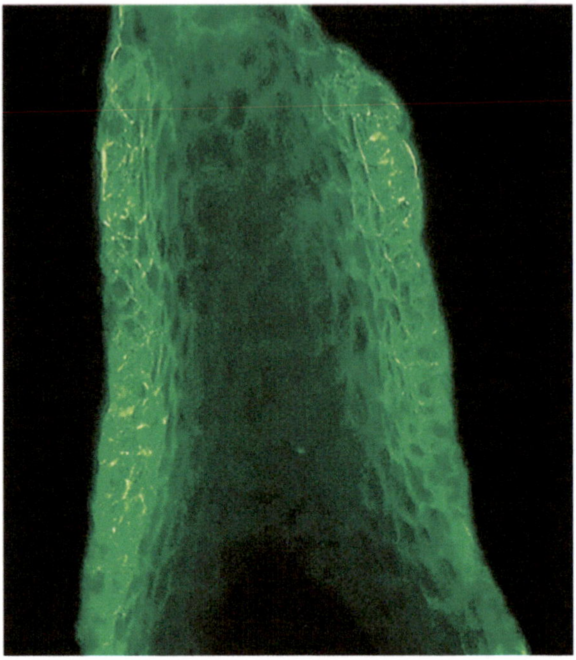

Fig. 8.6 Positive direct immunofluorescence with chicken wire pattern within outer hair root sheath of plucked anagen hair in pemphigus

The term neurotic excoriations refer to patients with self-inflicted excoriations of the scalp in the absence of an underlying specific dermatologic disease condition. The inflicted lesions are rather nonspecific. Varying in size from a few millimeters to several centimeters in the well-developed case, lesions are seen in all stages of evolution, from small superficial excoriations through deep scooped-out skin lesions. The underlying mental disorders of neurotic excoriations are varied with the necessity of making a specific diagnosis for an individual therapeutic approach [53–55]. In mild and transient cases, it may be a response to stress, mainly in someone with obsessive-compulsive personality traits. In the more severe and sustained cases, psychiatric evaluation may reveal a generalized anxiety disorder, depression, or obsessive-compulsive disorder.

Since other dermatologic conditions can lead to similar lesions as neurotic excoriations of the scalp, clinicians must be careful not to make this diagnosis based on the morphology of the skin lesions alone. Specifically, pruritic skin conditions of dermatologic or other origin need to be excluded. Examples include atopic dermatitis, folliculitis necrotica, chronic cutaneous lupus erythematosus, pemphigus vulgaris, pemphigoid, parasitic infestation, neurologic disorders, and other psychiatric disorders, such as cocaine intoxication, delusions of parasitosis, and factitial dermatitis (see Chap. 11).

Summary

- DAE is characterized by extensive anagen hair loss.
- Direct damage to the rapidly dividing of the bulb matrix cells is the common pathogenesis linking the various etiologies of DAE.
- Causes of this condition include: antineoplastic drugs, X-ray irradiation, environmental or occupational exposure to toxins, or immunologic injury.
- Observational data suggest that hair loss due to chemotherapy may be the most traumatic aspect of anticancer therapy and the reason for withdrawal.
- Although chemotherapy or radiotherapy-induced DAE cannot be completely avoided, the condition is reversible. The key steps in managing this type of hair loss remain predicting, accepting the inevitability, and controlling hair loss.
- Patients with chemotherapy or radiation-induced alopecia will benefit from psychological counseling and the wearing of wigs or the use of hair replacement systems.

References

1. Trüeb RM. Chemotherapy-induced alopecia. Curr Opin Support Palliat Care. 2010a;4(4):281–4.
2. Trüeb RM. Chemotherapy-induced alopecia. Semin Cutan Med Surg. 2009;28(1):11–4.
3. Trüeb RM. Chemotherapy-induced anagen effluvium: diffuse or patterned? Dermatology. 2007;215(1):1–2.
4. Trüeb RM. Chemotherapy-induced hair loss. Skin Therapy Lett. 2010b;15(7):5–7.
5. Baker B, Wilson C, Davis A, et al. Busulphan/cyclophosphamide conditioning for bone marrow transplantation may lead to failure of hair regrowth. Bone Marrow Transplant. 1991;7:43–7.
6. Vowels M, Chan LL, Gir N, et al. Factors affecting hair regrowth after bone marrow transplantation. Bone Marrow Transplant. 1993;12:347–50.
7. Miteva M, Misciali C, Fanti PA, Vincenzi C, Romanelli P, Tosti A. Permanent alopecia after systemic chemotherapy: a clinicopathological study of 10 cases. Am J Dermatopathol. 2011;33(4):345–50.
8. McGarvey EL, Baum LD, Pinkerton RC, et al. Psychological sequelae and alopecia among women with cancer. Cancer Pract. 2001;9:283–9.
9. Rosman S. Cancer and stigma: experience of patients with chemotherapy-induced alopecia. Patient Educ Couns. 2004;52:333–9.
10. Poot F. Le retentissement psychologique des pathologies chroniques du cheveu [Psychological consequences of chronic hair diseases]. Revue Médicale de Bruxelles (in French). 2004;25(4):A286–8.
11. Grevelman EG, Breed WPM. Prevention of chemotherapy-induced hair loss by scalp cooling. Ann Oncol. 2005;16:352–8.
12. Betticher DC, Delmore G, Breitenstein U, Anchisi S, Zimmerli-Schwab B, Müller A, von Moos R, Hügli-Dayer AM, Schefer H, Bodenmann S, Bühler V, Trüeb RM. Efficacy and tolerability of two scalp cooling systems for the prevention of alopecia associated with docetaxel treatment. Support Care Cancer. 2013;21(9):2565–73.
13. Wang J, Lu Z, Au JLS. Protection against chemotherapy-induced alopecia. Pharm Res. 2006;23:2505–14.
14. Tran D, Sinclair RD, Schwarer AP, et al. Permanent alopecia following chemotherapy and bone marrow transplantation. Austral J Dermatol. 2000;41:106–8.

15. Freites-Martinez A, Shapiro J, Chan D, Fornier M, Modi S, Gajria D, Dusza S, Goldfarb S, Lacouture ME. Endocrine therapy-induced alopecia in patients with breast cancer. JAMA Dermatol. 2018;154:670–5.
16. Kluger N, Jacot W, Frouin E, et al. Permanent scalp alopecia related to breast cancer chemotherapy by sequential fluorouracil/epirubicin/cyclophosphamide (FEC) and docetaxel: a prospective study of 20 patients. Ann Oncol. 2012;23:2879–84.
17. Trüeb RM. Minoxidil for endocrine therapy-induced alopecia in women with breast cancer-Saint Agatha's blessing? JAMA Dermatol. 2018;154(6):656–8.
18. Gröber U, Holzhauer P, Kisters K, Holick MF, Adamietz IA. Micronutrients in oncological intervention. Nutrients. 2016;8:163.
19. Micke O, Bruns F, Glatzel M, Schönekaes K, Micke P, Mücke R. Predictive factors for the use of compelentary and alternative medicine (CAM) in radiation oncology. Eur J Integr Med. 2009;1:22–30.
20. Lawenda BD, Kelly KM, Lasas EJ, et al. Should supplemental antioxidant administration be avoided during chemotherapy and radiotherapy? J Natl Cancer Inst. 2008;100:773–83.
21. Gröber U, Mücke R, Adamietz IA, Holzhauer P, Kisters K, Büntzel J, Micke O. Komplementärer Einsatz von Antioxidanzien aund Mikronährstoffen in der Onkologie—Update 2013. Der Onkol. 2013;19:136–43.
22. Moss RW. Should patients undergoing chemotherapy and radiotherapy be prescribed antioxidants? Integr Cancer Ther. 2006;5:63–82.
23. Tong H, Isenring E, Yates P. The prevalence of nutrition impact symptoms and their relationship to quality of life and clinical outcomes in medical oncology patients. Support Care Cancer. 2009;17:83–90.
24. Krasovec M, Trüeb RM. Temporary roentgen epilation after embolization of a cerebral arteriovenous malformation. Hautarzt. 1998;49(4):307–9.
25. Piérard GE. Toxic effects of metals from the environment on hair growth and structure. J Cutan Pathol. 1979;6:237–42.
26. Bratel J, Haraldson T, Meding B, et al. Potential side effects of dental amalgam restorations. An oral and medical investigation. Eur J Oral Sci. 1997;105:234–43.
27. Furhoff AK, Tomson Y, Ilie M, Bågedahl-Strindlund M, Larsson KS, Sandborgh-Englund G, Torstenson B, Wretlind K. A multidisciplinary clinical study of patients suffering from illness associated with release of mercury from dental restorations. Medical and odontological aspects. Scand J Prim Health Care. 1998;16:247–52.
28. Langworth S, Björkman L, Elinder CG, Järup L, Savlin P. Multidisciplinary examination of patients with illness attributed to dental fillings. J Oral Rehabil. 2002;29:705–13.
29. Bailer J, Rist F, Rudolf A, Staehle HJ, Eickholz P, Triebig G, Bader M, Pfeifer U. Adverse health effects related to mercury exposure from dental amalgam fillings: toxicological or psychological causes? Psychol Med. 2001;31:255–63.
30. Lindberg NE, Lindberg E, Larsson G. Psychologic factors in the etiology of amalgam illness. Acta Odontol Scand. 1994;52:219–28.
31. Sundström A, Bergdahl J, Nyberg L, Bergdahl M, Nilsson LG. Stressful negative life events and amalgam-related complaints. Community Dent Oral Epidemiol. 2011;39:12–8.
32. Bågedahl-Strindlund M, Ilie M, Furhoff AK, Tomson Y, Larsson KS, Sandborgh-Englund G, Torstenson B, Wretlind K. A multidisciplinary clinical study of patients suffering from illness associated with mercury release from dental restorations: psychiatric aspects. Acta Psychiatr Scand. 1997;96:475–82.
33. Feldman J, Levisohn DR. Acute alopecia: clue to thallium toxicity. Pediatr Dermatol. 1993;10:29–31.
34. Daniel CR 3rd, Piraccini BM, Tosti A. The nail and hair in forensic science. J Am Acad Dermatol. 2004;50(2):258–61.
35. Gross M. Beethoven's ringlets—from a medical point of view. [Article in German]. Dtsch Med Wochenschr. 2013;138:2633–8.
36. Kintz P, Ginet M, Cirimele V. Multi-element screening by ICP-MS of two specimens of Napoleon's hair. J Anal Toxicol. 2006;30:621–3.

37. Mulinari-Brenner F. Psychosomatic aspects of alopecia areata. Clin Dermatol. 2018;36(6):709–13.
38. Trüeb RM, Dias MFRG. Alopecia areata: a comprehensive review of pathogenesis and management. Clin Rev Allergy Immunol. 2018;54(1):68–87.
39. Serbina I, Andrashko Y, Galnykina S, Kadigrob I, Khobzei K, Liadova T, Litus O, Sviatenko T, Svistunov I, Syzon O, Vozianova S, Ovcharenko Y. Clinical guidelines of the Ukraine Hair Research Society. Diagnosis and treatment of alopecia areata. Actual problems of modern medicine. 2023;12P:45–67 https://doi.org/10.26565/2617-409X-2023-12-06.
40. Trüeb RM, Cavegn B. Trichotillomania in connection with alopecia areata. Cutis. 1996;58:67–70.
41. Cipriani R, Perini GI, Rampinelli S. Paroxetine in alopecia areata. Int J Dermatol. 2001;40:600–1.
42. Ricciardi A, Ruberto A, García-Hernández MJ, et al. Alopecia areata with comorbid depression: early resolution with combined paroxetine-triamcinolone treatment. J Eur Acad Dermatol Venereol. 2006;20:1000–1.
43. Abedini H, Farshi S, Mirabzadeh A, Keshavarz S. Antidepressant effects of citalopram on treatment of alopecia areata in patients with major depressive disorder. J Dermatolog Treat. 2014;25(2):153–5.
44. Willemsen R, Haentjens P, Roseeuw D, Vanderlinden J. Hypnosis and alopecia areata: Long-term beneficial effects on psychological well-being. Acta Derm Venereol. 2011;91(1):35–9.
45. Hay IC, Jamieson M, Ormerod AD. Randomized trial of aromatherapy. Successful treatment for alopecia areata. Arch Dermatol. 1998;134(11):1349–52.
46. Van den Biggelaar FJ, Smolders J, Jansen JF. Complementary and alternative medicine in alopecia areata. Am J Clin Dermatol. 2010;11(1):11–20.
47. Montgomery K, White C, Thompson A. A mixed methods survey of social anxiety, anxiety, depression and wig use in alopecia. BMJ Open. 2017;7(4):e015468.
48. Delmonte S, Semino MT, Parodi A, Rebora A. Normal anagen effluvium: a sign of pemphigus vulgaris. Br J Dermatol. 2000;142(6):1244–5.
49. Hamm H, Traupe H. Loose anagen hair of childhood: the phenomenon of easily pluckable hair. J Am Acad Dermatol. 1989;20:242–8.
50. Tosti A, Peluso AM, Misciali C, et al. Loose anagen hair. Arch Dermatol. 1997;133:1089–93.
51. Trüeb RM. Differential diagnosis in pediatric dermatology: trichotillomania/battered child syndrome. Eur J Pediatr Dermatol. 1993;3:134–9.
52. Schaerer L, Trüeb RM. Direct immunofluorescence of plucked hair in pemphigus. Arch Dermatol. 2003;139:228–9.
53. Fruensgaaard K. Neurotic excoriations: a controlled psychiatric examination. Act Psychiatr Scand Suppl. 1986;69:1–52.
54. Fruensgaaard K. Psychotherapeutic strategy and neurotic excoriations. Int J Dermatol. 1991a;30:198–203.
55. Fruensgaaard K. Psychotherapy and neurotic excoriations. Int J Dermatol. 1991b;30:262–5.

Androgenetic Alopecia

9

Yuliya Ovcharenko, Kuzma Khobzei,
and Nino Lortkipanidze

Introduction

The high level of clinical interest in androgenetic alopecia (AGA) is explained by its prevalence in both men and women. Genetic polymorphism and pathogenetic multifactorial nature of AGA are manifested by a variety of clinical forms of the disease.

Progressive miniaturization in the predisposed hair follicles (HF), followed by a shortening of the subsequent growth phases, leading to a gradual transformation of pigmented terminal hair into vellus-like shafts, clinically significant reduction in hair density, and hair thinning in different distribution patterns.

Despite the researchers' interest in this condition, the pathophysiology of AGA remains unclear, and current therapies have limited efficacy in many patients. The active search for possible cofactors of the AGA complex etiology contributes to our understanding of the nosology and identifies new therapeutic targets promoting evolution of therapy.

The current study of AGA is a prerequisite for the implementation of the most progressive and ambitious strategies of HF cells neogenesis and reprogramming. Besides the development of basic research on AGA, data from modern clinical observations reveal correlations between the age-related manifestation of AGA, comorbidity with the clinical subtype and prognosis, and identify possible clinical and pathogenetic variants of the disease, and the research results of the genetically

Y. Ovcharenko (✉)
V. N. Karazin Kharkiv National University, University Clinic "Trichology Institute", Kharkiv, Ukraine

K. Khobzei
Department of Infectious Diseases and Clinical Immunology of the V. N. Karazin Kharkiv National University, Khobzei Clinic, Kyiv, Ukraine

N. Lortkipanidze
Department of Dermatology and Venereology at D. Tvildiani Medical University, Tbilisi, Georgia

Y. Ovcharenko et al. (eds.), *Psychotrichology*,
https://doi.org/10.1007/978-3-031-64083-4_9

related conditions put AGA in a broader medical and biological context (Ovcharenko 2021) [1].

An important aspect in the study of AGA patients is the high degree of negative impact on the quality of life (QoL), which significantly exceeds the clinical severity of the condition itself. The prevailing stereotype assumes that balding men are less attractive in terms of physical, personal, and social qualities. Men with AGA often present with lower self-esteem, depression leading to increased introversion, and dissatisfaction with their own appearance, especially in case on an early onset condition. However, studies on the AGA effect on QoL in women revealed greater emotional distress.

These observations are of high clinical significance and contribute to the individual therapeutic route planning, both taking into account gender, age, clinical form and severity, and on the basis of patient's somatic comorbid pathology and psychostatus.

Epidemiology

The true prevalence of AGA is difficult to determine due to a lack of universally accepted diagnostic criteria. It is generally agreed that the frequency of AGA varies among different population groups.

While precise statistics are lacking, some studies claim that the incidence in Caucasians is close to 100% (Dawber 1998) [2]. According to other sources, approximately half of men and women over the age of 40 have AGA (Olsen 1994) [3]. These figures are markedly different in other races, where baldness is much less common.

In most people of Chinese ethnicity, the prepubertal hairline maintains after puberty, baldness is less common, less extensive, and develops later in life [4]. The incidence rate in Japanese men is also lower, balding begins about 10 years later than in Caucasians (Takashima et al. 1981), and the proportion of men of African descent who keep a full head of hair are four times the number of Caucasians [5]. The reason for these major racial differences is not clear, but it is likely to be genetic, since differences persist regardless of the region of living.Similarly, to the lower incidence and severity of AGA in African men compared to Caucasians (Smith and Wells 1964; [6]), differences in women were also discovered. In Caucasian women, the prevalence of AGA increases with age, from 3–12% in the third to fourth decade to 14–28% in the 50s, and 29–56% in those over 70 [7–9]. Asian women have a similar age-related trend in AGA as Caucasian women, but the incidence is lower. A study of 4601 Korean women conducted in 2001 discovered an overall prevalence of 5.6% (Paik) [10]. In 2010, a Chinese study of 8446 women discovered the same rate (Wang) [4]. The largest study, with 26,226 women, was conducted in Taiwan in 2013. It showed a total prevalence of 11.8% (Su) [11].

Etiology and Pathogenesis of Androgenetic Alopecia

Currently, AGA is considered to be a multifactorial trait with a complex genetic structure. This likely reflects the complexity of the biological pathways associated with AGA.

Based on a clearly defined genetic component, significant progress has been made in understanding the basic elements of the involved androgen's metabolism [12]. HFs on the scalp are classified as androgen-sensitive or androgen-independent. It was hypothesized that genetically predisposed HFs in affected areas undergo a gradual androgen-dependent transformation from pigmented terminal hairs to barely visible depigmented vellus hairs. The process is distinguished by a progressive shortening of subsequent phases in the hair growth cycle, resulting in a reduction in anagen hair count at a given time point and progressive follicular miniaturization.

Androgen-dependent processes occur predominantly due to dihydrotestosterone (DHT) binding to the androgen receptor (AR). DHT-dependent cell functions are determined by the conversion of testosterone into a more powerful metabolite by 5-reductase (type II), low enzymatic activity of androgen-deactivating enzymes, and the presence of large amounts of functionally active AR on the scalp area lead to increased susceptibility to AGA.

The mechanism of androgen action involves testosterone conversion to DHT by type II 5-reductase, followed by DHT binding to androgen-sensitive dermal papilla (DP) receptors and activating androgen-dependent genes in genetically predisposed follicles. The conversion of testosterone to DHT in the DP is important in AGA, with androgen-regulated factors produced by DP cells influencing the growth of other HF components. An increase in the local concentration of DHT causes anagen shortening and progressive miniaturization of the HF due to a sharp decrease in the DP and the dermal sheath cells.

Inhibiting Type II 5-reductase has been shown to be effective in the treatment of male pattern baldness, highlighting the role of DHT in the pathogenesis of AGA. Men who are castrated before puberty do not go bald, but they do develop baldness if they are exposed to testosterone. Furthermore, men with congenital type II 5-reductase deficiency and androgen insensitivity syndrome never develop AGA. Moreover, it was discovered that the number of androgen receptors in AGA patients is higher than in men who do not have patterned hair loss.

In some women, AGA probably involves androgen-mediated mechanisms but the evidence is less conclusive than in men with AGA. Only one-third of women with AGA show abnormal androgen levels [13]. Most women with AGA have increased HF sensitivity to normal androgen levels, but the disease can develop even in the absence of androgens, suggesting an androgen-independent mechanism. In women, as a rule, a decrease in the activity of aromatase, which converts blood circulating ovarian testosterone into 17ß-estradiol, plays a major role. There have been reports of male pattern AGA in women caused by the use of aromatase inhibitors. Estrogens may play a protective role in AGA. It is supported by the increased prevalence of AGA after menopause, the prolongation of anagen during pregnancy

[14], increased hair thinning in women taking tamoxifen or aromatase inhibitors for breast cancer, and documented hair regrowth in transsexuals with AGA taking estrogens [15, 16].

Research is currently focused on identifying the androgen-regulating factors. Candidates include Wnt signaling [17] activated by 5α-dihydrotestosterone in balding DP cells. The Wnt/ß-catenin signaling pathway prolongs the anagen phase and regulates the DP cells' activity. This suggests that the Wnt/ß-catenin-signaling pathway may play a key role in the effect of androgens on the hair life cycle and, in general, in the pathogenesis of AGA.

Prostaglandins may be one of the regulators of the interaction between androgens and the Wnt/ß-catenin-signaling pathway, according to recent research. Increased levels of prostaglandin D2 (PG-D2) have been shown to affect the miniaturization process by inhibiting hair growth in human and mouse hair follicles extracted from affected scalp, though this has only been confirmed in males [18].

In addition to androgen-dependent changes in the pathogenesis of AGA, the involvement of follicular microinflammation with the formation of fibrosis, provoked by the presence of bacterial flora, toxins, and oxidative stress, has been proven.

Although AGA is not an inflammatory alopecia, the early histological changes show nonspecific focal perivascular basophilic degeneration in the lower third of the follicle dermal sheath, followed by mild or moderate perifollicular lymphocytic infiltrate at the level of the sebaceous duct. Multinucleated giant cells may form as the condition progresses.

Hair Follicle Microinflammation and Fibrosis in Androgenetic Alopecia

Several independent studies have suggested that microscopic follicular inflammation plays a role in the pathogenesis of AGA. In areas of actively progressive alopecia, early studies reported an inflammatory infiltrate of activated T-cells and macrophages in the upper third of the hair follicle, accompanied by an overgrowth of the follicular dermal sheath composed of collagen streamers (perifollicular fibrosis) [19]. Horizontal sections of scalp biopsies revealed mild perifollicular fibrosis with loose concentric layers of collagen (Whithing 1993) [20]. The term "microinflammation" was proposed because the process is slow, subtle, and indolent, as opposed to the inflammatory and destructive process seen in classical inflammatory scarring alopecias (Mahe 2000) [21].

Inflammation is regarded as a multistage process that starts from a primary event. The perifollicular infiltrate in the upper part of the follicle near the ostium suggests that the main inflammation-triggering event may occur in this location. Under the condition of such localization and colonization of the follicular ostium by microbes Propionibacterium spp., Staphylococcus spp., Malassezia spp., or other nonresident flora, it can be assumed that microbial toxins or antigens may be involved in an inflammatory response. Furthermore, the production of porphyrins by Propionibacterium spp. bacteria in the pilosebaceous unit is also considered a possible cofactor of this initial pro-inflammatory stress.

In the search for mechanisms regulating the activation and progressive development of AGA, it has been established that oxidative stress is an important factor with its negative contribution to baldness [22]. Keratinocytes respond to chemical stress caused by irritants, pollutants, and UV radiation by producing reactive oxygen species and nitric oxide as well as releasing intracellularly stored IL1-a. This pro-inflammatory cytokine has been shown to inhibit the growth of individual HF in culture, with neighboring fibroblasts responding as well. As a result, if pathogens are not inhibited, persistent inflammation develops, accompanied by connective tissue modification caused by collagenases such as matrix metalloproteinases, also transcriptionally driven by pro-inflammatory cytokines. Collagenases are most likely involved in tissue changes in perifollicular fibrosis.

Additional factors supporting this hypothesis were the results of the study analyzing the DP cell sensitivity to oxidative stress. DP cells from the balding region of the scalp in men were discovered to have a significantly higher sensitivity to oxidative stress than cells from the occipital area that are unaffected by alopecia. Reactive oxygen species levels rose along with decreased proliferation and migration in DP cells isolated from the scalp region affected by alopecia. According to the available data, AGA can be categorized as an organ-specific accelerated aging process with increased HF fibroblast sensitivity to oxidative stress.

In a study by Miao et al., increased expression of key inflammatory regulatory genes (AP-1 family, TLRs, PTGS, EGRs, AREG, HSPA1B) was found indicating the possible significance of inflammatory processes in the pathogenesis of AGA [23].

Thus, the "oxidative stress-microinflammation-fibrosis" cascade of successive reactions can be considered as non-androgenic cofactors in the pathobiology of AGA.

The role of other organs in close proximity to the HF has recently received special attention. For example, the arrector pili muscle was identified as a new player in the pathogenesis of AGA. It is hypothesized that in AGA the loss of connection between the arrector pili muscle and the follicular unit regulates the miniaturization process and results in its irreversibility, in contrast to the reversible process observed in alopecia areata, in which the connection between the muscle and the follicular unit is preserved. It has been suggested that the arrector pili muscle is replaced by adipose tissue, and this event may lead to depletion of stem or progenitor cells in the follicle mesenchyme [24].

Furthermore, the sebaceous glands have been proposed as potential factors in the pathogenesis of AGA. It has been demonstrated that in AGA patients, the size of the sebaceous glands increases significantly, as does the number of lobes. It has been proposed that the close relationship between DHT and sebaceous gland functional activity results in their expansion, which can cause an early transition of HF to the catagen or telogen phase.

Although the role of the environment in the development of AGA is still debatable, it is likely to have played a much smaller role than the genetic component. There is only a marginal correlation between smoking and alcohol use and the severity of alopecia. Our understanding of the nosology and the development of targeted treatments for this condition will be aided by further research into the cofactors of the complex etiology of AGA.

Genetic Impact

It is a "well-known" fact that AGA often develops in relatives. However, thorough studies of AGA in generations of families are lacking. Family analysis has established a high level of disease coincidence in twins, and sons of fathers suffering from baldness have increased risk of early AGA. In the study of 476 monozygotic and 408 dizygotic twins, a heritability index was 0.81, while smaller studies of twins showed a concordance rate from 92 to 100% in monozygotic twins and from 50 to 69% in dizygotic twins. Until the 1980s, it was believed that the AGA phenotype was inherited in an autosomal dominant pattern. Kuster and Happle challenged this theory by showing that the polygenic model better explains the inheritance pattern, and by suggesting that some degree of maternal predisposition is more important than paternal inheritance.

Scientists have concluded that AGA is characterized by a complex genetic structure However, the involvement of one major gene appears to be acceptable, because predisposition to AGA can be passed down from a father or mother in many families, affecting approximately half of the children. In this case, the "usual suspect" gene on the "androgenic side" is the AP gene on the X chromosome. Its X chromosome location may explain the maternal transmission of AGA.

Indeed, the association between AR and AGA has been strongly confirmed, and variations at this locus have been found to represent up to 0.46 etiological fraction (very high risk for a single gene in a multifactorial trait). First of all, a single nucleotide polymorphism (SNP) in exon 1 (rs6152, StuI RFLP, E211 G>A) was associated with AGA. This marker is located on the border of two triplet repeat polymorphisms: polyglutamine repeat (CAG) and polyglycine repeat (GGN). However, a later study failed to show an association between GGN and AGA, and revealed only a weak association between CAG and AGA. It's interesting to note that shorter triplet repeats have been linked to androgen-dependent prostate cancer and precocious puberty. Recently, a genetic screening test for AGA was created using the SNP rs6152. The estimated test sensitivity and specificity are 93% and 25%, respectively.

The relationship between AGA and other "usual suspect" genes encoding type I and type II 5′-reductases (SRD5A1 and SRD5A2, respectively) has not been proven. However, it would be beneficial to reassess these genes in light of recent developments in genetic association analysis techniques. Genetically speaking, the involvement of androgen genes alone cannot fully account for AGA. Therefore, a thorough search for potential non-androgenic genes linked to the condition should be made. Understanding the genetic underpinnings of AGA has been greatly aided by the genome-wide association studies of the disease.

Two studies in European populations discovered a susceptibility locus at 20p11.22. It was discovered that one in every seven men carried risk alleles on chromosome 20p11.22 and AR, and that the risk of developing AGA in this population is increased sevenfold. Variants in 20p11 may affect the expression of Pax1, which is found near this region and is actively expressed in scalp skin. A recent genome-wide association study on European populations identified HDAC9 at 7p21.2 as a novel candidate gene for AGA, and a German population study discovered a susceptibility locus at 3q26.

Additional loci associated with monogenic hair disorders (autosomal recessive woolly hair/hypotrichosis and hereditary hypotrichosis simplex, respectively) were identified in a study on the German population, including the LIPH and APCDD1 genes. A direct link between these genes and AGA has yet to be established, but it is possible that they have a cumulative effect on the development of AGA. A locus near AR, at Xq11-12 (EDA2R), associated with AGA was recently discovered in a male Sardinian population. The EDA2R gene was discovered to be expressed in mouse hair follicles and linked to the NF-kB signaling pathway or c-jun, both of which are required for AR transactivation. Six additional susceptibility loci were identified in a recent meta-analysis of seven genome-wide association studies in early-onset AGA. Using a genotypic score based on known AGA susceptibility loci, researchers discovered that people in the highest risk quartile were six times more likely to develop early-onset AGA.

Recent genetic studies of this disease have brought the role of inheritance to the forefront. In a German case-control study of AGA, it was shown that a pronounced polygenic component was the reason for the genetic risk of developing AGA. In this regard, a recent analysis of published AGA genetic studies revealed a new association of AGA and rs7349332 located in the intron region of WNT10A, thus suggesting the involvement of WNT signaling in the AGA etiology.

Recently, additional genes linked to AGA have been discovered. For instance, it has been shown that women with PCOS (polycystic ovarian syndrome) and their brothers who have early-onset androgenetic alopecia share a linkage to a single allele of the steroid metabolism gene CYP17. Adrenoleukodystrophy has also been linked to early-onset severe AGA in males who have a gene on the X chromosome and low testosterone levels.

Our knowledge of the genetic basis for AGA is obviously far from complete, and additional factors, such as environmental and epigenetic ones, are likely to play a significant role in the etiology of the disease.

Additionally, it needs to be noted that the majority of genetic research conducted to date has been based on the population of Europe. Additionally, the definition of AGA is still not entirely clear, and there is no clear connection between the male AGA and its female "analogue."

Redler et al. [25] provided an overview of recent genetic studies carried out to identify main genes provoking this disease. The scientists conclude that none of the published genetic studies show a clear overlap in susceptibility loci between male and female pattern baldness. Although the disease may have the same pathology and in some cases female pattern baldness androgens may be involved, the data from these genetic studies clearly indicate the presence of several non-androgenic factors that lead to female pattern alopecia. We hope that a better understanding of the AGA etiology will drive the development of targeted therapies for the condition.

Diagnosis

The diagnosis of AGA is usually based on the history and clinical examination of the affected area of the scalp, which demonstrates a typical alopecia distribution pattern. The trichoscopy results will help confirm the diagnosis. Histological examination may be required in doubtful cases. For comorbid pathology, laboratory and instrumental studies may be recommended. Assessment of the patient's psychoemotional status may require interdisciplinary consultations. The measurement of quantitative trichoscopic parameters will provide useful information in the patient's subsequent management.

A family history plays a very important role in prognosis, which will also be useful in assessing the disease onset, duration, and progressing.

Pull test could be positive in the androgen-dependent zone and in the initial phases of AGA, showing telogen roots. In long-standing cases, it is usually negative.

Clinical Phenomenology

AGA is a continuous protracted process, rather than a series of individual phases of the disease, and is characterized by progressive miniaturization of the HF, accompanied by the transformation of pigmented terminal hair into vellus-like hair, an increase in the telogen/anagen ratio, a reduction in the duration of subsequent growth phases leading to a clinically significant decrease in hair density, and thinning in the scalp area prone to the condition.

Genetic polymorphism and pathogenetic multifactorial nature of AGA are manifested by a variety of the disease clinical forms. Clinical observations reveal correlations between the age-related manifestation of AGA, comorbidity with the clinical subtype, and prognosis.

The frontotemporal region and the crown are affected in AGA with typical male manifestations (Norwood-Hamilton pattern) (Fig. 9.1a). As the disease progresses, alopecia can merge, leaving only a line of normal growth on the sides and back of the scalp. Furthermore, males can experience diffuse hair thinning on the crown and central-parietal area while maintaining the frontal hairline, similar to female pattern alopecia (Fig. 9.1b).

AGA in women is distinguished by slower progression, lower severity, and a broader range of therapeutic responses. If left untreated, it causes a slow progressive hair thinning of the scalp, but not complete baldness, as it does in men.

In women with AGA, "typical distribution" is much less pronounced than in men, and is manifested by: diffuse thinning of the central parietal region while maintaining the frontal hairline (Ludwig pattern) (Fig. 9.2a); thinning and distribution to the central part of the scalp along with damage of the frontal hairline (Olsen's "Christmas tree" pattern) (Fig. 9.2b). Atypical thinning similar to male pattern baldness, associated with bitemporal hair recession and sometimes thinning of the crown (Norwood-Hamilton pattern) (Fig. 9.2c) as a rule is observed in women with severe androgenization [26–28].

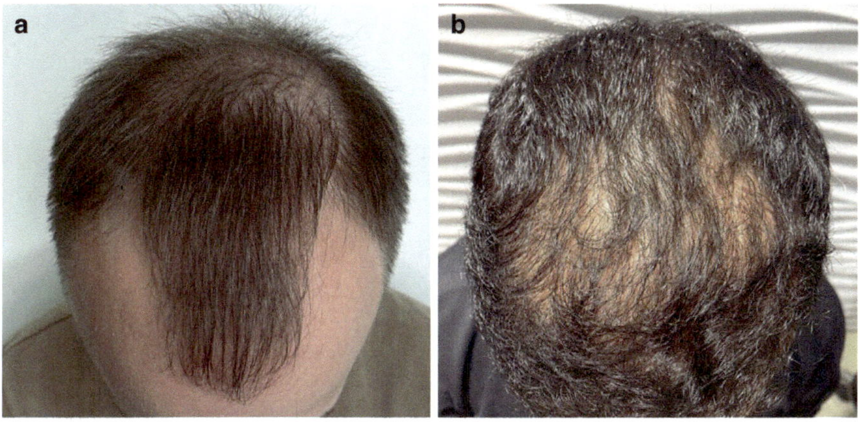

Fig. 9.1 A typical manifestation of AGA in a man with affected frontotemporal region and vertex (**a**). Patient showing an atypical pattern of AGA (diffuse thinning of hair on the crown and in central parietal zone with the sparing of the frontal hairline (**b**)

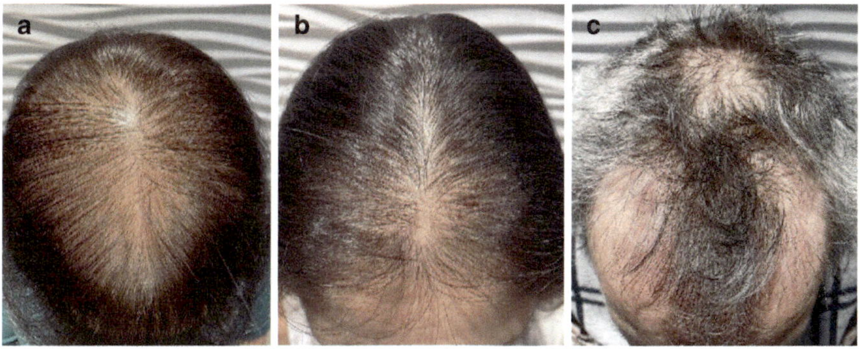

Fig. 9.2 Clinical patterns of AGA presenting in women. Diffuse thinning of the central parietal region while maintaining the frontal hairline (Ludwig pattern) (**a**); thinning and distribution to the central part of the scalp along with damage of the frontal hairline (Olsen's "Christmas tree" pattern) (**b**); thinning similar to male pattern baldness, associated with bitemporal hair recession and thinning of the crown (Norwood-Hamilton pattern) (**c**)

AGA may develop at any age after puberty, and in rare cases before. The first signs of AGA appear in both men and women during puberty, and the frequency and severity increase with age. The clinical phenotype with distribution in the central scalp in women may be due to: a hereditary androgen-dependent condition that manifests in young women, i.e., the female counterpart of male AGA; or an age-dependent condition that may or may not have a hereditary component and is likely associated with hormonal changes caused by menopause, adrenopause, and somatopause; or a nonheritable androgen-driven process, which can occur at any age (Olsen 2005) [29].

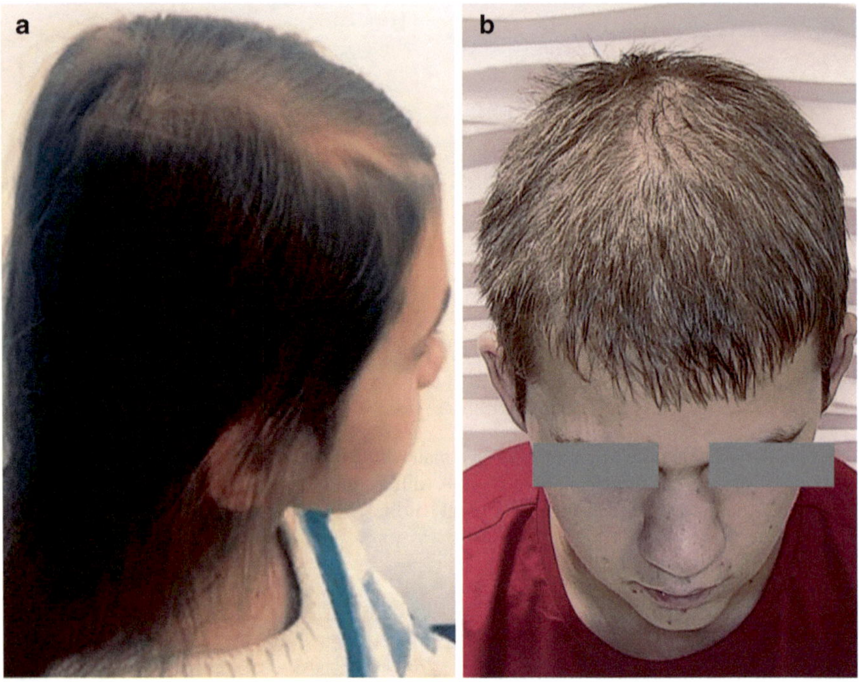

Fig. 9.3 AGA clinical presentation in an 8-year-old girl (**a**) and a 12-year-old boy (**b**)

AGA with clinical signs manifesting between the ages of 10 and 20 years is called premature or early alopecia (alopecia prematura). In children, of both sexes, the disease before puberty presents exclusively as a Ludwig pattern and is characterized by a strong family history (Fig. 9.3a, b). This type of AGA is associated with the most unfavorable prognosis, rapid formation of severe forms, and resistance to therapy [30–32].

Furthermore, extremely severe AGA or early onset AGA may be a symptom of a complex genetic disease, such as trichorhinophalangeal syndrome (Fig. 9.4), progeria, or Laron syndrome, in rare cases.

AGA is associated with involutional alopecia (IA), which is clinically similar to AGA and characterized by a decrease in growth rates, in hair shaft diameter, and by the initiation and duration of kenogen. Probably, the concept of "involutional alopecia" as presented by Kligman (1988) overlaps with the type of late-onset AGA [33]. However, an inflammatory component pronounced in AGA is not observed in IA. Additionally, in IA there is no marked heterogeneity of hair diameters, vellus hair and yellow dots as a rule are absent. Such similarities and differences suggest that AGA and IA are two separate conditions, however belonging to the same spectrum and representing different mechanisms of the general follicle miniaturization phenotype.

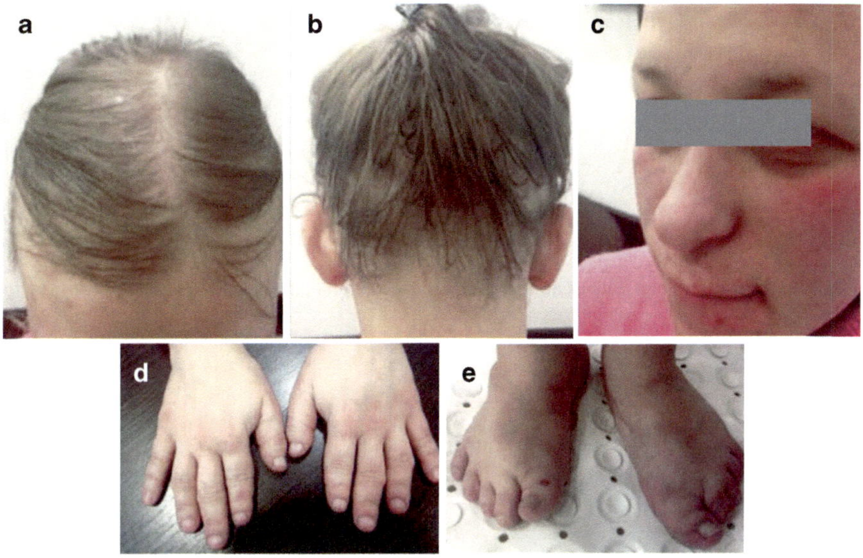

Fig. 9.4 Female patient with trichorhinophalangeal syndrome (TRPS 1). Short and sparse hair growth on the scalp with affected frontal-temporal, parietal areas (**a**) and central occipital region, where the condition has presented in a unique triangular shape (**b**). Additional features include: a beak-like nose with long philtrum, lateral thinning of the eyebrows (**c**), thickened proximal interphalangeal joints (**d**), short toes (**e**)

Patients with AGA frequently (to varying degrees) have erythematous scalps, with erythema showing up as a diffuse or patchy distribution. In most cases, erythema is related to comorbid seborrheic dermatitis, and is accompanied by complaints of itching. Trichodynia, which is thought to be a marker of inflammatory activity, is more frequently reported than scalp pruritus in AGA associated with active telogen effluvium (TE).

Trichoscopy

Trichoscopy for male and female AGA demonstrates the similarity of trichoscopic features and reflects pathophysiological processes corresponding to the disease severity. Early stages are characterized by: heterogeneity of hair diameters with more than 20% of follicular miniaturization, perifollicular pigmentation, predominance of single follicular units, yellow dots indicating the presence of empty follicles, and more than 10% increase in the vellus hair ratio (Fig. 9.5a). At later stages, small areas of atrichia may show other nonspecific signs, such as fine wavy hair and honeycomb hyperpigmentation (Fig. 9.5b) [34–36].

Rakowska et al. in 2009, proposed major and minor trichoscopic criteria for diagnosing AGA in women. The diagnosis is made with the presence of two major criteria or one major plus two minor criteria [36].

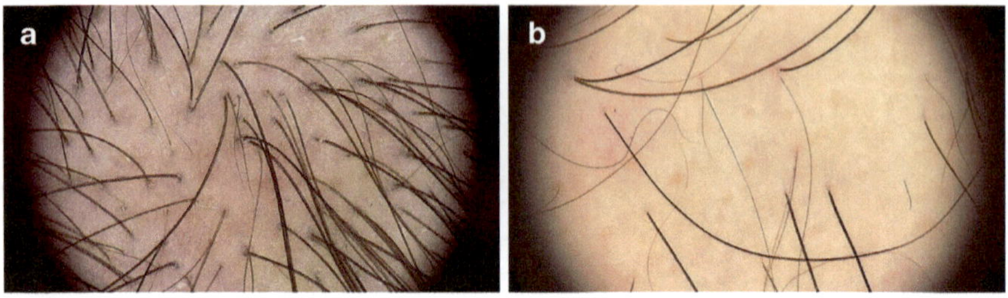

Fig. 9.5 Trichoscopic picture of an early stage (**a**) (×20) and late stage (**b**) (×20) of androgenetic alopecia

Major criteria include:

- More than four yellow dots in four images in the frontal area
- Lower average hair thickness in the frontal area compared to the occipital area
- >10% of thin hairs (<0.03 mm) in the frontal area

Minor criteria include:

- Increased frontal to occipital ratio of single-hair follicular units (greater than 2:1)
- Increased frontal to occipital ratio of vellus hairs (greater than 1.5:1)
- Increased frontal to occipital ratio of perifollicular discoloration (greater than 3:1)

Visualization of comparative trichoscopic picture of two regions (frontal and occipital) will allow demonstrating the patient hair changes characteristic of AGA and discuss the goals and possibilities of therapy (Fig. 9.6a, b).

However, practically, a frequent dilemma with the differential diagnosis in trichology practice is the early detection of AGA. It is known that in AGA the hair cycle pathodynamics involves a gradual replacement of terminal hairs with vellus-like hairs, shortening of subsequent growth phases with an increase in telogen hairs ratio, and presence of follicles in the kenogen phase. This suggests that the symptom of the increased telogen hair loss clinically characterizes the onset of this stepwise process, while accompanying it as AGA develops. This symptom sometimes complicates the early diagnosis of AGA, and is also a risk of missing the coexistence of AGA and TE that developed due to another cause.

In this context, objectifying the patient's hair condition based on quantitative hair growth parameters in androgen-dependent and androgen-independent areas can confirm the diagnosis of AGA and allows more accurate follow-up of the dynamics of the patient's condition for both the doctor and the patient.

The classic TrichoScale® phototrichogram (see Chap. 7) provides a set of numerical parameters of diagnostic value. The table presents the comparison of changes characteristic of the androgen-dependent androgen-independent areas in AGA (Table 9.1).

At the initial stages, there may be changes only of some parameters shown in the table, such as an increase in the fine hair count and a decrease in the average hairs

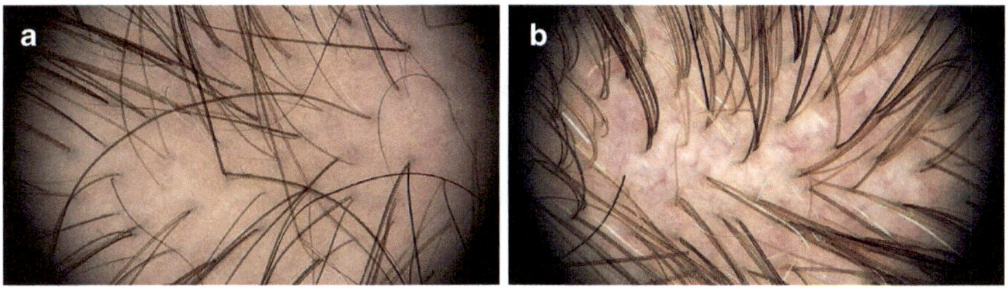

Fig. 9.6 Trichoscopic images from androgen-independent (**a**) and androgen-dependent (**b**) areas. The androgen-dependent area shows signs of anisotrichosis, an increase in the number of fine vellus-like hairs, single hair units (×20). Trichoscopy of the occipital area is normal (×20)

Table 9.1 Comparison of the numerical parameters of hair in androgen-dependent and androgen-independent areas in androgenetic alopecia

Parameter	Androgen-dependent area	Androgen-independent area
Hair growth density per 1 cm^2	Decreased	Normal
Average hair diameter	Decreased	Normal
Single follicular unit quantity	Increased	Normal
Triple and more follicular unit quantity	Decreased	Normal
Fine (vellus-like) hair count[a]	Increased	Normal
Thin (terminal) hair count[a]	Decreased	Normal
Anagen hair count[b]	Decreased	Normal
Telogen hair count[b]	Increased	Normal

[a] To differentiate vellus-like from terminal hairs the program algorithm uses a threshold of 40 μm
[b] To obtain these parameters, a two-stage phototrichogram is required

thickness. Nevertheless, it is important to understand the particular value of dynamic comparison of studies, which is recommended every 6–12 months.

The authors of the chapter use in their practice the advanced program of the new generation of quantitative calculations TrichoLAB Trichoscale DX, available to users of digital dermatoscopic systems Fotofinder. Among its advantages is the combination in one program of two basic options of quantitative hair measurement: quantitative trichoscopy without shaving with the ability to evaluate and monitor the average diameter, hair density, vellus/thinning/terminal ratio, unit hierarchy and the classic phototrichogram with shaving. This is the optimal option for fast automatic calculation with the ability to perform manual correction, which the doctor can independently perform during the appointment.

The classical phototrichogram and the method of quantitative trichoscopy without shaving in TrichoLAB Trichoscale DX synergize the diagnostic capabilities for obtaining quantitative parameters and monitoring observations in clinical practice. An additional advantage of the method of obtaining quantitative hair growth parameters without shaving is the higher accuracy of measurements. The assessment is made on images taken with 50x magnification, which ensures greater reliability of the result than in the case of 20x magnification.

Secondly, for research using a classic phototrichogram, it is necessary to shave hair in the area of interest, even for one-stage phototrichogram. This requirement alone is extremely negatively perceived by patients, even if the need for the procedure is justified by diagnostic purposes.

Pathology

When cicatricial alopecia or alopecia areata is suspected or when the clinical evaluation cannot make a conclusive diagnosis, a scalp skin biopsy may be helpful. It is advised to perform a 4-mm punch biopsy with the dermis under trichoscopy guidance. The temporal area should be avoided as this region may have miniaturized hairs without AGA. It is best to perform both vertical and horizontal sectioning. The evaluation of the number of HF per field of view is made possible by horizontal sections. When compared to a normal scalp, the ratio of terminal to vellus-like HF is typically 3:1 in AGA patients (Whiting et al.) [20]. Around the upper part of the HF, there may be perifollicular fibrosis and low levels of mild perifollicular inflammation. Other typical histopathological features are an increase of telogen/anagen ratio (Vujovic) [37].

Differential Diagnosis

Ludwig's AGA model suggests a differential diagnosis with other nosologies showing a diffuse distribution pattern: TE, diffuse form of alopecia areata and alopecia areata incognita; as well as scarring hair loss: fibrosing alopecia with pattern distribution, central centrifugal cicatricial alopecia. Frontal fibrosing alopecia is the differential diagnosis in Norwood-Hamilton AGA pattern in both men and women. Simple isolated hypotrichosis and ectodermal dysplasia are the differential diagnoses for premature alopecia.

It should also be noted that because AGA is so common, it can coexist with other hair diseases.

Comorbidity

Assessment of comorbid pathology is a serious diagnostic stage in the examination of a patient with AGA. It indicates possible clinical and pathogenetic disease variants; the comorbidity causal relationship with clinical subtype highlights clinical prognosis and dictates an individual therapeutic route for the patient (Ovcharenko 2021) [1].

Recent studies have further strengthened the link between AGA and the risk of cardiovascular disease and metabolic syndrome in men [38]. It is emphasized that these diseases are more consistent with early-onset AGA affecting the crown area. According to the data, inflammatory markers like fibrinogen and C-reactive protein are risk factors for cardiovascular disease in AGA. AGA has also been linked to increased arterial rigidity, even in asymptomatic young adults. Furthermore, AGA has been shown to be an independent predictor of diabetes mellitus and cardiovascular disease mortality.

An association between AGA and benign prostatic hyperplasia (BPH) has also been established. Patients with BPH have been shown to have a higher degree of AGA severity. There was also a link between BPH, AGA, and the AR gene polymorphism (SNP rs6152 G>A). According to a recent meta-analysis, AGA distribution over the crown is associated with a significant increase in prostate cancer risk unlike other types of AGA distribution.

Furthermore, greater severity of hair loss in men with AGA, particularly in cases of early onset, was significantly associated with a high body mass index (BMI).

AGA in women is associated with a variety of endocrine disorders. Polycystic ovarian syndrome (PCOS), hyperprolactinemia, adrenal hyperplasia, and, in rare cases, ovarian and adrenal tumors are among the most frequently implicated conditions characterized by the development of hyperandrogenism [39]. However, changes in androgen metabolism have been reported in only a subset of women with AGA, and these changes are frequently minor. Only 29% of women with AGA had an increase in free testosterone, according to Moltz study [40].

AGA has been linked to insulin resistance, hypertension, diabetes mellitus, and an increased risk of cardiovascular disease in women. Waist circumference and arterial hypertension have been shown to correlate with disease severity in women with AGA. Higher levels of aldosterone, C-protein, D-dimers, and insulin in women with AGA could be one explanation for these associations.

Other endocrine disorders, such as thyroid disease and a decrease in melatonin and somatotropin levels, were observed beyond the androgenic horizon.

Laboratory and Instrumental Evaluation

The above observations emphasize the essential role in determining the status of those organ and body systems, disorders in which most often correlate with AGA. Laboratory and instrumental research methods are prescribed according to indications (complaints, clinical manifestations), as well as for therapy planning.

A hyperandrogenic state should be considered in women with AGA who have signs of androgen excess (e.g., hirsutism, irregular menstruation, acne, hyperprolactinemia, acanthosis nigricans), which are not common in all women with AGA. The following parameters should be examined: The free androgen index test (FAI = total testosterone·[nmol L1]·100/sex hormone-binding globulin [SHBG]) and prolactin to screen for ovarian hyperandrogenism, and DHEA and 17-hydroxyprogesterone (17-OH-P) to screen for androgen-producing tumors and adrenal congenital hyperplasia.

Note that testing of androgen levels should be done during the follicular phase, between the fourth and the seventh day of the cycle, and that oral contraceptives should be discontinued for at least 2 months prior to this testing. Ultrasound of the ovaries and adrenal glands should be performed to rule out the presence of ovarian cysts, androgen-producing tumors, or congenital adrenal hyperplasia. It is recommended to rule out metabolic syndrome and/or cardiovascular disease in female patients with early-onset AGA.

Given the recently described correlations of oligospermia in patients with moderate and severe AGA, the development of BPH and prostate cancer in patients with severe AGA, when planning the AGA treatment with 5α-reductase inhibitors in men, AGA should be considered as a marker for the early detection and control of these conditions prior the prescription of therapy. Laboratory testing of PSA levels prior to treatment is critical, because finasteride at 1 mg/day lowers PSA levels, therefore mimicking early symptoms of prostate cancer.

Patients with first signs of AGA before puberty should consult an endocrinologist and be examined for precocious puberty. For the evaluation and treatment of other conditions that may affect hair regrowth in AGA, it is informative to study the anemiogram, levels of vitamin D, zinc, and thyroid function.

Depending on the findings, an interdisciplinary approach may be necessary.

Psychcomorbidity

> AGA affects not only humans, but also other primates such as orangutans, chimps, and stump-tailed macaques. This possibly can indicate the natural development of secondary sexual characteristics, and not a disease. In an era when life expectancy was short, pronounced AGA would distinguish older male survivors as leaders. Male gorillas that develop a silver saddle of hair on their backs as they age, or large antlers in older deer, are examples from the animal world [41, 42]. Whatever the possible benefits of this condition, the lower incidence of baldness in African men suggests evolutionary selection pressure to preserve scalp hair for protection from direct sunlight [6].

Although AGA is widely common, not life threatening, does not have physical symptoms, and does not disrupt physical functioning, it is a significant source of stress. This is not surprising, since throughout centuries hair has had major symbolic significance. History teaches us that hair plays an important, albeit often overlooked, role in human social and sexual life, regardless of genetic or cultural background (see Chap. 1). The relationship of baldness with aging have a negative connotation in the culture of developed countries. Although the original biological role of hair has lost its importance in the industrialized world, AGA frequently causes psychological distress and a decrease in QoL in both men and women [43].

Several published studies show that, when compared to men without hair loss, men with male pattern baldness have a less favorable first impression. The dominant stereotype holds that balding men are less attractive in terms of physical, personal, and social qualities [44].

The first thing we notice about a new person is their hair. The condition of a person's hair has a large influence on whether or not they are perceived as physically attractive. Furthermore, studies conducted over the last 20 years have confirmed that the perception of a person as "attractive" by cultural standards has been the most advantageous in most human relationships. An adverse social position, on the other hand, is associated with a person's image as "unattractive," particularly if such an image is caused by a dermatological disease [45]. The consequences of this attitude can extend beyond personal isolation and reach extremes, such as direct discrimination in employment.

Selective sociological data on the **phenomenon of physical attractiveness**, which is influenced in part by hair condition, can be presented as generalized data from the social sciences specializing in hair research. The fundamental principles underlying the phenomenon of physical attractiveness, according to Patzer [46], are as follows:

- Physical attractiveness serves as a signal for obtaining extensive information about a person.
- Phenomenon is comprehensive and powerful.

In several studies of this phenomenon, hair has been rated as an "important," "very important," and "essential" component. Another study found that the mouth was the most important component of attractiveness, followed by the eyes, hair, and nose. This suggests that hair, first and foremost, is a determining factor in physical attractiveness, and secondly, an additional element of enhancing positive qualities and diverting attention away from negative ones.

A neat haircut, pleasant smell, and clean hair are also of great importance. In a study conducted in [47] by Graham, 41 men and women were asked to rate female professionals under four experimental conditions: before and after cosmetic care routine, as well as before and after hair care routine. Women were rated as more caring, kind hearted, sincere, reliable, even-tempered, tenacious, kind, sensitive, and organized after having their hair styled.

An article published by Girman [48] examined scores related to the scalp hair count (normal, balding, and hairless), as well as hair color, length, and quality. The results showed that a person with normal amount of hair was perceived to be the most attractive, masculine, strong, active, and intelligent. A balding person was rated as the least strong, weak, narrow-minded, and inactive, and a bald person was found to be unfriendly and unpleasant.

Given the psychological and symbolic significance of hair, as well as the fact that hair removal was used as a punishment in many cultures, it is not surprising that baldness can affect a person's QoL. Unfortunately, those who are not affected frequently underestimate or even ignore the negative impact. Many studies have confirmed the importance of the psychological issues that men with AGA face. It has been suggested that physicians who counsel such patients be familiar with both the physical and psychological aspects of AGA.

According to published studies, there is a significant negative correlation between male AGA and QoL, which is frequently secondary to significant psychological problems.

Reduced self-esteem, feelings of physical unattractiveness, depression, emotional distress, increased feelings of embarrassment, anxiety, and psychosocial maladjustment have all been reported as negative effects of AGA. Furthermore, AGA patients express dissatisfaction with their own appearance, preoccupation with hair loss, anxiety about other people's opinions and judgments, and fear of social rejection [49].

According to the findings of Cash's study, more than 25% of men find their hair loss extremely unpleasant, and 62% experience moderate emotional distress. Baldness was reported to cause significant preoccupation, moderate stress or distress, and the many coping efforts. These effects were especially noticeable in men with more extensive balding, as well as in younger men, single men, and men whose hair loss began earlier. Balding men had lower body image satisfaction than controls.

In a study of mentally stable men [50], 20% reported feeling awkward in the presence of women, feeling less attractive, and feeling much older. Almost a quarter of participants were concerned about baldness and considering a hair transplant, more than 30% were annoyed by baldness jokes, and 41% felt that others underestimated their hair problems. Surprisingly, only 37% of bald patients sought medical treatment.

The findings of a questionnaire-based survey of general practitioners on patients who had recently seen them for scalp or hair problems were published by de Koning et al. [51]. Almost 34% of patients went back multiple times. About half of the male patients reported having psychological issues. Low self-esteem (26%) and depression (9%) were the most frequently mentioned issues among men. Regarding the treatment options provided to male patients, the AGA was explained to 58% of patients, minoxidil was prescribed to 30% of them, and 28% were given dermatologist referrals. A psychologist wasn't recommended for any patients. This study demonstrates the prevalence of psychological issues among men who seek medical attention for hair loss and the severe lack of psychological care provided to these patients.

In a [52] study by Wells et al., 182 men between the ages of 19 and 73 were divided into three groups based on their hair condition: unaffected, balding, and bald. A questionnaire about psychosocial aspects of life, such as self-esteem, depression, psychotism, introverted neuroticism, and feelings of unattractiveness, was filled out by participants. According to the findings, baldness was linked to lower self-esteem, more depression and introversion, neuroticism, and feelings of unattractiveness. Young men with AGA were more likely to feel unattractive, have high levels of introversion, and have low self-esteem in this study. The authors state that premature hair loss significantly affects intimate relationships, social life, self-confidence, self-esteem, and professional growth.

Another point of view suggests that the likelihood of developing psychological problems in a patient with alopecia is determined by the existence of a personality disorder. Depending on whether the balding man has a personality or psychological disorder, the same severity of alopecia will be tolerated differently [53].

The low referral rate of patients with severe AGA, as compared to patients with minimal or early frontotemporal alopecia, who urgently seek assistance from a trichologist, is an interesting finding. These visits might conceal a high level of anxiety, personal dissatisfaction, or hidden depression [54, 55]. This observation may be the basis for the conclusion that apparently only patients with mental disorders will seek advice from AGA

In the context of the psychotrichological approach to patients with AGA, it is important to discuss a recent phenomenon known as **post-finasteride syndrome (PFS).** Finasteride is recognized as a significant breakthrough in the treatment of male pattern baldness based on understanding of the underlying AGA pathophysiology. Clinical studies have demonstrated both efficacy and a favorable safety profile of finasteride, making it a first-line treatment for AGA in men.

PFS has been claimed to occur in men who have taken oral finasteride to treat hair loss or benign prostatic hyperplasia. The condition was characterized by sexual dysfunction, somatic symptoms, and psychological disturbances that persisted after finasteride treatment was discontinued.

In [56], Trüeb et al. described the first case of PFS in a patient treated with oral finasteride for male pattern baldness and provided circumstantial evidence that PFS may be a delusional disorder of a somatic type, possibly secondary to hysterical personality disorder and with the potential for mass psychogenic illness due to its media and social media coverage. The authors drew analogies with controversial "mysterious syndromes," such as amalgam disease (ecosyndrome), multiple chemical sensitivity, Morgellons disease: the symptoms cannot be adequately explained biologically, and the frequency of consultations for the relevant condition is consistent with media coverage, indicating a high degree of suggestibility.

Obviously, practicing trichologists may note that PFS has become a problem that needs to be addressed exclusively in the professional community. Since there are no predictive risk factors for developing PFS, it is advisable to obtain history of preexisting mental health problems, such as depression or histrionic personality disorder and conduct strict selection of patients before starting finasteride treatment. Moreover, treatment for PFS should focus on the underlying psychopathological disorder [56].

In [57], Camacho conducted a retrospective study of 100 cases of female AGA and 100 cases of male AGA to describe the psychological characteristics of the disease. Based on the results of the study, it was concluded that anxiety was more common in female AGA (92%/30%), and aggressiveness was more frequent in male AGA (8%/6%).

A study by Biondo and Sinclair [58] examined the psychological impact of AGA on Australian women using a questionnaire (Health-Related Quality of Life (HRQoL)). The study showed that women with AGA had lower QoL than women without hair loss. This conclusion is consistent with previously obtained data that AGA in women can be psychologically debilitating and suggests that woman's self-esteem is closely related to her appearance. However, all women in this study sought and received treatment. The study revealed those aspects of hair problems that were perceived by women as the most disturbing or having the greatest impact on daily life. For women with AGA, of the most important was the ongoing hair loss. Other important aspects were dissatisfaction with appearance, inability to style hair, and anxiety about central hair part and exposing the scalp. Patients were also concerned about emotional aspects associated with hair loss. These included feelings of jealousy/envy of people with thick hair, feelings of unattractiveness, inability to stop hair loss, and frustration. Women with AGA were less preoccupied with other problems, such as feelings of discomfort from interacting with people and the opposite sex (or with the same sex).

Because the majority of studies described are cross-sectional, it is impossible to establish a temporal relationship between AGA and psychosocial correlates. It is unknown whether AGA is a cause of low self-esteem, depression, introversion, and feelings of self-unattractiveness, or whether these issues existed prior to the onset of baldness.

In summary, it is absolutely not important when a psychological disorder appeared in patients suffering from alopecia: before or after hair loss. The patient who visits the clinic is both balding and experiencing psychological difficulties. In our opinion, the psychotrichological approach with the simultaneous use of trichotropic and mental medications appears to be the most beneficial for the majority of patients.

Therapeutic Concepts

Interestingly, over the past decades and today the study of AGA is a prerequisite for the most progressive and ambitious projects—development of models of neogenesis/reprogramming of HF cells in order to create a method that can become an alternative/addition to the existing hair transplantation.

However, patients' expectations for treatment outcomes do not always match the reality. Among the main therapeutic strategies are antiandrogens and agents with direct effect on follicles. To increase efficacy and reduce side effects, existing methods have been improved with new dosage form, different delivery methods, and experimental use of related group drugs. However, most of them are prescribed off-label, and the therapy is aimed at stabilizing the process, increasing hair diameter and density.

5α Reductase Inhibitors

5α-reductase inhibitors interact with the androgen receptor due to their structural similarity to DHT. Although they have been recommended since the 1990s, their use remains a subject of ongoing debate.

Finasteride 1 mg is an approved treatment for AGA in men. The drug is a selective inhibitor of type II 5α-reductase, which is responsible for the development of AGA. It also inhibits type III 5α-reductase, which does not have any known effect in androgenetic alopecia. Several studies and meta-analyses have confirmed the efficacy of finasteride. As with most approaches used in patients with AGA, the crown and central scalp areas respond better to finasteride therapy. The studies of the finasteride efficacy have shown that patients aged 30–40 with hair loss less severe than stage 4 on the Norwood-Hamilton scale are the best candidates for therapy. The maximum improvement is observed after 2 years of use. In a retrospective study, the treatment duration of 5 years or more provided better results without diminishing efficacy over time. In general, finasteride shows process stabilization in 90% of patients [59, 60].

Due to its teratogenicity, the US Food and Drug Administration (FDA) recommends that patients taking finasteride should not donate blood during treatment and within a month after drug discontinuation. Finasteride may have rare sexual side effects that have been documented. Reduced libido, erectile dysfunction, and decreased ejaculate volume are among the symptoms. Gynecomastia may develop and persist for a long time after treatment is stopped in rare cases. According to the literature, approximately 2% of patients taking finasteride reported one or more sexual adverse effects, compared to 1% of patients in the placebo group. Sexual side effects may resolve on their own without the need to stop taking the medication. Nevertheless, information about the risk of developing post-finasteride syndrome in patients with AGA treated with 1 mg finasteride has raised concerns both in patients and dermatologists, as persistent sexual side effects and depression in patients have been discussed. Finasteride 1 mg daily for 48 weeks had no adverse effect on sperm parameters in a double-blind, placebo-controlled study of 181 otherwise healthy male patients. Nonetheless, it is recommended that finasteride be discontinued or avoided entirely in patients who have changes in sperm analysis or fertility problems. It should be noted that the finasteride level in sperm is very low, and male drug use has no negative effects on pregnancy or the fetus.

A double-blind, placebo-controlled fertility study in 181 otherwise healthy patients showed that finasteride 1 mg daily for 48 weeks had no adverse effect on sperm parameters. Although finasteride does not affect the fertility of young healthy men, data from centers for family planning and reproduction indicate that finasteride should be discontinued or not used at all in patients who have changes in semen analysis or fertility problems. The finasteride level in semen is very low, and the drug administration by men does not have adverse effects on pregnancy or the fetus [61].

Despite classical guidelines advising patients with a history of depression to avoid medication, the authors' experience has shown that this is not always easy to do due to the high frequency of patients with psychocomorbidity at trichological consultation. It is critical for doctors to provide patients with information about the condition; otherwise, the patient will research potential side effects on the Internet and forego treatment.

Prostate specific antigen (PCA) serum levels are reduced by about 50% with finasteride 1 mg/day. Therefore, finasteride therapy may mask signs and postpone early prostate cancer detection. Thus, the, PCA levels in men over 50 should be assessed prior to starting treatment and then followed up on annually. Patients should also inform their urologist that they're taking the medication.

Finasteride in women. Finasteride in women with AGA is used off-label. Positive results were observed in pre- and postmenopausal women at 2.5–5.0 mg of finasteride in clinical cases, case series, and uncontrolled studies. In contrast to the increasing effectiveness of finasteride therapy in men, in women the maximum effect develops after 6 months of treatment; this period is prognostic for further efficacy in women (Oliveiro-Soares et al. 2013) [62].

However, in both men and women, the duration and severity of the disease, as well as age over 70 years, are associated with a poor prognosis, possibly indicating the ineffectiveness of 5-reductase inhibitor therapy at the stage of fibrosis. Because finasteride can cause feminization of a male fetus, women of reproductive age who use it must use birth control. Aside from the teratogenic effect, finasteride has been linked to estrogen-mediated malignancies such as breast cancer due to its ability to produce excess estrogen. As a result, if the patient has a personal or family history of breast cancer, finasteride should not be prescribed.

Dutasteride is approximately three times more effective than finasteride in inhibiting type I 5-reductase and 100 times more effective in inhibiting type II 5-reductase. Dutasteride 0.5 mg/day has been shown to reduce serum DHT levels by more than 90%, while finasteride 5 mg daily reduces DHT levels by 70%. Dutasteride 0.5 mg/daily is used to treat BPH all over the world. In Korea, Japan, and Mexico, dutasteride is approved for the treatment of AGA in men. A series of clinical cases demonstrated that dutasteride treatment of AGA in men who did not respond to finasteride therapy was effective.

According to available data, the safety profile and side effects of dutasteride are comparable to those of finasteride. However, because the available dutasteride studies are not long term, the possibility of long-term side effects is unknown.

Dutasteride is prescribed at a dose of 0.5 mg per day. It may be a treatment option for men who have failed to respond to finasteride therapy after a year of use. In 2020, a group of Spanish researchers published their findings on the use of low-dose oral dutasteride as a treatment for AGA in men. According to the findings, taking

2–3 capsules of 0.5 mg dutasteride per week can be effective and safe for men with early forms of AGA, or as a maintenance therapy for men who have already improved (Vano-Galvan et al. 2020) [63].

Compared with finasteride, treatment with dutasteride in women with AGA showed a statistically significant increase in the group under 50 years of age. Due to the long half-life of the drug, women of childbearing potential should use effective methods of contraception during and at least 6 months after treatment (Boersma et al. 2014) [64].

Topical 5α reductase inhibitors. Main efforts are aimed at the creation of finasteride/dutasteride delivery methods targeted at HF with minimal systemic absorption. **Topical finasteride** has been studied for the past several years as an alternative to oral finasteride. According to a study by Piraccini et al. topical finasteride produced a statistically significant improvement when compared to placebo and its action is similar to oral finasteride. Finasteride can be applied topically in concentrations ranging from 0.25 to 1%. But, since topical finasteride can be absorbed systemically, there remains the question of the safety of its use in women of childbearing age [65].

Mesotherapy with dutasteride also demonstrated positive results in men and women. In 2022, Spanish scientists announced the results of a multicenter retrospective study in the largest cohort of patients receiving mesodutasteride (Duta Ox, Skymedic). In 84.3% of patients, after injections of 0.01% dutasteride by mesotherapy once every 3 months for a year, clinical improvement was observed in 34.8%. Pain at the administration site, as well as TE, local edema, and headache as a result of edema were the most commonly reported adverse effects. This method is recommended by the authors as an alternative to oral finasteride, or as maintenance therapy to preserve the effect achieved with the systemic drug (David Caseda-Corallo et al.) [66].

Antiandrogens

This class of drugs is mostly prescribed off-label for the treatment of AGA in women, and its use is still debatable. The majority of studies have been conducted in postmenopausal women due to their teratogenic potential. The low rate of hyperandrogenism in women with AGA may explain why antiandrogens have limited efficacy. According to the authors, they should be used in conjunction with minoxidil in patients with hyperandrogenism.

Spironolactone is a potassium-saving diuretic that is primarily used to treat heart failure, hypertension, and hyperaldosteronism. It is also approved to treat hirsutism. Patients with AGA associated with hirsutism or acne may benefit from switching to spirolactone instead of finasteride. Spironolactone's mechanisms of action are complicated because they are mediated both directly by acting as an antagonist of aldosterone on androgen receptors and indirectly by reducing hyperandrogenism and systemic inflammation. The medication activates aromatase, inhibits 5′-reductase and 17-hydroxysteroid dehydrogenase at the ovarian and adrenal level, and increases SHBG. It also partially inhibits ovarian and adrenal steroidogenesis. The initial dose is 50 mg daily for the first month, followed by 100–200 mg daily after that. To determine its effectiveness, it should be continued for at least 6–9 months.

There is limited evidence that spironolactone is effective in AGA. A total of 80 women with AGA aged 12–79 years were included in the study by Sinclair et al. and were given oral antiandrogen therapy for a minimum of 12 months. Spironolactone 200 mg was given to 40 women daily, while cyproterone acetate was given to 40 women (50 mg daily if postmenopausal or 100 mg for 10 days per month if pre-menopausal). The results showed 88% of women receiving oral antiandrogens can experience a halt of progression of their AGA, or even a clinical improvement with no significant differences between spironolactone and cyproterone acetate. During the treatment period, 35 (44%) of the women experienced hair regrowth, 35 (44%) had no distinguishable change in hair density before and after treatment, and 10 (12%) experienced ongoing hair loss [67].

The side effects of spirolactone, which include headaches, decreased libido, irregular menstruation, orthostatic hypotension, breast tenderness, and hyperkalemia, are generally well tolerated. Pure liquorice pastilles may be helpful for women who experience orthostatic hypotension because they can lessen the negative effects of spironolactone's diuretic activity. The addition of 2.5 mg nomegestrol for 4–5 days starting on the 14th day of the menstrual cycle can stop intermenstrual bleeding in some cases, and after a few cycles of treatment, the bleeding may stop completely.

The antiandrogen **cyproterone acetate (CPA)** works by blocking androgen receptors and reducing the release of luteinizing hormone and follicle-stimulating hormone. It is approved to treat hirsutism, acne, and AGA in Europe and Canada. Its effectiveness is comparable to spironolactone, as was already mentioned. CPA had a lower efficacy when compared to minoxidil 2% in a 1-year trial with 66 AGA patients [68]. Women who experience irregular menstruation seem to react more positively than those who experience regular menstruation. In oral contraceptive pills, CPA is typically prescribed in conjunction with an estrogen. For the treatment of AGA in premenopausal women, the following regimens are advised: 100 mg/day on days 5–15 of the menstrual cycle, along with 50 g of ethinyl estradiol on days 5–25, or 50 mg/day on days 1–10, and 35 g of ethinyl estradiol on days 1–21. The recommended dosage for postmenopausal women is 50 mg per day.

Menstrual cycle irregularities, weight gain, breast tenderness, decreased libido, depression, and nausea are some of the side effects. Patients with liver diseases shouldn't be prescribed the medication. Patients taking oral contraceptives containing estrogen run a higher risk of developing venous thromboembolism, which can then be exacerbated in patients using CPA-containing contraceptives.

Flutamide, which inhibits testosterone action by binding to androgen receptors, has been approved by the FDA for the treatment of prostate cancer. Flutamide is used off-label for AGA at doses ranging from 62.5 to 250 mg daily. Despite being more effective than finasteride and spironolactone, it is not commonly prescribed due to the risk of hepatotoxicity. Flutamide should not be given to patients who have impaired hepatic function. Flutamide treatment necessitates serum transaminase monitoring at baseline, monthly for the first 4 months, and on an ongoing basis. Other minor side effects include a reduction in libido and hot flushes.

Two recent studies demonstrated the efficacy of **bicalutamide** in the treatment of AGA in women while also demonstrating a favorable safety profile in this group of drugs. The authors also highlighted the drug's effectiveness against other androgenic dermatopathies (seborrhea and acne), which are frequently combined with AGA [69].

Agents with Direct Effect on Follicles

Topical minoxidil (TM) is approved by the US FDA as a first-line therapy for the treatment of AGA in women. It is used off-label in various trichopathies and in the absence of an alternative, in some cases, it becomes a trichological prosthesis for some patients. However, less than 40% of patients regrow hair, apparently, follicular sulfotransferase activity is a key step in the medication's effectiveness.

Minoxidil is a potassium channel blocker that was originally used as an oral hypotensive with the unusual side effect of increasing hair regrowth. From the moment of its creation the mechanism of action is being studied, some hypotheses include enhanced vasodilatation and proliferative, anti-androgenic and anti-inflammatory effects [70]. The final result is to prolong the anagen phase of the hair follicle and induce an enlargement of miniaturized follicles, leading to the conversion of miniaturized hair follicles to terminal hair follicles.

TM efficacy has been confirmed in double-blind placebo-controlled trials. Minoxidil 2% solution applied twice daily shows similar efficacy to minoxidil 5% solution or foam applied once daily [71, 72]. Patients should be informed about: transitory increase in telogen hair shedding during the first months of treatment; topical minoxidil efficacy could be observed after 6–12 months of treatment; if successful, it should be continued indefinitely; its withdrawal will lead to a TE because of the simultaneous transition to hair telogen with a minoxidil-dependent prolonged anagen phase [73]. Hypertrichosis is the most concerning side effect in women. It can be due to personal sensitivity or, more commonly, incorrect application with local spreading. Irritant or allergic contact dermatitis may occur, which is usually caused by propylene glycol and not by minoxidil. If patch testing confirms contact dermatitis, a switch to 5% foam that does not contain propylene glycol or oral minoxidil can be made. Although TM is not recommended for pregnant women, the American Academy of Pediatrics approved its use during lactation. Despite the proven effectiveness and high safety profile of TM, according to the authors' experience, some patients may be afraid of using it.

In recent years, there has been a large number of publications devoted to improving the effectiveness of TM. The benefit of combining TM with microneedling over monotherapy has been demonstrated in several studies [74]. The method of using TM with enhancers has become a valuable idea of increasing minoxidil response in previously unresponsive patients. In 2019, Sharma demonstrated that in the interaction of retinoids and minoxidil, topical application of tretinoin affects the expression of follicular sulfotransferase [75]. Another suggested strategy with low ferment activity of sulfotransferase was to provide therapeutic effect with almost no increase in frequency of adverse effects by increasing the dose of TM. The data was published by Ghonemy et al., according to which 5% of TM was moderately superior to 10% TM and placebo in increasing hair regrowth opposite to the expected, the irritation was marked for 10% TM [76].

However, the leader among new therapeutic strategies in AGA treatment has become the brave idea of using **oral minoxidil** (OM) [77]. If patients' hair loss does not respond to TM or if the topical medication becomes intolerable, they may be candidates for OM. The introduction of this FDA-approved potent arteriolar vasodilator for the treatment of severe hypertension has been limited since 1979 due to serious dose-related side effects including postural hypotension, fluid retention, and hypertrichosis.

Use of low-dose oral minoxidil (LDOM), ranging from 0.25 to 5 mg/day, overcomes many of these therapeutic limitations and has recently become more popular with several studies published, devoted to finding a balance between its efficacy and safety. Ramos and co-authors compared the efficacy of 1 mg daily oral minoxidil (OM) to 5% topical minoxidil solution and found that by week 24, OM was as effective as the topical treatment in women. An added benefit of using OM was a greater improvement in hair shedding scores related to telogen effluvium, along with reduced local irritation [78]. A retrospective study by Rodrigues-Barata determined a mean dose of 1 mg of OM in women to be an effective treatment for AGA in women with about 80% achieving clinical improvement. The authors noted an interesting observation—response to therapy was more significant in patients with more advanced AGA [79]. Lueangarun et al., investigated the efficacy of oral minoxidil 5 mg once daily in men. After 24 weeks, photographs showed 100% improvement, total hair count showed an increase, which is only slightly higher compared to topical administration, but with a longer duration of treatment, more patients showed remarkable improvement [80]. These observations are supported by the results of a meta-analysis published by Gupta in 2022 in which LDOM at 5 mg/day was significantly more effective in increasing terminal hair count at 24 weeks than 0.25 mg/day, topical minoxidil, and various doses of 5ARIs [81]. In a review of 16 studies, Randolph and Tosti reported that low-dose OM is generally well tolerated, with mild, dose-dependent side effects [82]. The most common was hypertrichosis, while less frequent side effects included postural hypotension or dizziness, lower limb edema, mild blood pressure fluctuations, and ECG abnormalities [83]. These studies demonstrate that LDOM is an effective and safe treatment alternative for AGA in men and women. However, oral minoxidil should be used carefully in patients with severe hypertension, cardiac failure, severe migraine, and several medications. To inform clinicians until high-quality evidence-based data becomes available, the results of the first international consensus statement on initiation and monitoring of low-dose oral minoxidil for different types of hair loss were published in 2024 [84].

In 2020, an article published by Sinclair et al. first described the use of **sublingual minoxidil (SM).** Compared to oral administration, sublingual route bypasses primary hepatic metabolism, thereby increasing its bioavailability; it therefore has the potential advantage of similar efficacy at a lower dose compared to OM [85]. In a randomized, phase IB trial, SM produced a dose-dependent increase in mean terminal hair count of the frontal and vertex scalp and an improvement in hair density without affecting blood pressure [86].

Alternative Molecules

As a cosmetic alternative to topical minoxidil, products based on the **aminexil** molecule, similar in structure to minoxidil, can be used. The results of a study conducted in Italy showed that aminexil acts on the thickening of the root sheath of HF by inhibiting lysyl hydroxylase, thereby reducing collagen reticulation and thickening of the fibronectin network. Among the advantages is a more pronounced proven antifibrotic effect, which justifies the use of aminexil in the complex therapy of AGA both in the early and late stages of typical thinning. Authors' experience suggests that aminexil can be used in pediatric practice, in cases of early manifestation of AGA, intolerance, or contraindications to minoxidil and/or propylene glycol. In patients afraid of taking minoxidil, it can be used as an external therapy in the complex treatment of AGA, for a synergistic effect in combination with a medicinal product.

Regenerative Medicine

Platelet-rich plasma (PRP) is obtained by centrifuging a patient's own blood and concentrating the platelets. Platelets that have been supplemented with growth factors, chemokines, and cytokines are then injected into the affected areas [87].

The mechanisms of HF action are still being debated. PRP stimulates DP cell proliferation and prevents apoptosis in vitro by increasing Akt and Bcl-2 expression. Furthermore, PRP helps to form hair epithelium and stem cell differentiation into hair follicle cells by upregulating β-catenin, which is expressed in the HF bulge area. An extended anagen phase of the hair cycle is determined by increased expression of FGF-7 (fibroblast growth factor-7). Furthermore, in AGA, PRP promotes bulge cell proliferation by releasing Ki-67. Finally, because it suppresses inflammatory cytokines, PRP appears to be a potent anti-inflammatory agent.

The efficacy of PRP in hair transplants has been studied, and significant improvements in the density and regrowth of transplanted hair follicles have been observed (Starace et al. 2019). According to recent studies, PRP proved to be a promising option for the treatment of AGA. A placebo-controlled, randomized, half-head trial that included 12 men and 13 women with AGA found a greater increase in hair density in sites treated with PRP compared with control sites 6 months after the first of 3 monthly PRP treatments (Alves and Grimalt 2016) [88].

Ovcharenko et al. presented the results of a clinical comparative randomized study of the effectiveness of a combination therapy with PRP and TM. According to the criterion of increasing hair density in a group of PRP in monotherapy (group 2), a result comparable to a group using monominoxidil (group 1) was observed 18 weeks after. According to the criterion for reducing perifollicular inflammation in group 2, the result was 2 TIMES superior to the result in group 1 using monominoxidil. The best result according to the two criteria was shown in group 3, using combined therapy with PRP with 5% topical minoxidil. Positive associations were mild AGA, absence of perifollicular inflammation and fibrosis, negative associations were disease duration of more than 10 years, moderate severity of AGA, and the presence of perifollicular inflammation and fibrosis. Among the 36 patients who continued therapy, authors observed that after 9 months, the rate of hair growth began to decrease in the 5% minoxidil group, but persisted in the combination treatment group [89].

Although studies may differ in methodology, patient selection, and treatment technique, regrowth rates have been reported after five local treatments of 3 mL of PRP at 2- to 3-week intervals. Pain and transient post-treatment edema and tenderness, persistent trichodynia, psoriasiform scalp reactions, telogen effluvium, secondary infections, and scarring are the most common side effects of PRP injections.

Today, there is intense debate about the amount of PRP required, the frequency of application, the exact site of administration, and the method/system of preparation used. According to the authors, factors to be considered for achieving better outcomes include the severity of AGA, the need for ongoing treatments, the potential for combination with other therapies, and patient preference. Considering that PRP allows to save the lost HF functionality, it is appropriate to start such treatment in the early stages of the development of the disease. And taking into account the known course and pathobiology of AGA, PRP therapy should be regularly and constantly used.

Based on data from the literature and the authors' experience, PRP demonstrates a pronounced synergistic effect with approved drugs and represents a viable option for patients who do not respond adequately to standard treatments or who are reluctant to use them. Further research is required to confirm the efficacy and develop standardized treatment protocols.

Laser Therapy

Following the first published report of paradoxical hair growth in patients treated with intense pulsed light for hair removal (phenomenon known as "paradoxical hypertrichosis"), there has been increased interest in the potential effects and applications of low-level laser light therapy (LLLT) to treat alopecia. Hypertrichosis is widely acknowledged to occur with all types of low-fluence lasers at an incidence rate ranging from 0.6 to 10%.

The mechanism by which LLLT influences hair growth is unknown; it is hypothesized that the light increases mitochondrial respiratory activity and adenosine triphosphate production. A number of LLLT devices have been approved by the FDA for the treatment of AGA. This therapy is generally well tolerated. Dryness, itching, tenderness, and a warm sensation are some of the side effects. A meta-analysis of randomized controlled trials on LLLT for adult AGA was recently published. The majority of studies found that LLLT therapy improved hair regrowth, thickness, and patient satisfaction. More controlled randomized clinical trials are needed to determine the efficacy of these treatments. According to the authors, LLLT is indicated for patients with AGA who have a significant inflammatory component.

Hair Restoration Surgery

Hair transplantation is the only radical surgical method for hair restoration. The essence of the procedure is the movement of one's own hair follicles from the donor zone to the recipient zone. Follicles retain all of their characteristics, as well as the type and quality of hair that they produce, in a recipient location. Patients with advanced stages of AGA are classic candidates for hair transplantation. Formed fibrosis negates the efforts of doctors to restore growth in these areas, limiting the effectiveness of treatment by improving the characteristics of only those follicles that have retained susceptibility to conservative methods of exposure. However, according to the authors experience, it is possible to achieve the maximum result in the synergy of surgical and therapeutic methods. Despite common guidelines recommending surgical intervention only when nonsurgical treatments for AGA are ineffective, the authors believe that in some cases, hair transplantation may be prescribed earlier as a psychotherapeutic approach to patients, particularly those who are extremely concerned about the condition of their hair.

Summary

- Clinical and research progress helped clarify some pathogenic stages leading to AGA. Apart from androgens and genetic imbalance, the role of additional cofactors, microbial flora, endogenous and exogenous stresses, micro-inflammation, and possibly other factors is hypothesized. And although other potential causes will obviously be identified, when considering the biological conditions contributing to AGA, it is necessary to take into account the individual variety of causative agents, as well as the sequence and combination of events.
- Data from modern clinical observations reveal correlations between the age-related manifestation of AGA, comorbidity with the clinical subtype and prognosis, and identify possible clinical and pathogenetic variants of the disease, and the research results of the genetically related conditions put AGA in a broader medical and biological context.
- AGA, although widely common, is not life threatening or painful, but is a source of stress. Published reports suggest a significant negative correlation between male and female AGA and QoL, often secondary to very serious psychological problems. Negative effects have been reported, including decreased self-esteem,

feelings of physical unattractiveness, depression, emotional distress, increased feelings of embarrassment, anxiety, and psychosocial maladjustment.

- The timing of psychological disorders in patients with alopecia—whether they begin before or after hair loss—is not the primary concern. The patient presenting to the clinic is both experiencing hair loss and psychological distress, which necessitates the simultaneous and equally prioritized treatment of both conditions. For most patients, this combined approach is likely to offer the greatest benefit.
- Most modern methods of AGA treatment are prescribed off-label and aimed at stabilizing the process, increasing hair diameter and density. There is a need for a paradigm shift from single-target to multi-target therapeutic approaches, directed not only at androgens, but also at inflammation, oxidative stress, aging, and increased stress mediators. And the individual therapeutic route should be based on gender, age, clinical form, and the degree of severity, as well as on somatic comorbid pathology and psychiatric status of the patients.

References

1. Ovcharenko Y, Salyenkova O. Modern concept of the etiology and pathogenesis of androgenetic alopecia. J VN Karazin Kharkiv Nat Univ Ser Med. 2021;(42) https://doi.org/10.26565/2313-6693-2021-42-11.
2. Dawber RPR, de Berker D, Wojnarowska F. Alopecia Ch 66, Disorders of hair. In: Champion RH, Burton JL, Burns DA, Breathnach SM, editors. Rook/Wilkinsson/Ebling, Textbook of dermatology, vol. 4. 6th ed. Oxford: Blackwell Science Publ; 1998. p. 2903–9.
3. Olsen EA. Androgenetic alopecia. In: Olsen EA, editor. Disorders of hair growth: diagnosis and treatment. New York: McGraw-Hill; 1994.
4. Wang TL, Zhou C, Shen YW, Wang XY, Ding XL, Tian S, et al. Prevalence of androgenetic alopecia in China: a community-based study in six cities. Br J Dermatol. 2010;162:843–7.
5. Takashima I, Iju M, Sudo M. Alopecia androgenetica — its incidence in Japanese and associated conditions. In: Orfanos CE, Montagna W, Stüttgen G, editors. Hair research. Berlin, Heidelberg: Springer; 1981. https://doi.org/10.1007/978-3-642-81650-5_42.
6. Setty LR. Hair patterns of the scalp of white and negro males. Am J Phys Anthropol. 1970;33:49–55.
7. Birch MP, Messenger JF, Messenger AG. Hair density, hair diameter and the prevalence of female pattern hair loss. Br J Dermatol. 2001;144:297–304.
8. Norwood OT. Incidence of female androgenetic alopecia (female pattern alopecia). Dermatol Surg. 2001;27:53–4.
9. Gan DC, Sinclair RD. Prevalence of male and female pattern hair loss in Maryborough. J Investig Dermatol Symp Proc. 2005;10:184–9.
10. Paik JH, Yoon JB, Sim WY, Kim BS, Kim NI. The prevalence and types of androgenetic alopecia in Korean men and women. Br J Dermatol. 2001;145:95–9.
11. Su LH, Chen LS, Chen HH. Factors associated with female pattern hair loss and its prevalence in Taiwanese women: a community-based survey. J Am Acad Dermatol. 2013;69:e69–77.
12. Inui S, Itami S. Androgen actions on the human hair follicle: perspectives. Exp Dermatol. 2013;22:168–71.
13. Futterweit W, Dunaif A, Yeh HC, Kingsley P. The prevalence of hyperandrogenism in 109 consecutive female patients with di use alopecia. J Am Acad Dermatol. 1988;19:831.
14. Lynfield YL. Effect of pregnancy on the human hair cycle. J Invest Dermatol. 1960;35:323.

15. Adenuga P, Summers P, Bergfeld W. Hair regrowth in a male patient with extensive androgenetic alopecia on estrogen therapy. J Am Acad Dermatol. 2012;67(3):e121–3.
16. Yeung H, Luk KM, Chen SC, Ginsberg BA, Katz KA. Dermatologic care for lesbian, gay, bisexual, and transgender persons: epidemiology, screening, and disease prevention. J Am Acad Dermatol. 2019;80(3):591–602.
17. Kitagawa T, Matsuda K, Inui S, Takenaka H, Katoh N, Itami S, Kishimoto S, Kawata M. Keratinocyte growth inhibition through the modification of Wnt signalling by androgen inbalding dermal papilla cells. J Clin Endrocrinol Metab. 2009;94:1288–94.
18. Garza LA, Liu Y, Yang Z, et al. Prostaglandin D2 inhibits hair growth and is elevated in bald scalp of men with androgenetic alopecia. Sci Transl Med. 2012;4:126ra134.
19. Jaworsky C, Kligman AM, Murphy GF. Characterization of inflammatory infiltrates in male pattern alopecia: implications for pathogenesis. Br J Dermatol. 1992;127(3):239–46. https://doi.org/10.1111/j.1365-2133.1992.tb00121.x.
20. Whiting DA. Diagnostic and predictive value of horizontal sections of scalp biopsy specimens in male pattern androgenetic alopecia. J Am Acad Dermatol. 1993;28:755–63.
21. Mahé YF, Michelet JF, Billoni N, et al. Androgenetic alopecia and microinflammation. Int J Dermatol. 2000;39:576–84.
22. Salenkova O, Danilyuk S, Ovcharenko Y. Immunohistochemical characteristics of the skin of patients with androgenetic alopecia. Int Med J. 2021:3.
23. Miao Y, Qu Q, Jiang W, Liu XM, Shi PL, Fan ZX, Du LJ, Wang GF, Liu XN, Guo ZH, et al. Identification of functional patterns of androgenetic alopecia using transcriptome profiling in distinct locations of hair follicles. J Invest Dermatol. 2018;138(4):972–5. https://doi.org/10.1016/j.jid.2017.10.027.
24. Sinclair R, Torkamani N, Jones L. Androgenetic alopecia: new insights into the pathogenesis and mechanism of hair loss. F1000Res. 2015;4(F1000 Faculty Rev):585.
25. Redler AG, Messenger R, Betz C. Genetics and other factors in the aetiology of female pattern hair loss. 2017.
26. Hamilton JB. Patterned loss of hair in man: types and incidence. Ann NY Acad Sci. 1951;53:708–28.
27. Ludwig E. Classification of the types of androgenetic alopecia (common baldness) occurring in the female sex. Br J Dermatol. 1977;97:247–54.
28. Olsen EA. The midline part: an important physical clue to the clinical diagnosis of androgenetic alopecia in women. J Am Acad Dermatol. 1999;40:106.
29. Olsen EA. Female pattern hair loss and its relationship to permanent/cicatricial alopecia: a new perspective. J Investig Dermatol Symp Proc. 2005;10(3):217–21. https://doi.org/10.1111/j.1087-0024.2005.10109.x.
30. Trüeb RM, Lee WS. Male alopecia. Guide to successful management. Cham, Switzerland: Springer International Publishing; 2014.
31. Tosti A, Iorizzo M, Piraccini BM. Androgenetic alopecia in children: report of 20 cases. Br J Dermatol. 2005;152:556–9.
32. Ovcharenko Y. Trichopathies in children. Kharkiv: Maidan; 2017. p. 264.
33. Kligman AM. The comparative histopathology of male-pattern baldness and senescent baldness. Clin Dermatol. 1988;6:108–18. https://doi.org/10.1016/0738-081x(88)90074-0.
34. de Lacharrière O, Deloche C, Misciali C, Piraccini BM, Vincenzi C, Bastien P, et al. Hair diameter diversity: a clinical sign refecting the follicle miniaturization. Arch Dermatol. 2001;137(5):641–6.
35. Hu R, Xu F, Han Y, et al. Trichoscopic findings of androgenetic alopecia and their association with disease severity. J Dermatol. 2015;42:602–7.
36. Rakowska A, Slowinska M, Kowalska-Oledzka E, et al. Dermoscopy in female androgenic alopecia: method standardization and diagnostic criteria. Int J Trichol. 2009;1(2):123–30.
37. Vujovic A, Del Marmol V. The female pattern hair loss: review of etiopathogenesis and diagnosis. Biomed Res Int. 2014;2014:767628. https://doi.org/10.1155/2014/767628. (Published online 2014 Apr 9)

38. Ertas R, Orscelik O, Kartal D, et al. Androgenetic alopecia as an indicator of metabolic syndrome and cardiovascular risk. Blood Press. 2015;20:1–8.
39. Carmina E, Azziz R, Bergfeld W, Escobar Morreale HF, Futterweit W, Huddleston H, et al. Female pattern hair loss and androgen excess: a report from the multidisciplinary androgen excess and PCOS Committee. J Clin Endocrinol Metab. 2019;104:2875. https://doi.org/10.1210/jc.2018-02548. Epub ahead of print
40. Moltz L. Hormonale Diagnostik der sog. androgenetischen Alopezie der Frau. Geburtsh Frauenheil. 1988;48:203–14.
41. Goodhart DB. The evolutionary significance of human hair patterns and skin coloring. Ad Sci. 1960;17:53–9.
42. Uno H, Imamura K, Pan H. Androgenetic alopecia in the stump-tailed macaque: an important model for investigating the pathology and antiandrogenic therapy of male pattern baldness. In: Camacho F, Randall VA, Price VH, editors. Hair and its disorders: biology, research and management. London: Martin Dunitz; 2000. p. 137–51.
43. Cash TF. The psychological effects of androgenetic alopecia in men. J Am Acad Dermatol. 1992;26:926–31.
44. Grimalt R. Psychological aspects of hair disease. J Cosmet Dermatol. 2005;4:142–7.
45. Grimalt R. In: Grimalt F, Cotterill J, editors. Aspectos psicológicos de la alopecia areata. Barcelona: Aula Médica; 2002. p. 277–82.
46. Patzer GL. Psychologic and sociologic dimensions of hair: an aspect of the physical attractiveness phenomenon. Psychol Sociol Dimen. 1988;6:93–101.
47. Graham JA, Jouhar AJ. The effects of cosmetics on person perception. In J Cosmet Sci. 1980;3:199–210.
48. Girman CJ, Hartmaier S, Roberts J, Bergfeld W, Waldstreicher J. Patient-perceived importance of negative effects of androgenetic alopecia in women. J Womens Health Gend Based Med. 1999;8:1091–5.
49. Cash TF. Losing hair, losing points? The effects of male pattern baldness on social impression formation. J Appl Soc Psychol. 1990;20:154–67.
50. Passchier J, van der Donk J, Dutree-Meulenberg ROGM, Stolz E, Verhage F. Psychological characteristics of men with alopecia androgenetica and effects of treatment with topical minoxidil: an exploratory study. Int J Dermatol. 1988;27:441–6.
51. de Koning EB, Passchier J, Dekker FW. Psychological problems with hair loss in general practice and the treatment policies of general practitioners. Psychol Rep. 1990;67:775–8.
52. Wells PA, Willmoth T, Russell RJH. Does fortune favour the bald? Psychological correlates of hair loss in males. Br J Psychol. 1995;86:337–44.
53. Maffei C, Fossati A, Rinaldi F, Riva E. Personality disorders and psychopathologic symptoms in patients with androgenetic alopecia. Arch Dermatol. 1994;130:868–72.
54. Grimalt R. Cabello e imagen. Piel. 2001;21:4–7.
55. Grimalt R. Trichopsychodermatology. Dermatol Psychosom. 2001;2:41–50.
56. Trüeb RM, Régnier A, Dutra Rezende H, Gavazzoni Dias MFR. Post-Finasteride syndrome: an induced delusional disorder with the potential of a mass psychogenic illness? Skin Appendage Disord. 2019;5(5):320–6.
57. Camacho FM. Aspectos psicológicos de la alopecia androgenética. Monogr Dermatol. 1998;1:53–60.
58. Biondo S, Sinclair R. Quality of life in Australian women with female pattern hair loss. Open Dermatol J. 2010;4:90–4.
59. Rossi A, Anzalone A, Fortuna MC. Multi-therapies in androgenetic alopecia: review and clinical experiences. 2016; https://doi.org/10.1111/dth.12390.
60. Boyapati A, Sinclair R. Combination therapy with finasteride and low-dose dutasteride in the treatment of androgenetic alopecia. Australas J Dermatol. 2013 Feb;54(1):49–51. https://doi.org/10.1111/j.1440-0960.2012.00909.x. Epub 2012 Jun 12. PMID: 22686691.
61. Overstreet JW, Fuh VL, Gould J, Howards SS, Lieber MM, Hellstrom W, Shapiro S, Carroll P, Corfman RS, Petrou S, Lewis R, Toth P, Shown T, Roy J, Jarow JP, Bonilla J, Jacobsen CA, Wang DZ, Kaufman KD. Chronic treatment with finasteride daily does not affect spermatogenesis or semen production in young men. J Urol. 1999;162(4):1295–300.

62. Oliveira-Soares R, Silva E, JM, Correia MP, André MC. Finasteride 5 mg/day treatment of patterned hair loss in normo-androgenetic postmenopausal women. Int J Trichol. 2013;5:22–5.
63. Vanó-Galván S, Saceda-Corralo D, Moreno-Arrones OM, Rodrigues-Barata R, Morales C, Gil-Redondo R, et al. Efectiveness and safety of oral dutsteride for male androgenetic alopecia in real clinical practice: a descriptive monocentric study. Dermatol Ther. 2020;33(1):e13182.
64. Boersma IH, Oranje AP, Grimalt R, Iorizzo M, Piraccini BM, Verdonschot EH. The effectiveness of finasteride and dutasteride used for 3 years in women with androgenetic alopecia. Indian J Dermatol Venereol Leprol. 2014;80(6):521–5. https://doi.org/10.4103/0378-6323.144162.
65. Piraccini BM, Blume-Peytavi U, Scarci F, et al. Topical Finasteride Study Group. Efficacy and safety of topical finasteride spray solution for male pattern hair loss: a phase III, randomized, controlled clinical trial. J Eur Acad Dermatol Venereol. 2022;36(2): 286–294.
66. Saceda-Corralo D, Moustafa F, Jaén-Olasolo P, Vañó-Galván S, Camacho FM. Mesotherapy with dutasteride for androgenetic alopecia: a retrospective study in real linical practice. J Drugs Dermatol. 2022;21:742.
67. Famenini S, Slaught C, Duan L, Goh C. Demographics of women with female pattern hair loss and the effectiveness of spironolac-tone therapy. J Am Acad Dermatol. 2015;73:705–6.
68. Vexiau P, Chaspoux C, Boudou P, Fiet J, Jouanique C, Hardy N, et al. Effects of minoxidil 2% vs. cyproterone acetate treatment on female androgenetic alopecia: a controlled, 12-month randomized trial. Br J Dermatol. 2002;146:992.
69. Fernandez-Nieto D, Saceda-Corralo D, Jimenez-Cauhe J, Moreno-Arrones OM, Rodrigues-Barata R, Hermosa-Gelbard A, et al. Bicalutamide: a potential new oral antiandrogenic drug for female pattern hair loss. J Am Acad Dermatol. 2020;83:355–6.
70. Messenger AG, Rundegren J. Minoxidil: mechanisms of actionon hair growth. Br J Dermatol. 2004;150:186–94.
71. Lucky AW, Piacquadio DJ, Ditre CM, Dunlap F, Kantor I, Pandya AG, et al. A randomized, placebo-controlled trial of 5% and 2% topical minoxidil solutions in the treatment of female pattern hair loss. J Am Acad Dermatol. 2004;50:541–53.
72. Blume-Peytavi U, Shapiro J, Messenger AG, Hordinsky MK, Zhang P, Quiza C, Doshi U, Olsen EA. Efficacy and safety of once-daily minoxidil foam 5% versus twice-daily minoxidil solution 2% in female pattern hair loss: a phase III, randomized, investigator-blinded study. J Drugs Dermatol. 2016;25:883–9.
73. Kanti V, Messenger A, Dobos G, Reygagne P, Finner A, Blumeyer A, et al. Evidence-based (S3) guideline for the treatmentof androgenetic alopecia in women and in men. Eur Acad Dermatol Venereol. 2018;32(1):11–22.
74. Dhurat R, Sukesh M, Avhad G, Dandale A, Pal A, Pund P. A randomized evaluator blinded study of effect of microneedling in androgenetic alopecia: a pilot study. Int J Trichol. 2013;5(1):6–11.
75. Sharma A, Goren A, Dhurat R, Agrawal S, Sinclair R, Trüeb RM, Vañó-Galván S, Chen G, Tan Y, Kovacevic M, Situm M, McCoy J. Tretinoin enhances minoxidil response in androgenetic alopecia patients by upregulating follicular sulfotransferase enzymes. Dermatol Ther. 2019;32(3):e12915. https://doi.org/10.1111/dth.12915. Epub 2019 Apr 23. PMID: 30974011.
76. Ghonemy S, Alarawi A, Bessar H. Efficacy and safety of a new 10% topical minoxidil versus 5% topical minoxidil and placebo in the treatment of male androgenetic alopecia: a trichoscopic evaluation. J Dermatolog Treat. 2021;32(2):236–41. https://doi.org/10.1080/09546634.2019.1654070. Epub 2019 Oct 21. PMID: 31403367.
77. Sinclair RD. Female pattern hair loss: a pilot study investigating combination therapy with low-dose oral minoxidil and spironolactone. Int J Dermatol. 2018;57(1):104–9.
78. Ramos PM, Sinclair RD, Kasprzak M, Miot HA. Minoxidil 1 mg oral versus minoxidil 5% topical solution for the treatment of female-pattern hair loss: A randomized clinical trial. J Am Acad Dermatol. 2020;82:252–3. https://doi.org/10.1016/j.jaad.2019.08.060.
79. Rodrigues-Barata R, Moreno-Arrones OM, Saceda-Corralo D, Jiménez-Cauhé J, Ortega-Quijano D, Fernández-Nieto D, et al. Low-dose oral minoxidil for female pattern hair loss: a unicenter descriptive study of 148 Women. Skin Appendage Disord. 2020;

80. Lueangarun S, Panchaprateep R, Tempark T, Noppakun N. Efficacy and safety of oral minoxidil 5 mg daily during 24-week treatment in male androgenetic alopecia. J Am Acad Dermatol. 2015;72(5):AB113.
81. Gupta AK, Bamimore MA, Foley KA. Efficacy of non-surgical treatments for androgenetic alopecia in men and women: a systematic review with network meta-analyses, and an assessment of evidence quality. J Dermatolog Treat. 2022;33(1):62–72.
82. Randolph M, Tosti A. Oral minoxidil treatment for hair loss: a review of efficacy and safety. J Am Acad Dermatol. 2021;84(3):737–46. https://doi.org/10.1016/j.jaad.2020.06.1009. Epub 2020 Jul 2. PMID: 32622136.
83. Vanó-Galván S, Pirmez R, Hermosa-Gelbard A, Moreno-Arrones OM, Saceda-Corralo D, Rodrigues-Barata R, et al. Safety of low-dose oral minoxidil for hair loss: a multicenter study of 1404 patients. J Am Acad Dermatol. 2021;84:1644–51.
84. Akiska YM, Mirmirani P, Roseborough I, Mathes E, Bhutani T, Ambrosy A, Aguh C, Bergfeld W, Callender VD, Castelo-Soccio L, Cotsarelis G, Craiglow BG, Desai NS, Doche I, Duque-Estrada B, Elston DM, Goh C, Goldberg LJ, Grimalt R, Jabbari A, Jolliffe V, King BA, LaSenna C, Lenzy Y, Lester JC, Lortkipanidze N, Lo Sicco KI, McMichael A, Meah N, Mesinkovska N, Miteva M, Mostaghimi A, Ovcharenko Y, Piliang M, Piraccini BM, Rakowska A, Salkey KS, Schmidt A, Shapiro J, Sibbald C, Sinclair R, Suchonwanit P, Taylor S, Tosti A, Vañó-Galván S, Wall DR, Fu JM. Low-dose oral minoxidil initiation for patients with hair loss: an international modified Delphi consensus statement. JAMA Dermatol. 2024; https://doi.org/10.1001/jamadermatol.2024.4593. Epub ahead of print. PMID: 39565602.
85. Sinclair R, Trindade de Carvalho L, Ferial Ismail F, Meah N. Treatment of male and female pattern hair loss with sublingual minoxidil: a retrospective case-series of 64 patients. J Eur Acad Dermatol Venereol. 2020, 34(12):e795–6. https://doi.org/10.1111/jdv.16616. Epub 2020 Jul 28. PMID: 32386429.
86. Bokhari L, Jones LN, Sinclair RD. Sublingual minoxidil for the treatment of male and female pattern hair loss: a randomized, double-blind, placebo-controlled, phase 1B clinical trial. J Eur Acad Dermatol Venereol. 2022;36(1):e62–6. https://doi.org/10.1111/jdv.17623. Epub 2021 Aug 30. PMID: 34420241.
87. Starace M, Alessandrini A, D'Acunto C, Melandri D, Bruni F, Patrizi A, Piraccini BM. Platelet-rich plasma on female androgenetic alopecia: tested on 10 patients. J Cosmet Dermatol. 2019;18(1):59–64.
88. Alves R, Grimalt R. Randomized placebo-controlled, double-blind, half-head study to assess the efficacy of platelet-rich plasma on the treatment of androgenetic alopecia. Dermatol Surg. 2016;42(4):491–7.
89. Ovcharenko Y, Salyenkova O. Autologous platelet-rich plasma: a review of scientific articles on the study of efficiency in treatment of androgenetic alopecia in men and women. J VN Karazin Kharkiv Natl Univ Ser Med. 2019;36:72–9.

Hirsutism and Hypertrichosis

10

Ralph Trüeb

Introduction

Throughout the history of civilized mankind, overgrowth of hair has been of significant concern, the object of superstition and mystery, as well as of cosmetic and medical interest. Excessive hair may cause cosmetic embarrassment, resulting in a significant emotional burden, particularly if extensive. Sometimes the complaint of excess hair may pose a vexing problem for nonspecialized physicians, who tend to trivialize the complaint, though an individual's perception of abnormality is important in determining whether or not medical care is sought. Besides significant racial and ethnic differences in normal hair growth patterns, the role of society is to set the threshold level for normality, which is much determined by advertisement for cosmetic treatments. A 1993 Market Survey of 25,000 women in the USA concluded that 41% of women remove unwanted hair and 22% remove facial hair on a weekly basis [1]. Finally, hair overgrowth may be a manifestation of a more general medical problem that needs systematic investigations.

Terminology

A number of dermatologic conditions cause stigmatization and significant emotional burden, which is why disrespectful terminology, such as the faun's tail or the werewolf syndrome, should be banned from medical terminology, and sensationalism should be replaced by compassion. Specifically, because of their derogative connotation, zoological epithets should be omitted in the description of medical conditions altogether. This holds particularly true to conditions with excessive hair

R. Trüeb (✉)
Center for Dermatology and Hair Diseases, Wallisellen, Zürich, Switzerland
e-mail: r.trueeb@derma-haarcenter.ch

Y. Ovcharenko et al. (eds.), *Psychotrichology*,
https://doi.org/10.1007/978-3-031-64083-4_10

growth, where the coarse and dark hair already have a negative psychosocial impact on the patient's life.

Congenital forms of generalized hypertrichosis are rare and a particularly dramatic familial disorder, with only 50 cases having been recorded since the Middle Ages, and fewer than 100 cases in the newer scientific publications and by the media. In olden times such individuals were sought after by sovereigns to adorn their courts, and later exhibited by showmen to satisfy the curiosity of the public.

Since the first well-documented observation concerning a man named Petrus Gonsalvus, born in 1556, and his family, whose portraits are shown in the castle of Ambras near Innsbruck, Austria, the term **Ambras syndrome** has been coined for the disorder, originally by Baumeister [2]. Petrus Gonsalvus' life has been well described as he became famous during his lifetime because of his condition. He and is family became an object of scientific inquiry by Italian naturalist Ulisse Aldrovandi (1522–1605) and others, including Swiss physician in Basel, Felix Platter (1536–1614). Gonsalvus first came to the court of Henry II (1519–1559), King of France in 1547, and was sent from there to the court of Margaret of Parma (1522–1586), regent of the Netherlands. He married while there, and later was moved into the court of Alexander Farnese (1545–1592), Duke of Parma. Four of his seven children were also afflicted with universal hypertrichosis and were painted. The Chamber of Art and Curiosities, Ambras Castle collection, originally exhibited paintings of Petrus Gonsalvus and of his family. Ultimately, it is believed that the marriage between Petrus Gonsalvus and Lady Catherine may have partially inspired the fairy tale of "Beauty and the Beast."

Ambras syndrome is characterized by excessive hair growth on the entire body, with the exception of the palms, soles, and mucous membranes. Hypertrichosis is most excessive on the face, ears, and shoulders. The forehead, eyelids, nose, cheeks, and preauricular regions are uniformly covered with hair. The fine silky hair is of the vellus type, the hair is fine and long, reaching a length of several decimeters if not cut. The hypertrichosis of the ears is typical; with long curls protruding from the external auditory canal (Fig. 10.1). Facial and dental abnormalities may also be

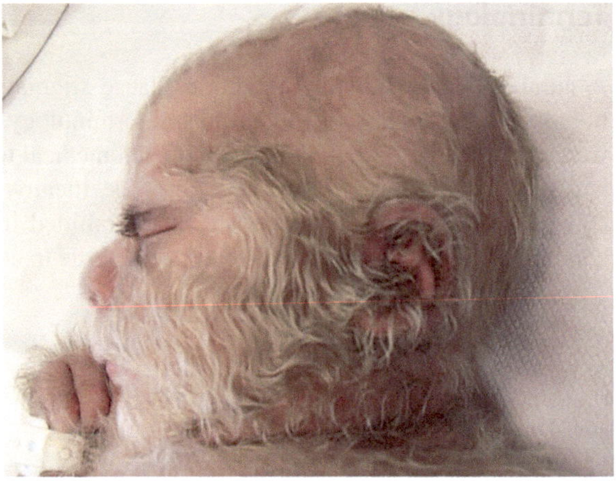

Fig. 10.1 Ambras syndrome (congenital universal hypertrichosis)

present. Ambras syndrome has been mapped to the short (q) arm of chromosome 8, and it appears to follow an autosomal dominant pattern of inheritance.

More recently, Chen et al. [3] put forth that the designation Ambras syndrome has historically been applied to various genetic types of congenital universal hypertrichosis with potential gene loci so far identified on 8q12, 17q24.2-q24.3, or Xq24-q27.1 that differ to such a degree that the term has no specific meaning, neither in the past nor in the future, and therefore should be rejected as misleading. The family portrayed in Ambras probably represented a syndromic type of congenital generalized terminal hypertrichosis with abnormal dentition, and autosomal dominant inheritance. While we cannot know with certainty in the case of Petrus Gonsalvus and his family, the discussion does not seem to be relevant, since in many instances a syndrome is not specific to only one condition, for example, toxic shock syndrome can be caused by various toxins, premotor syndrome can be caused by various brain lesions, and premenstrual syndrome is not a disease but simply a set of symptoms. Moreover, eponyms have a long-standing tradition in Western medical terminology. Traditionally, syndromes have been named after the physician who originally identified the condition. Nevertheless, the term eponym is to be regarded in a broader sense, since—by definition—an eponym is a person, place, or thing for whom or for which something is named. Accordingly, some eponymous syndromes do not refer to the physician who originally reported the condition, but alternatively to the indicator patient, a geographic location, a historical, a literary, or a mythological context, in the case of congenital generalized hypertrichosis after the castle of Ambras, where the portraits of Petrus Goncalvus and his family were originally displayed.

The recent past has seen a shift toward naming conditions descriptively by symptoms rather than eponymously. When the syndrome name is formed as an abbreviation from the initial letters of the symptoms, it is referred to as an acronym. The use of acronyms has become particularly popular, and is often taught as mnemonic device, or used as mental checklist [4]. However, the use of eponyms confers historical, literary, and cultural information that reaches beyond and therefore conveys the dignity of a broader educational background and understanding [5]. In its most extreme form, acronymophilia has reduced the respective acronym to a single letter, such as the H syndrome (for hypertrichosis, hyperpigmentation hepatosplenomegaly, heart anomalies, hearing loss, hypogonadism, low height, and hyperglycemia/diabetes mellitus) [6], despite the three simple rules recommended for creating an acronym: (1) the acronym must have at least three letters and be easily pronounceable, (2) it has to make the communication easier, (3) and to be more readily recognized by the reader compared to the original phrase, with familiarity as the most important characteristic [7].

Beyond the Ambras syndrome, **congenital generalized hypertrichosis** has been associated with a number of abnormalities, such as gingival fibromatosis, osteochondrodysplasia, or congenital amaurosis, or may be a symptom of a more complex syndromic disorder, such as the Cornelia de Lange syndrome, the mucopolysaccharidoses, and porphyries [8]. In these cases, excessive body and facial hairs is either present at birth or develops during early infancy or puberty, and usually involves terminal hairs.

Originally, the nineteenth century circus freak Julia Pastrana (1834–1860) was believed to have universal congenital hypertrichosis or hypertrichosis lanuginosa congenita, however, the generalized terminal hypertrichosis associated with her gingival hyperplasia indicates that her condition was *generalized terminal hair hypertrichosis with gingival hyperplasia* [9]. The responsible gene defect (deletion) maps to 17q24.2-q24.3. Julia Pastrana earned her living as circus sideshow performer traveling throughout the USA as the bearded lady being promoted as having distinct human and animal traits, and capturing the attention of many artists. One medical doctor, Alexander B. Mott, certified that she was the offspring of the mating between a human and an Orangutan [10]. She is portrayed as having dark extensive hairs distributed equally throughout the surface of her body, even on the palms of her hands. People with hair often found jobs as circus performers, making the best of their unusual appearance. Fedor Jeftichew (1868–1904) called "Jo-Jo the Dog-faced Boy," Stephan Bibrowski (1890–1934) or "Lionel the Lion-faced Man," Annie Jones (1865–1902) the "the bearded woman," and Alice Elizabeth Doherty (1887–1933) "The Minnesota Woolly Girl," and Jesús "Chuy" Aceves the "Wolfman" (born 1968) all had hypertrichosis. In 2011, Supattra Sasupan (Thai: สุพัตรา สะสุพันธ์; born 2000), a then 11-year-old girl from Thailand with hypertrichosis was named the world's hairiest girl by the Guinness Book of World Records (as Supatra Sasuphan) [11].

Among the complex metabolic disorders associated with hypertrichosis are the mucopolysaccharidoses and the porphyries.

Again, the term gargoylism for the condition characterized by coarsened facial surface and distorted features with thickened gums and upturned nose associated with *Hurler's syndrome* (mucopolysaccharidosis I-H) [12] should be omitted. In architecture, the gargoyle is a carved or formed grotesque with a spout designed to convey water from a roof and away from the side of a building, thereby preventing rainwater from running down masonry walls and eroding the mortar between. The term originates from the French "gargouille," which in English is likely to mean throat, gullet, or similar words derived from the root "gar," "to swallow," which represented the gurgling sound of water. The term gargoyle is most often applied to medieval work, the most famous example being the Notre Dame de Paris. The primary use of the gargoyle was to illustrate evil through the form of the gargoyle.

In the twelfth century, eminent French abbot of the Cistercian Order St. Bernard of Clairevaux (1090–1153) was notorious for speaking out against gargoyles: *"What are these fantastic monsters doing in the cloisters before the eyes of the brothers as they read? What is the meaning of these unclean monkeys, these strange savage lions, and monsters? To what purpose are here placed these creatures, half beast, half man, or these spotted tigers? I see several bodies with one head and several heads with one body. Here is a quadruped with a serpent's head, there a fish with a quadruped's head, then again an animal half horse, half goat... Surely if we do not blush for such absurdities, we should at least regret what we have spent on them"* [13].

Finally, in 1985 Canadian biochemist and internationally recognized expert in porphyrin chemistry and biochemistry David Dolphin (born 1940) proposed a link between porphyria, specifically *congenital erythropoetic porphyria (Günther's disease)*, and vampire folklore. Noting that the condition is treated by intravenous haem, he suggested that the consumption of large amounts of blood may result in haem being transported somehow across the stomach wall and into the bloodstream. Thus, vampires were merely sufferers of porphyria seeking to replace haem and alleviate their symptoms [14]. The theory has been rebuffed medically as suggestions that porphyria sufferers crave the haem in human blood, or that the consumption of blood might ease the symptoms of porphyria, are based on a misunderstanding of the disease. Furthermore, Dolphin was noted to have confused fictional (bloodsucking) vampires with those of folklore, many of whom were not noted to drink blood. Similarly, a parallel is made between sensitivity to sunlight by sufferers, yet this was associated with fictional and not folkloric vampires. In any case, Dolphin did not go on to publish his work more widely [15]. Despite being dismissed by experts, the link gained media attention and entered popular modern folklore.

Rather, patients should receive adequate medical counseling regarding the origins, prognosis, and heredity of their condition, medical support, and guidance to successful coping strategies.

Patterns of Excessive Hair

With respect to the pattern of excessive hair growth, a distinction is made between hirsutism in women and hypertrichosis. Hirsutism is further classified depending on its severity (mild, moderate, severe), and hypertrichosis on the age of onset (congenital or acquired), the extent of distribution (generalized or circumscribed), the site involved, and associated anomalies [8].

Hirsutism is defined as excessive growth of terminal hair that appears in women in a pattern more characteristic of adult men. The androgen-dependent areas of hair growth include the chin, upper lip, chest, breasts, abdomen, back, and anterior thighs (Fig. 10.2a–e). Objective assessment of hirsutism is obtained by evaluation and grading of hair growth and distribution according to the Ferriman-Gallwey (F-G) scale [16]. The F-G score quantitates the extent of hair growth in nine key anatomic sites, which is graded using a scale from 0 (no terminal hair) to 4 (complete and heavy cover), for a maximum score of 36. Hirsutism is defined by a score of 8 or more. A F-G score of 8–15 is considered mild, and a F-G score of more than 15 moderate or severe. Approximately 5–10% of women of reproductive age in the general population are hirsute, assessed as having a F-G score of 8 or more [17].

Far from being only a cosmetic problem, hirsutism may be a marker for an underlying hormonal disorder, and identification of the underlying etiology helps to detect patients at risk for infertility, diabetes, cardiovascular disease, and endometrial carcinoma [18].

Hypertrichosis is the term used for the growth of hair on any part of the body in excess of the amount usually present in persons of the same age, race, and sex,

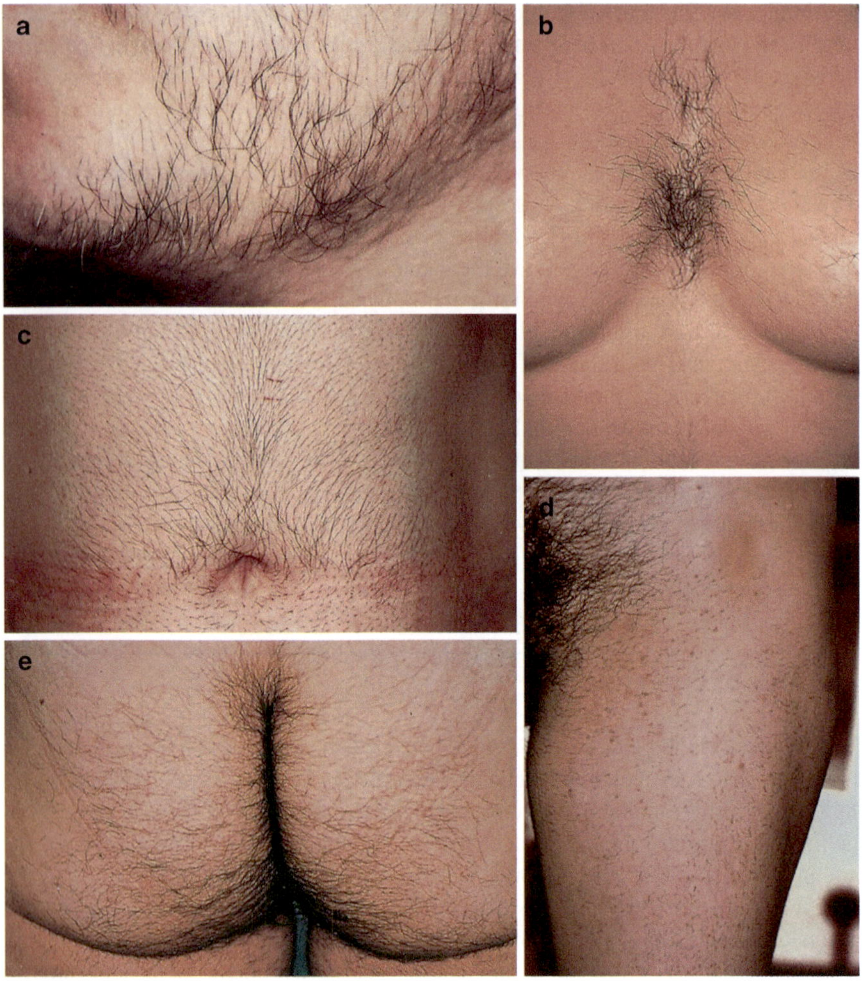

Fig. 10.2 Hirsutism: excessive growth of terminal hairs in androgen-dependent areas: chin (**a**); chest (**b**); abdomen (**c**); thigh (**d**); buttocks (**e**)

excluding androgen-dependent hair growth [8]. It may involve lanugo (in hypertrichosis lanuginosa), vellus (in congenital universal hypertrichosis), or terminal hairs (in generalized terminal hair hypertrichosis), and may be generalized or circumscribed [8]. In both, its generalized and circumscribed forms, hypertrichosis may be an isolated finding, or be associated with other abnormalities [8]. For instance, *lumbosacral hypertrichosis* (Fig. 10.3) frequently indicates occult spinal defects, or the *hair collar sign* (Fig. 10.4) may be a marker for underling ectopic neural tissue in the scalp and/or underlying central nervous system malformations. Therefore, it is essential that this possibility is investigated early, if neurologic sequels are to be prevented.

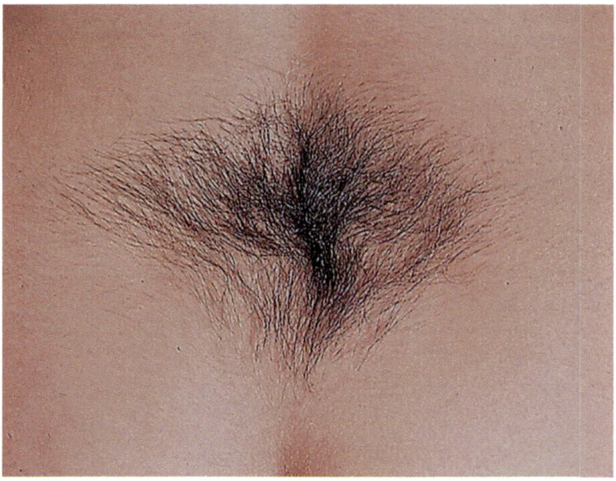

Fig. 10.3 Lumbosacral hypertrichosis

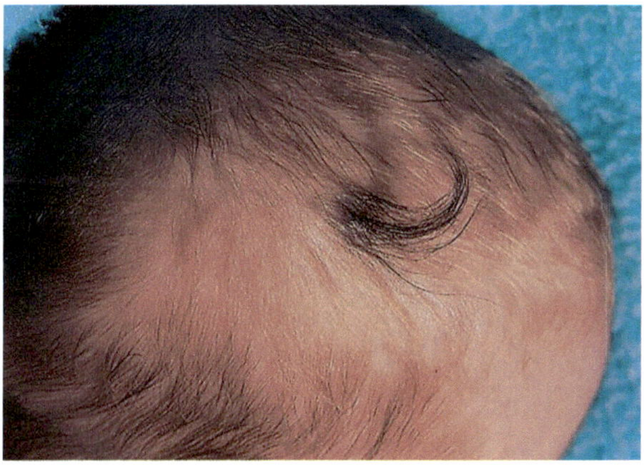

Fig. 10.4 Hair collar sign

Evaluation of the Patient with Excessive Hair

The first step in the evaluation of the patient with excessive hair is to clarify the problem: hirsutism must be distinguished from hypertrichosis. Accurate classification of excess hair must precede any treatment and includes [8]:

- Characterization of the type of hair involved (lanugo, vellus, terminal)
- Characterization of the pattern of hair growth (generalized or circumscribed hypertrichosis, hirsutism)
- Age at initial manifestation (congenital, acquired)
- Patient history with regard to systemic disorders or drug intake
- Physical examination for associated abnormalities
- Family history, including ethnic and racial background
- Psychological impact of the disorder

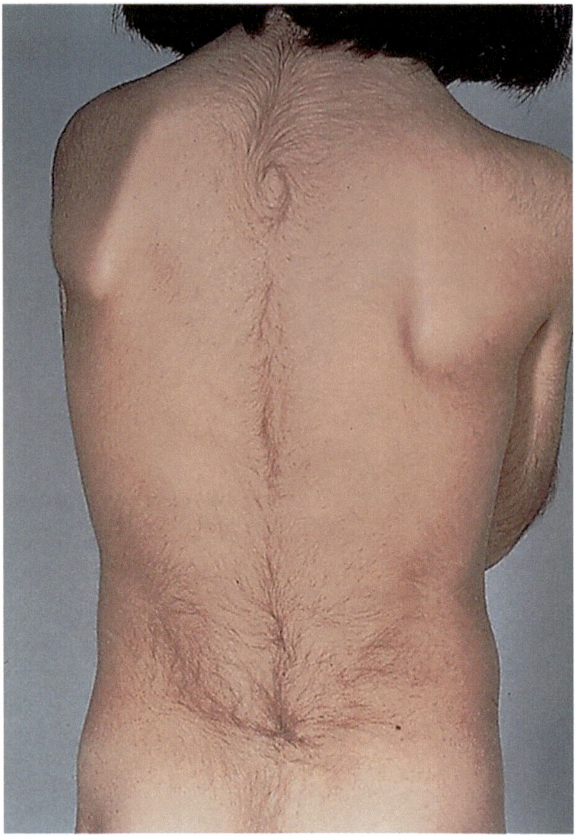

Fig. 10.5 Prepubertal hypertrichosis

The two distinct types of hypertrichosis are generalized hypertrichosis, which occurs over the entire body, and localized hypertrichosis, which is restricted to a specific area, with the exception of androgen-dependent hair in women (see hirsutism). The disorder can be either congenital or acquired later in life.

Prepubertal hypertrichosis (Fig. 10.5) is a common disorder affecting healthy children that is characterized by a generalized terminal hair hypertrichosis [19]. There is hair growth on the temples spreading across the forehead, bushy eyebrows, and marked growth of hair on the upper back and proximal limbs. The condition is usually noted at birth, increases in severity during early childhood, and is not rare. It probably often has been confused with racial hirsutism, though it is not limited to a specific race, nor androgen-mediated.

A variety of underlying pathologic states may give rise to **acquired generalized hypertrichosis**. These include: head injuries and other cerebral disturbances, malnutrition and anorexia nervosa, juvenile hypothyroidism, and juvenile dermatomyositis [8]. Besides acquired trichomegaly (overgrowth of eyelashes, Fig. 10.6), also a more generalized form of hypertrichosis has been observed in patients with AIDS [20].

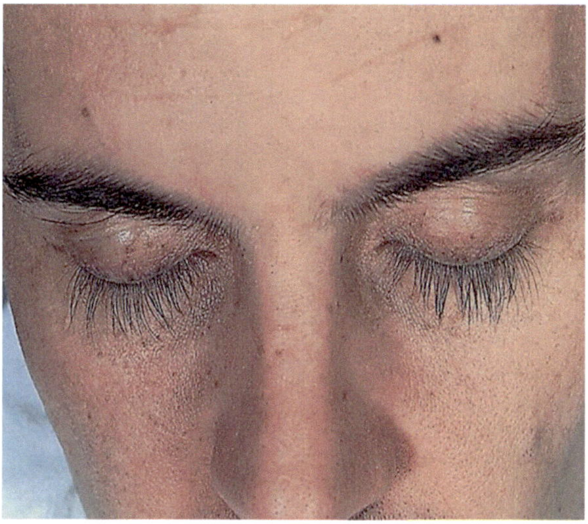

Fig. 10.6 Acquired eyelash trichomegaly

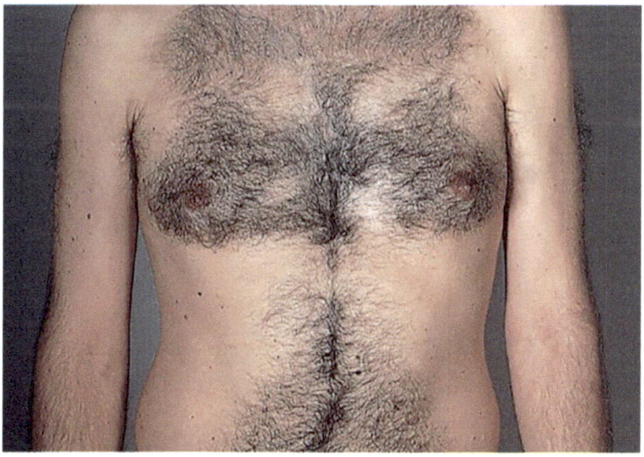

Fig. 10.7 Acquired generalized terminal hair hypertrichosis in POEMS syndrome

Acquired hypertrichosis lanuginosa describes the sudden onset and rapid growth of long, fine, lanugo-type, white-yellow downy hairs over a large area of the body in association with an underlying malignancy. While this presentation represents an exceedingly rare event, it is now becoming clear that the less conspicuous growth of lanugo (malignant down), particularly on the face of patients with malignant disease is not so uncommon [21]. The lanugo may develop a few weeks or up to 2 years before an underlying malignancy is diagnosed.

Yet another form of paraneoplastic hypertrichosis may be found in the **POEMS syndrome** (Fig. 10.7), an acronym for the major constellation of signs including peripheral neuropathy, organomegaly, endocrine dysfunction, monoclonal gammopathy, and skin changes [22]. The hypertrichosis is of the terminal hair type and most common on the extensor surfaces, malar areas, and forehead.

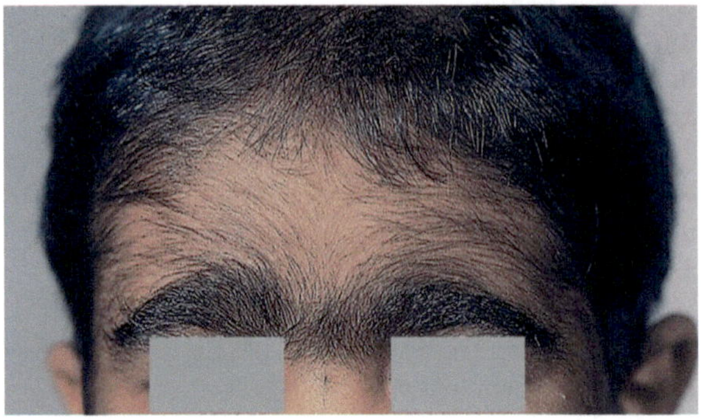

Fig. 10.8 Drug-induced acquired generalized hypertrichosis in a child due to cyclosporin

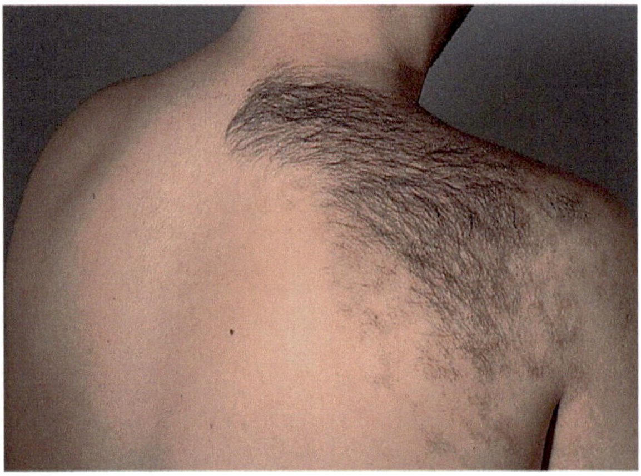

Fig. 10.9 Nevoid hypertrichosis (Becker's pigmentary hamartoma)

Finally, several therapeutic agents are well-known to cause significant drug-induced generalized hypertrichosis, the most frequent currently being: corticosteroids, phenytoin sodium, cyclosporin A (Fig. 10.8), and minoxidil [8]. Discontinuation of the offending drug leads to resolution of drug-induced hypertrichosis within several months to 1 year, depending on the hair cycling characteristics of the affected site (face: 3 months; arms: 1 year). In summer 2019, at least 17 Spanish children have developed the so-called "werewolf syndrome," Spain's health ministry has said. Instead of being treated with omeprazole, a drug that helps with gastric reflux, they had received a treatment of minoxidil. How the laboratory FarmaQuimica Sur, based in Malaga, made the mistake, is not yet clear.

Circumscribed forms of hypertrichosis include: **nevoid hypertrichosis** (Fig. 10.9), **familial hypertrichosis of the elbows** (Fig. 10.10), **hairy pinnae** (Fig. 10.11), hypertrichosis associated with spinal dysraphism, and the hair collar sign.

Hypertrichosis may sometimes be mistakenly classified as hirsutism. Hirsutism is a type of hypertrichosis exclusive to women and children, resulting from an excess of androgen-sensitive hair growth. Therefore, female patients with hirsutism exhibit patterns of adult male hair growth.

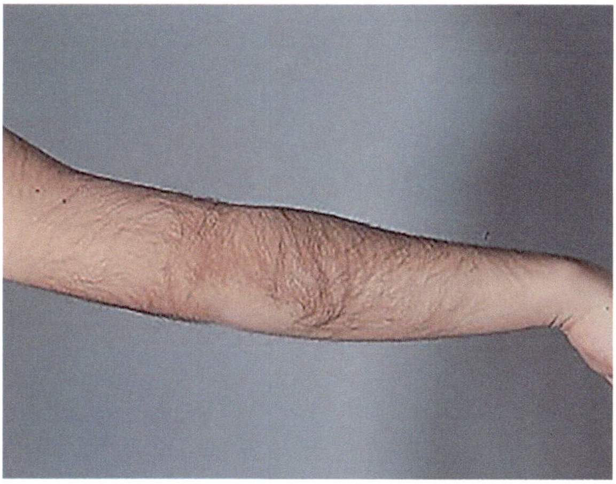

Fig. 10.10 Hairy elbow

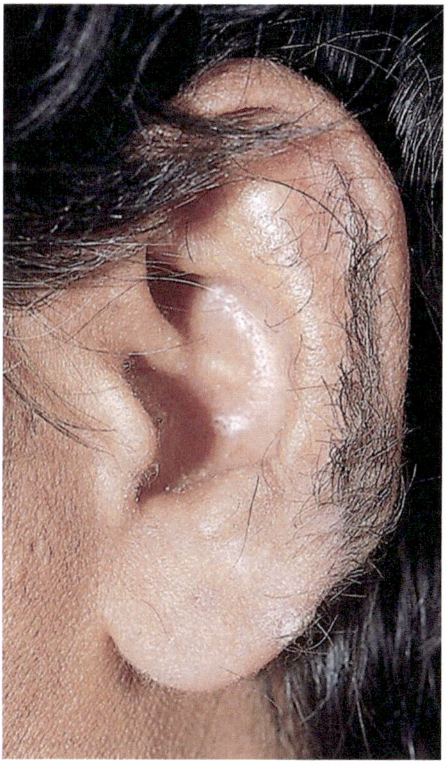

Fig. 10.11 Hairy pinna of the ear

Hirsutism results from either an exogenous or endogenous increase in circulating androgens or from increased sensitivity (metabolism) of the hair follicle to normal serum androgen levels. There is thought to be considerable heterogeneity of responses among androgen-dependent follicles in different individuals [23].

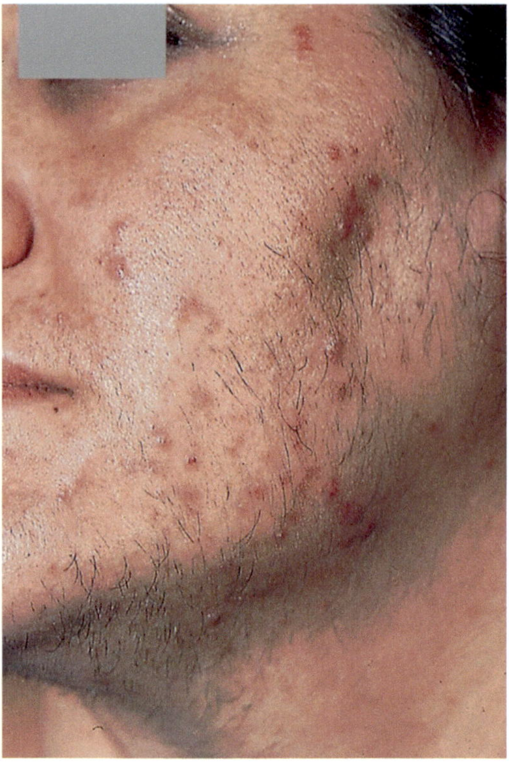

Fig. 10.12 SAHA syndrome

Therefore, the clinical severity of hirsutism does not always correlate well with expected levels of circulating androgens. Nevertheless, most women with a twofold or greater increase in their androgen levels have some degree of hirsutism or correlating symptoms, such as seborrhea, acne, and alopecia (**SAHA syndrome**, Fig. 10.12).

Exogenous sources of androgens include: androgenic medications, such as oral contraceptives with androgenic progestins (norgestrel, levonorgestrel, norethindrone), anabolic steroids (danazol), high-dose glucocorticoids, androgen therapy (testosterone), and valproic acid (raises plasma testosterone).

Endogenous androgens in women arise from the ovary or adrenal glands, and peripherally from the skin and fat. Seventy to eighty percent of patients with androgen excess demonstrate hirsutism. Androgenic causes are responsible in up to 80% of patients [24], and include polycystic ovary syndrome (PCOS) in about 70–80% of hirsute women, **hyperandrogenic insulin-resistant acanthosis nigricans syndrome** (**HAIR-AN syndrome**, Fig. 10.13) affecting about 3%, (21-OH-deficient) late onset congenital adrenal hyperplasia in 2–8% of patients, and rarely, pituitary, ovarian, or adrenal tumors (Fig. 10.14).

Originally described by Irving Stein and Michael Leventhal in 1935 in a case series of seven women with anovulation and polycystic ovaries discovered during surgery [25], the **polycystic ovary syndrome (PCOS)** has more recently been

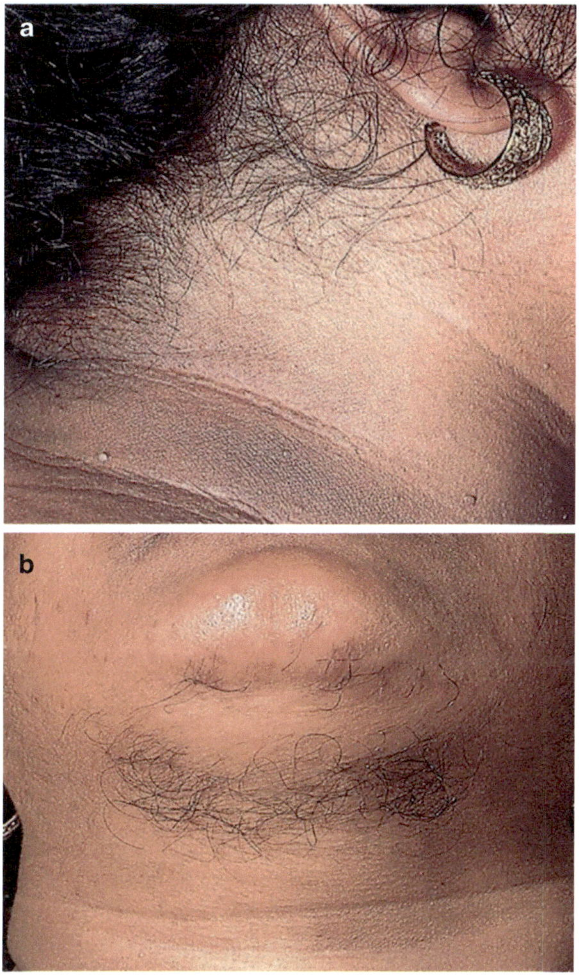

Fig. 10.13 HAIR-AN syndrome: (**a**) acanthosis nigricans, (**b**) facial hirsutism

defined by the Rotterdam criteria (Table 10.1) [26]. Given the broad definition described by the Rotterdam criteria, the prevalence of PCOS in women has been estimated to range from 15 to 18% [27].

PCOS represents a complex disorder with several aberrant hormonal and metabolic pathways. Hyperandrogenism is one of the most important clinical features of the syndrome and the most relevant to the role of the dermatologist in diagnosis and management of the condition. The prevalence of hirsutism in PCOS ranges from 70 to 80%, versus 4 to 11% in women in the general population [28], frequently seen on the upper lip, chin, areola, chest, back, lower abdomen, and thighs [29]. Acne is another common cutaneous manifestation of hyperandrogenism in PCOS, and originates or persists into adulthood while being refractory to conventional treatment (Fig. 10.15) [30].

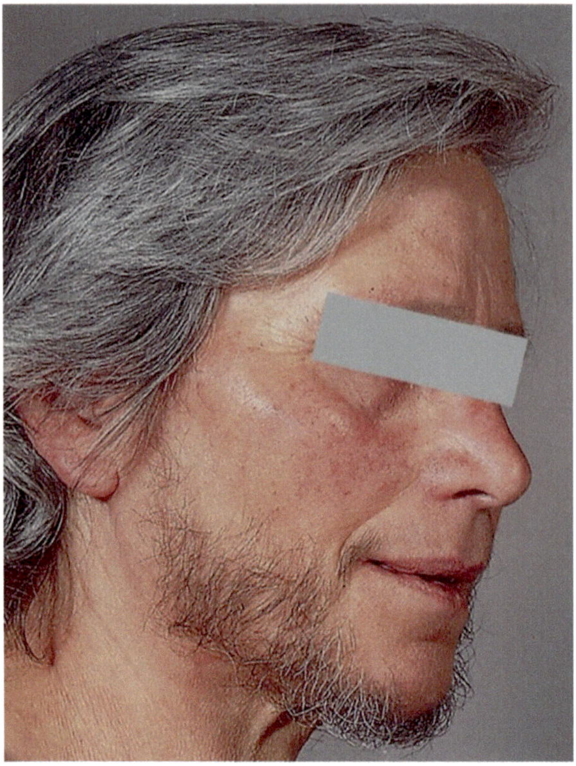

Fig. 10.14 Facial hirsutism from androgen-producing ovarian carcinoma

Most importantly, PCOS presents with potentially serious systemic long-term implications, including risks of metabolic syndrome and of endometrial carcinoma [31]. PCOS is associated with several metabolic complications, including obesity, metabolic syndrome, and insulin resistance. Obesity is present in 75% of women with PCOS, and up to 47% of women with PCOS have metabolic syndrome. Insulin resistance is common among patients with PCOS independent of obesity. Insulin plays an important role in the development of anovulation and hyperandrogenism, which explains the ability of insulin-sensitizing agents, such as metformin, to lower androgen levels and induce ovulation. Women with PCOS have an increased risk of cardiovascular disease, however it is not clear whether PCOS is an independent risk factor or whether cardiovascular disease results from the comorbidities associated with PCOS. In general, patients should be closely monitored and managed for obesity with weight loss and exercise, diabetes with insulin-sensitizing drugs such as metformin, hyperlipidemia, and hypertension. Although combined oral contraceptive pills are widely considered as first-line therapy in PCOS, a drawback may be the metabolic side effects, and risk of thromboembolism. The current recommendation suggests low-dose ethinyl estradiol (<50 µg), avoiding androgenic progestins, and addition of metformin to offset insulin resistance.

Table 10.1 2003 Rotterdam criteria for the diagnosis of polycystic ovary syndrome (PCOS)

1. **Oligo- or anovulation:**
   - <9 menses a year or missed menses for >3 months
2. **Clinical and/or biochemical signs of hyperandrogenism:**
   - hirsutism, acne, alopecia
   - serum levels of androgens, including androstenedione and testosterone may be elevated. The free testosterone level is thought to be the best measure, with ca. 60% of patients demonstrating elevated levels. Some other blood tests are suggestive but not diagnostic. The ratio of LH (luteinizing hormone) to FSH (follicle-stimulating hormone), when measured in international units, is elevated. Common cutoffs to designate abnormally high LH/FSH ratios are 2:1 or 3:1 as tested on day 3 of the menstrual cycle
3. Echogenic evidence of polycystic ovaries and exclusion of other causes of hyperandrogenism and anovulation:
   - polycystic ovaries on ultrasound are defined by the presence of >12 follicles in each ovary (each follicle measuring 2–9 mm in diameter) and/or increased ovarian volume of >10 mL
   - differential diagnosis of PCOS (laboratory evaluation): pregnancy (elevated serum or urine HCG), premature ovarian failure (elevated FSH and LH, low-normal estradiol levels), hypothyroidism (elevated TSH, low thyroxine levels), hyperprolactinemia (elevated prolactin level), late-onset congenital adrenal hyperplasia (elevated day 5 morning level of 17-hydroxyprogesterone), virilizing ovarian/adrenal tumor (total testosterone >200 ng/dL, DHEAS >700 µg/L, and elevated androstenedione), Cushing's syndrome (elevated 24-h urine free cortisol level, unsuppressed morning serum cortisol during the low-dose dexamethasone suppression test, and elevated midnight salivary cortisol)

Requires 2 out of 3 for diagnosis of PCOS

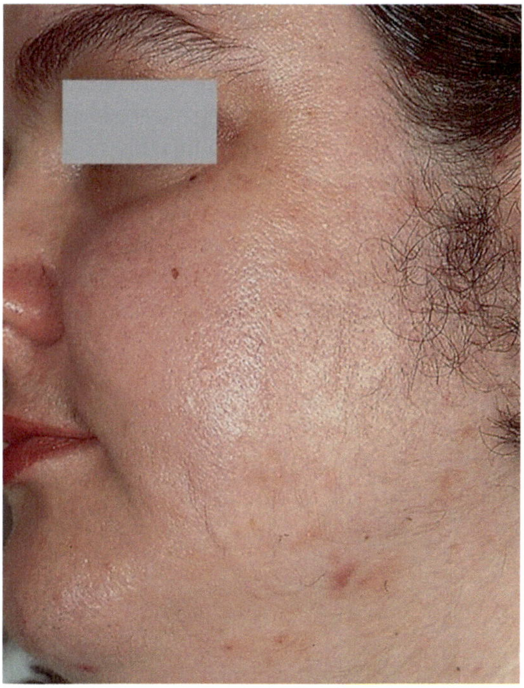

Fig. 10.15 Facial hirsutism in patient with PCOS

In a population of Iranian women aged 15–49 years diagnosed with PCOS, hirsutism was reported to have the strongest impact on the patients' health-related quality of life, followed in descending order by body mass index, irregular menses, and infertility. The relative level of hirsutism was directly proportional to decrease in health-related quality of life score [32].

Idiopathic hirsutism develops in the absence of detectable androgen excess and in conjunction with regular ovulation. It accounts for less than 20% of hirsute women [17]. The definition of idiopathic hirsutism has been an evolving concept, since normal androgen levels have been defined by conventional laboratory tests, while more sophisticated testing methods may uncover occult ovarian or adrenal functional hyperandrogenism in a large number of these patients [33].

Finally, an association of hirsutism with obesity has been reported early in as yet ill-defined, such as the Achard-Thiers syndrome and the Morgagni-Stewart-Morel syndrome, and is a frequent feature of the PCOS. Therefore, calculating the Body Mass Index (BMI = weight/height^2) should be part of the investigation.

Achard-Thiers syndrome [34, 35] is a rare disorder that occurs primarily in postmenopausal women and is characterized by type 2 diabetes mellitus, facial hirsutism, and a receding hair line, thus the synonymous term of the diabetic bearded woman syndrome (Fig. 10.16). The constellation of clinical androgen excess and hyperinsulinemia is now commonly identified earlier in a woman's life, typically during adolescence and young adulthood, as polycystic ovary syndrome (PCOS).

Morgagni-Stewart-Morel syndrome [36] is a disorder characterized by thickening of the frontal bone of the skull (internal frontal hyperostosis) causing headaches, in combination with obesity and excessive body hair growth. While individuals with Morgagni-Stewart-Morel syndrome nearly always have internal frontal hyperostosis, the finding may be incidental on X-ray films, computed tomography, or magnetic resonance imaging of the head in 12–37% of women, and by itself is not indicative of any specific disease. The cause of Morgagni-Stewart-Morel is unknown, although some have suggested that a hormonal imbalance due to genetic and environmental factors may be causative.

Testing of androgen levels is recommended in women with moderate to severe hirsutism (F-G score of 15 or more), and in women with any degree of hirsutism

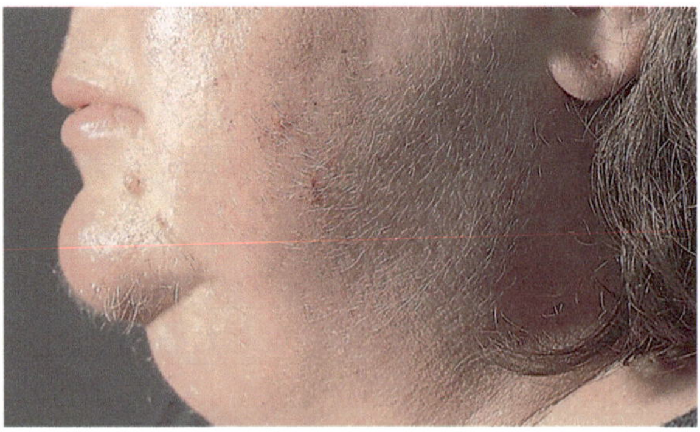

Fig. 10.16 Achard-Thiers syndrome

when it is sudden in onset, rapidly progressive, or when it is associated with any of the following: menstrual irregularity, central obesity, acanthosis nigricans, or clitoromegaly [37]. The initial laboratory investigations include free testosterone index (FAI) to assess biochemical hyperandrogenemia, thyroid function tests, prolactin, 17 hydroxyprogesterone, and a 24 h urine cortisol to rule out Cushing's syndrome, if there is a clinical suspicion.

Total testosterone measurements have a low sensitivity when used to diagnose PCOS. Sex hormone-binding globulin (SHBG) levels may influence total testosterone levels when increased, for instance, with the use of oral contraceptive pills, or decrease, for example, in obesity and insulin resistance. Measurement of SHBG level enables calculation of the FAI (FAI = total testosterone divided by SHBG × 100).

High testosterone levels more than 1.5–2 times the upper limit of normal are more likely to be associated with an androgen secreting tumor, and measurement of dehydroepiandrosterone sulfate (DHEAS) and androstenedione are warranted to identify an adrenal or ovarian source of hyperandrogenemia, respectively.

Ultimately, ultrasonographic examination of ovaries, the adrenal glands, or both represent a useful screening procedure if symptoms suggest presence of a neoplasm. Transvaginal ultrasound is the preferred mode if PCOS is suspected to fulfil the diagnostic criteria, but if the patient is a virgin or anatomically small, or slim, then transabdominal ultrasound may be sufficient.

Excessive hair often causes cosmetic embarrassment, resulting in significant emotional burden. The psychological burden of excessive hair should be addressed, since the condition is frequently associated with depression, social phobia, or body dysmorphic disorder.

The best way to relieve the patient from the psychological burden related to excessive hair is to effectively treat it. On the other hand, psychological symptoms should be investigated to evaluate if additional counseling or psychotherapy is necessary.

Therapeutic Strategies

From the Midrash Book of Proverbs (Hebrew: מִדְרָשׁ): The queen (of Sheba) was brought before him, and when she saw the king (Solomon) sitting in his glass house, she thought within herself that the king sat upon water, and so proceeded to draw up the hem of her dress so that she could pass over without getting wet. The king then saw her legs that they were full of hair, and when the queen had sat down beside him, he said unto her, *"Thy beauty is the beauty befitting women, but thy hairs are the hairs befitting men. Hair on a man's body is comely, but uncomely on a woman's."* Now the king greatly desired her beauty, but was taken aback by the hair upon her legs, and so it was that he devised a method by which unwanted hairs may be removed, that is, by taking an admixture of lime and water and orpiment (arsenic trisulfide), which the king himself discovered and made known its usage abroad, calling it neskasir. When the queen had bathed herself that night in its solution, the hair upon her legs fell off, and she found favor in the eyes of the king [38].

No single method of hair removal is appropriate for all body locations or patients; therefore, patients should be adequately advised of the available treatment modalities for temporary or permanent hair removal. The method adopted for removal of unwanted hair will depend on the cause, the character, area and amount of excessive hair growth, as well as on the age of the patient and personal preference.

The current available treatment methods for removal of unwanted hair include: cosmetic procedures, medical treatment, and hair removal using lasers and light sources. These may be combined [39].

Cosmetic Procedures for Removal of Excessive Hair

Unwanted hair may be masked by bleaching or removed by a variety of physical methods such as trimming of the hair, shaving, plucking or tweezing, and waxing, or chemical procedures (depilatories), and electrosurgical epilation [40].

Bleaching is a quick, easy, and painless process that can make unwanted hair less apparent through the partial or total removal of natural hair pigment, lightening the hair to a yellowish hue. A home bleach is made by mixing 40 mL hydrogen peroxide with 7 mL 20% ammonia. This is left in contact with the hair until the color is removed, usually 5–10 min. Bleaching can last up to 4 weeks. This method is best for treatment of localized excess pigmented hair on the face or arms of fair-skinned patients, because yellow bleached hair may emphasize the hair when viewed against the skin of more darkly pigmented patients. Occasionally, bleaching results in skin irritation. The addition of a persulfate to boost the peroxide bleach in commercial products may occasionally result in anaphylaxis in the sensitized individual [41]. ***Trimming*** of hair is a recommended option for young children with either localized or generalized hypertrichosis, making the hair of involved areas less noticeable, while not resulting in acceleration of hair regrowth.

Shaving. While unacceptable for removing facial hair to many women, the majority accepts to shave excess body hair. It is perceived as being fast, effective, easy, and cheap. Contrary to popular belief, shaving does not affect the width or rate of regrowth of individual hairs [42], though the perception of the stubble as it grows out without the finer tapered end of unshaven hair may give this impression. As a consequence, daily shaving must be undertaken or the cosmetic result is worsened. The disadvantages of shaving are the need to shave daily and skin irritation. Although dry or electrical shaves are not as close as wet shaves, a dry electric razor has been effectively used to treat generalized hypertrichosis during the neonatal period [43]. ***Plucking*** is an effective temporary hair removal method, but it is slow, tedious, and painful. It is only appropriate for individual, small groups, or scattered coarse hair and is performed with tweezers (tweezing). Adverse reactions of plucking include hyperpigmentation, folliculitis, scarring, ingrown hairs, and distorted follicles. A variation of plucking for treatment of more diffuse hypertrichosis acts as mechanized tweezers using a rotating, fine, coiled spring that grasps the hair shaft and pulls it out. The device is hand-held and moved over the skin like a shaver. A drawback of this method is that it is painful.

Waxing is performed with cold, warm, or hot wax. The wax is applied to hair-bearing areas, and stripped off, epilating the embedded hairs. Waxing methods are an efficient way of plucking vellus hairs in all areas of the body, and inexpensive when performed at home. The major disadvantages are discomfort, poor removal of short hair, and skin irritation or folliculitis. The method is too painful for use on children with hypertrichosis. As with hair plucking, the regrowth period is longer than that for shaving, and it requires to be repeated only every 2–6 weeks.

The Oriental techniques of *sugaring* (Halawa) [44] and *threading* [45] remove hair in much the same manner. Instead of using wax, the hairs are plucked out by a caramelized sugar and lemon mass or the scissoring action of a twisted thread, respectively.

Chemical depilatories function by damaging the hair to the point where it breaks at the skin surface. Substituted thiols form the basis of practically all contemporary preparations. Depilatories contain detergents to remove the protective sebum from the hair, adhesives that aid the depilatory in sticking to the hair shaft, swelling agents for better penetration of the bond breaking agent, pH adjusters, and disulfide bond-breaking agents (thioglycolic acid, calcium thioglycolate). Thioglycolates are used in a concentration of 2–4%, and act within 5–15 min. Since thioglycolates attack keratin, and the hair shaft and skin are similar in their keratin composition, most chemical depilatories hold a high irritancy potential and may have adverse effects on the skin if the manufacturers' recommendations are not carefully followed. Additional adverse effects from the use of thioglycolates include allergic contact dermatitis and, with inadvertent eye contact, corneal alkali burns [46, 47]. Their application is messy, they have an unpleasant odor, and are relatively expensive, especially if treating larger areas. Chemical depilatories are most appropriate for weekly hair removal from small areas. In children with extensive hypertrichosis, treatment with chemical depilatories should be limited to localized sites because of a theoretical risk of additional toxicity from systemic thioglycolate absorption [48].

Electrosurgical epilation. In contrast to the other cosmetic procedures for hair removal electrosurgical epilation represents a permanent mode of hair removal. Treatment involves the insertion of a disposable, fine wire needle into the hair follicle. Through this instrument a regulated and controlled electric current is transmitted from a highly sophisticated apparatus known as an epilator. The procedure is performed by a highly trained professional. Three techniques are available: galvanic electrolysis, thermolysis, and the blend method [49, 50]. Galvanic electrolysis uses galvanic current to destroy the hair growing cells of the hair follicle. This involves a direct current process that produces an electrochemical formation of sodium hydroxide, which congeals the hair follicle. Thermolysis uses high-frequency electrocoagulation that cauterizes the hair follicle. Galvanic electrolysis is slower, but destroys more follicles in one treatment, while thermolysis is quicker, but more regrowth is seen with this method. The blend method combines both galvanic and high-frequency current from a single machine, and is considered by most users to be the most effective method of electrosurgical epilation. Disadvantages of electrosurgical epilation are the length and the number of treatments required for permanent removal of hair in a particular body site, and discomfort during treatment, which is why the method is poorly tolerated in children. Generally, operators can only deal with 25–100 hairs per session, and individual treatments last from 15 min to 1 h. Problems that may occur are perifollicular inflammation, postinflammatory hyper- or hypopigmentation, and less frequently, punctate scarring. The method is most suitable for treatment of localized, coarse hair, for example, in nevoid hypertrichosis.

Medical Treatment

Since abnormal hair growth in hirsutism is either stimulated by excess androgens, or is related to hair follicle sensitivity to androgens, hormonal treatment of hirsutism is based upon suppressing androgen production or counteracting the biologic activity of androgens.

Today, for the majority of women with hirsutism, a monotherapy with oral contraceptive pills (OCPs) that have antiandrogenic activity is recommended as first-line treatment.

Antiandrogens may be the first-line therapy for postmenopausal women, or may be indicated in conjunction with OCPs in premenopausal women if clinical improvement is insufficient after 6 or more months of monotherapy. The choice between the different antiandrogens depends on patient preferences regarding efficacy, side effects, and costs [51]. Antiandrogens including spironolactone, cyproterone acetate, and flutamide, or the 5-alpha reductase inhibitors such as finasteride, should not be used in women of childbearing age unless they are strictly combined with a safe contraception method due to their potential feminizing effect on the male fetus.

In women with hirsutism, hyperandrogenism, and insulin resistance, insulin sensitizers such as metformin and rosiglitazone are effective for the hirsutism as well as the hyperinsulinemia, hyperandrogenism, and infertility, but there is no convincing evidence that they are effective for hirsutism alone [52].

Topical eflornithine *cream* is a medical treatment for slowing excessive hair growth and not removing excess hair [53]. The compound is a specific and irreversible inhibitor of the enzyme ornithine decarboxylase present in hair follicles that is important in hair growth. In clinical studies in women with facial hirsutism, twice daily application of eflornithine hydrochloride monohydrate 15% cream (Vaniqa®, Bristol-Myers Squibb) was superior to placebo in reducing hair growth, as demonstrated by objective and subjective methods, after 2–8 weeks treatment. After 24 weeks treatment, 58% of eflornithine and 34% of placebo recipients had at least some improvement, and 32 versus 8% of patients were judged to be successfully treated (at least marked improvement) [54]. Hair growth returned to pretreatment rates within 8 weeks of stopping treatment. Local irritation, characterized by burning, stinging, and/or tingling, occurred more frequently in eflornithine-treated patients. Use of eflornithine cream in combination with other therapies, including laser epilation, can be effective and results in a more rapid, visible hair reduction compared to laser monotherapy [55].

The safety and efficacy of topical eflornithine treatment for widespread hypertrichosis and children have not been established.

Hair Removal Using Lasers and Light Sources

The need for a rapid, noninvasive method for hair removal has led to the development of various laser and light sources for this purpose. An array of devices is now available. All are based on the principle of selective photothermolysis: Melanin pigment in the hair follicle provides the chromophore for selective targeting of hair follicles, while the surrounding dermis is spared. Therefore, at deeply penetrating wavelengths in the 600–1100 nm range, melanin absorption may be used for selective photothermolysis of hair follicles [56].

Several hair removal systems have been shown to be effective in this setting: long-pulsed ruby lasers (wavelength: 694 nm; pulse duration: 1–3 ms), long-pulsed alexandrite lasers (755 nm; 2–20 ms), diode lasers (800 nm; 5–400 ms), long-pulsed neodymium:yttrium-aluminum-garnet (Nd:YAG) lasers (1064 nm; 5–250 ms), and intense pulsed light (IPL) sources (590–1400 nm; 2.5–5 ms) [57–60]. The physical parameters (wavelength, pulse duration, fluence, spot size, repetition rate) and cooling systems used with each system vary considerably.

Regardless of the type of laser or light source used, all systems have been shown to temporarily reduce hair growth. Long-term, controlled hair counts have shown an

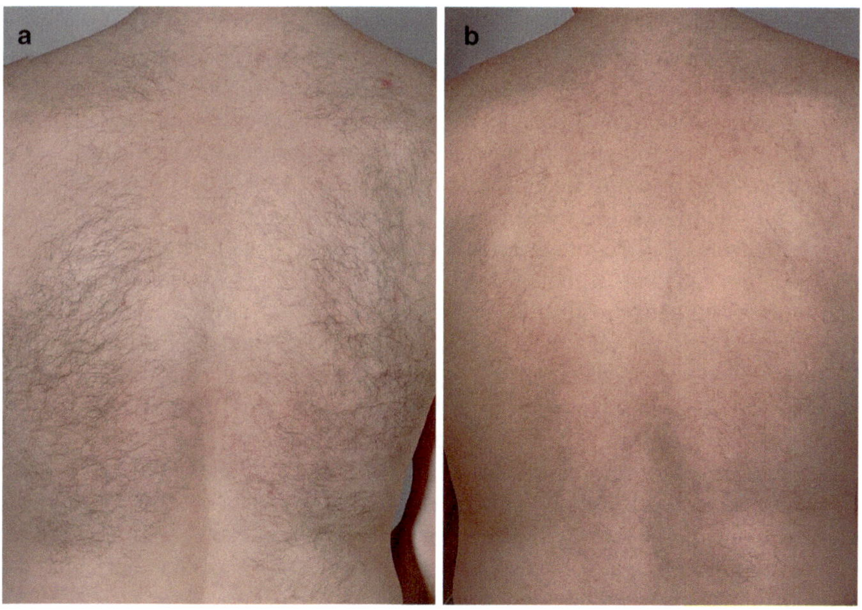

Fig. 10.17 Terminal hair growth of the back in a male patient before (**a**) and 6 months after fifth in-office IPL treatment (delivered at 2-month intervals) (**b**)

average of 20% hair loss with each treatment, indicating the need for multiple treatments to achieve satisfactory results. Research indicates that in 80% of patients, significant hair reduction can be achieved (Fig. 10.17), while 20% will fail [57]. Effectiveness for long-lasting hair reduction is strongly correlated with hair color. Blond, red, or white-haired patients are unlikely to experience a permanent reduction. In contrast, the patient with dark hair and fair skin may experience long-term hair removal after a single treatment [58]. Often, regrowing hairs are thinner and lighter in color, contributing to the improvement in the overall appearance. Although there is no obvious advantage of one laser system over another in terms of treatment outcome, laser parameters may be important for choosing the ideal laser for a patient [59]. A major drawback to using shorter wavelengths, for example, 694 nm ruby, is that a more deeply pigmented epidermis impedes laser radiation penetration of the dermis. The amount of light that reaches the hair bulb is therefore reduced with decreased efficacy. At the same time, unwanted epidermal injury may occur. Patients with darker skin tones should therefore receive laser treatment with either lower fluences of alexandrite and diode laser or with a long-pulsed Nd:YAG laser.

Adverse effects include commonly erythema and perifollicular edema, while crusting and vesiculation of treatment site, hypopigmentation and hyperpigmentation are less frequent, and depending on skin color and other factors. Most complications are usually temporary, and their incidence can be reduced by lightening of the skin and sun avoidance prior to laser treatment, effective cooling of the skin during treatment, and sun avoidance and protection following treatment [59]. Shaving the hair-bearing site is performed preoperatively in order to prevent conduction of thermal energy to the adjacent epidermis from overlying hairs.

One peculiar unwanted effect of laser-assisted hair removal is the stimulation of new hair growth within previously treated areas or in close proximity. This "paradoxical effect" has been seen following treatment with each of the laser and light hair removal systems, and its development has been attributed to activation of previously dormant hair follicles by either the application of subthreshold fluences or the conduction of heat to surrounding areas [61, 62].

As with traditional electrosurgical epilation, laser epilation is uncomfortable, which limits its usefulness in children with widespread hypertrichosis.

Since removing hair with in-office laser- or light-based treatments is expensive and requires multiple treatments sessions, recently, a novel, low-energy, pulsed-light device for home-use hair removal (Silk'nTM, Home Skinovations Ltd., Yokneam, Israel) has been developed to overcome these disadvantages. The device is composed of two flashlamps in a hand-held applicator (optical filter 475–1200 nm, fluences up to 5 J/cm^2). A study was performed with 20 women with Fitzpatrick skin phototypes I-IV and dark terminal hair in non-facial sites (axilla, forearms, inguinal region, legs) who self-administered three treatments at 2-week intervals using the device. Matched untreated skin sites were compared. Hair counts and clinical photographs were obtained pretreatment and at 1, 3, and 6 months after the third treatment, side effects and patient satisfaction scores were recorded. All patients showed a positive clinical response to treatment, with reduction of unwanted hair, while no hair reduction was noted in untreated matched areas. Hair counts were reduced 37.8–53.6% 6 months after the three treatments. Lower legs exhibited greater hair reduction than arms, inguinal, and axillary areas. Mild erythema was experienced in 25% of patients, but no other unwanted effects were encountered. Patient satisfaction scores were high, with all patients stating that they would purchase the device for future home use [63].

Quality-of-Life Benefits

Hirsutism has a negative impact on women's quality of life (QoL) due to cosmetic and psychosexual implications. Higher levels of hair growth are significantly correlated with a lower level of QoL and symptoms of both anxiety and depression [64, 65], as well as lower self-esteem in adolescent females [66]. Hair removal with laser therapy can improve the QoL in hirsute women [67]. Laser hair removal also supplies some functional QoL benefits up to 30 months post-treatment in facial hirsutism. Emotional benefits are less sustainable. Further laser hair removal treatment is required to maintain QoL benefits [68]. A modified Dermatology Life Quality Index (DLQI) provides a valid scoring system to assess the efficacy of laser epilation [69].

Summary

- Removal of unwanted hair is the most popular esthetic treatment worldwide. Excessive hair may cause cosmetic embarrassment, resulting in significant emotional burden.
- A number of dermatologic conditions cause stigmatization, which is why disrespectful terminology, specifically zoological epithet and sensationalism, should be banned for their derogative connotation.
- Sometimes the complaint of excess hair may pose a vexing problem for nonspecialized physicians. However, patient's individual perception of hair problems is the criteria for seeking medical assistance. Moreover, it must always be kept in mind that hair overgrowth, either hypertrichosis or hirsutism, may be a marker for a more general medical problem that may need serious investigation.
- The dermatologist seeing a patient with hypertrichosis or hirsutism must be prepared to look for the physical clues and perform the work-up that help both define the extent of excess hair and suggest the presence of associated physical and/or psychological disorders, specifically depression, social phobia, and body dysmorphic disorder.
- The best way to relieve the patient from the psychological burden related to excessive hair is to effectively treat it. No single method of hair removal is appropriate for all patients or body locations. The method adopted will depend on the cause, the character, area and amount of excessive hair growth, as well as on the age of the patient and personal preference.
- The best treatment of hirsutism is often a combination of medical therapy and the physical removal of unwanted hair.

- Over the recent past, hair removal using various efficacious lasers and light sources have been advocated for use in an office setting, although most people continue to remove unwanted hair with a variety of temporary physical methods in a home setting, presumably due to cost and convenience factors.
- Hair removal with laser therapy can improve the quality-of-life in hirsute women. A modified Dermatology Life Quality Index provides a valid scoring system to assess the efficacy of laser epilation.

References

1. Somani N, Harrison S, Bergfeld WF. The clinical evaluation of hirsutism. Dermatol Ther. 2008;21:376–91.
2. Baumeister FAM, Egger J, Schildhauer MT, et al. Ambras syndrome: delineation of a unique hypertrichosis universalis congenital and association with a balanced pericentric inversion (8) (p11.2;q22). Clin Genet. 1993;44:121–8.
3. Chen W, Ring J, Happle R. Congenital generalized hypertrichosis terminalis: a proposed classification and a plea to avoid the ambiguous term—Ambras syndrome. Eur J Dermatol. 2015;25:223–7.
4. Patel CB, Rashid RM. Averting the proliferation of acronymophilia in dermatology: effectively avoiding ADCOMSUBORDCOMPHIBSPAC. J Am Acad Dermatol. 2009;60:340–4.
5. Trüeb RM. Value of eponyms in dermato-trichological nomenclature. Skin Appendage Disord. 2018;4(2):71–7.
6. Molho-Pessach V, Agha Z, Aamar S, Glaser B, Doviner V, Hiller N, Zangen DH, Raas-Rothschild A, Ben-Neriah Z, Shweiki S, Elpeleg O, Zlotogorski A. The H syndrome: a genodermatosis characterized by indurated, hyperpigmented, and hypertrichotic skin with systemic manifestations. J Am Acad Dermatol. 2008;59:79–85.
7. Wren JD, Garner HR. Heuristics for identification of acronym-definition patterns within text: towards an automated construction of comprehensive acronym-definition dictionaries. Methods Inf Med. 2002;41:426–34.
8. Trüeb RM. Causes and management of hypertrichosis. Am J Clin Dermatol. 2002;3:617–27.
9. Bondeson J, Miles AE. Julia Pastrana, the nondescript: an example of congenital, generalized hypertrichosis. Am J Med Genet. 1993;47(2):198–212.
10. Bondeson J. The strange story of Julia Pastrana. A cabinet o medical curiosities. 1997; I. B. Tauris. p. 219. isbn:1860642284.
11. 11-year-old 'delighted' after being named world's hairiest girl. Fox News. 2011. Accessed 7 Mar 2011.
12. Cockayne E. Gargoylis (chondro-osteo-dystrophy, hepatosplenomegaly, deafness) in two brothers. Proc R Soc Med. 1936;30:104–7.
13. Clairevaux B St. Apologia ad Guillelmum abbatem. In: Leclercq J, Rochais HM, editors. Tractatus et Opuscula. S. Bernardi Opera. 3. Rome: Editiones cistercienses; 1963.
14. Dolphin D. Werewolves and vampires. Annual meeting of American Association for the Advancement of Science; 1985.
15. Cevil A. Did vampires suffer from the disease porphyria—or not?" The Straight Dope. Chicago Reader; 1999.
16. Ferriman D, Gallwey JD. Clinical assessment of body hair growth in women. J Clin Endocrinol Metab. 1961;21:1440–7.
17. Azziz R, Carmina E, Sawaya ME. Idiopathic hirsutism. Endocr Rev. 2000;21:347–62.
18. Trüeb RM. Hormone und Haarwachstum [Hormones and hair growth]. Hautarzt. 2010;61(6):487–95. German. https://doi.org/10.1007/s00105-009-1890-2. PMID: 20502852

19. Barth JH, Wilkinson JD, Dawber RPR. Prepubertal hypertrichosis: normal or abnormal? Arch Dis Child. 1988;63:666–8.
20. Prose NS, Abson KG, Scher RK. Disorders of the nails and hair associated with human immunodeficiency virus infection. Int J Dermatol. 1992;31:453–7.
21. Fretzin DF. Malignant down. Arch Dermatol. 1967;95:294–7.
22. Perniciario C. POEMS syndrome. Sem Dermatol. 1995;14:162–5.
23. Rosenfield RL. Hirsutism and the variable response of the pilosebaceous unit to androgen. J Investig Dermatol Symp Proc. 2005;10:205–8.
24. Azziz R. The evaluation and management of hirsutism. Obstet Gynecol. 2003;101:995–1007.
25. Azziz R, Adashi EY. Stein and Leventhal: 80 years on. Am J Obstet Gynecol. 2016;214:247.e1–e11.
26. Rotterdam ESHRE/ASRM-Sponsored PCOS Consensus Workshop Group. Revised 2003 consensus on diagnostic criteria and long-term health risks related to polycystic ovary syndrome (PCOS). Hum Reprod. 2004;19:41–7.
27. Ding T, Hardiman PJ, Petersen I, Wang FF, Qu F, Baio G. The prevalence of polycystic ovary syndrome in reproductive-aged women of different ethnicity: a systematic review and meta-analysis. Oncotarget. 2017;8:96351–8.
28. Spritzer PM, Barone CR, Oliveira FB. Hirsutism in polycystic ovary syndrome: pathophysiology and management. Curr Pharm Des. 2016;2016(22):5603–13.
29. Wong M, Zhao X, Hong Y, Yang D. Semiquantitative assessment of hirsutism in 850 PCOS patients and 2,988 controls in China. Endokrynol Pol. 2014;65(5):365–70.
30. Franik G, Bizoń A, Włoch S, Kowalczyk K, Biernacka-Bartnik A, Madej P. Hormonal and metabolic aspects of acne vulgaris in women with polycystic ovary syndrome. Eur Rev Med Pharmacol Sci. 2018;22:4411–8.
31. Gilbert EW, Tay CT, Hiam DS, Teede HJ, Moran LJ. Comorbidities and complications of polycystic ovary syndrome: an overview of systematic reviews. Clin Endocrinol (Oxf). 2018;89:683–99.
32. Bahri Khomami M, Tehrani FR, Hashemi S, Farahmand M, Azizi F. Of PCOS symptoms, hirsutism has the most significant impact on the quality of life of Iranian women. PLoS One. 2015;10(4):e0123608.
33. Rossi R, Tauchmanovà L, Luciano A, Valentino R, Savastano S, Battista C, Di Martino M, Lombardi G. Functional hyperandrogenism detected by corticotropin and GnRH-analogue stimulation tests in women affected by apparently idiopathic hirsutism. J Endocrinol Invest. 2001;24:491–8.
34. Malaisse W, Lauvaux JP, Franckson JR, Bastenie PA. Diabetes in bearded women (Achard-Thiers-Syndrome). A clinical and metabolic study of 20 cases. Diabetologia. 1966;1:155–61.
35. Lubowe I. Achard-Thiers syndrome. Arch Dermatol. 1971;103:544–5.
36. Gracia-Ramos AE. Morgagni-Stewart-Morel syndrome. Case report and review of the literature. Rev Med Inst Mex Seg Soc. 2016;54:664–9.
37. Martin KA, Chang RJ, Ehrmann DA, et al. Evaluation and treatment of hirsutism in premenopausal women: an endocrine society clinical practice guideline. J Clin Endocrinol Metab. 2008;93:1105–20.
38. Tobi Y. Queen of Sheba. Encyclopaedia Judaica, vol. 16. 2nd ed. Gale; 2007. p. 765.
39. Liew SH. Unwanted body hair and its removal: a review. Dermatol Surg. 1999;25:431–9.
40. Draelos ZK. Cosmetics in dermatology. New York: Churchill Livingstone; 1990. p. 99.
41. Wagner RF. Physical methods for the management of hirsutism. Cutis. 1990;45:19–26.
42. Lynfield YL, MacWilliams P. Shaving and hair growth. J Invest Dermatol. 1970;55:170–2.
43. Partridge JW. Congenital hypertrichosis lanuginosa: neonatal shaving. Arch Dis Child. 1987;62:623–5.
44. Lim V, Simmons BJ, Maranda EL, Afifi L, Kallis PJ, Jimenez J. Sugaring-modern revival of an ancient Egyptian technique for hair removal. JAMA Dermatol. 2016;152(6):660.
45. Scott MJ, Scott MJ III, Scott HM. Epilation. Cutis. 1990;46:216–7.
46. Yamasaki R, Dekio S, Jidio J. Allergic contact dermatitis to ammonium thioglycolate. Contact Dermatitis. 1984;11:255.

47. Smith RS, Shear G. Corneal alkali burns arising from accidental instillation of a hair straightener. Am J Ophthalmol. 1975;79:602–5.
48. Freeman MV, Draize JH, Smith PK. Some aspects of the absorption, distribution and excretion of sodium thioglycolate. J Pharm Exp Ther. 1956;118:296–303.
49. Hobbs ER, Ratz JL, James B. Electrosurgical epilation. Dermatol Clin. 1985;5:437–44.
50. Richards RN, Meharg GE. Electrolysis: observation from 13 years and 140000 hours of experience. J Am Acad Dermatol. 1995;33:662–6.
51. Swiglo BA, Cosma M, Flynn DN, et al. Antiandrogens for the treatment of hirsutism: a systematic review and metaanalyses of randomized controlled trials. J Clin Endocrinol Metab. 2008;93:1153–60.
52. Cosma M, Swiglo BA, Flynn DN, et al. Insulin sensitizers for the treatment of hirsutism: a systematic review and metaanalyses of randomized controlled trials. J Clin Endocrinol Metab. 2008;93:1135–42.
53. Barman Balfour JA, McCellan K. Topical eflornithine. Am J Clin Dermatol. 2001;2:197–201.
54. Wolf J Jr, Shander D, Huber F, et al. Randomized, double-blind clinical evaluation of the efficacy and safety of topical eflornithine HCl 13.9% cream in the treatment of women with facial hair. Int J Dermatol. 2007;46:94–8.
55. Smith SR, Piacquadio DJ, Beger B, Littler C. Eflornithine cream combined with laser therapy in the management of unwanted facial hair growth in women: a randomized trial. Dermatol Surg. 2006;32:1237–43.
56. Ross EV, Ladin Z, Kreindel M, et al. Theoretical considerations in laser hair removal. Dermatol Clin. 1999;17:333–55.
57. Dierickx C, Alora MB, Dover JS. A clinical overview of hair removal using lasers and light sources. Dermatol Clin. 1999;17:357–66.
58. Olsen EA. Methods of hair removal. J Am Acad Dermatol. 1999;40:143–55.
59. Liew SH. Laser hair removal. Guidelines for management. Am J Clin Dermatol. 2002;3:107–15.
60. Wanitphakdeedecha R, Alster TS. Physical means of treating unwanted hair. Dermatol Ther. 2008;21:392–401.
61. Alajlan A, Shapiro J, Rivers JK, et al. Paradoxical hypertrichosis after laser epilation. J Am Acad Dermatol. 2005;53:85–8.
62. Lolis MS, Marmur ES. Paradoxical effects of hair removal systems: a review. J Cosmet Dermatol. 2006;5:274–6.
63. Alster TS, Tanzi EL. Effect of a novel low-energy pulsed-light device for home-use hair removal. Dermatol Surg. 2009;35:483–9.
64. Sonino N, Fava GA, Mani E, Belluardo P, Boscaro M. Quality of life of hirsute women. Postgrad Med J. 1993;69(809):186–9.
65. Palmetun Ekbäck M, Lindberg M, Benzein E, Årestedt K. Health-related quality of life, depression and anxiety correlate with the degree of hirsutism. Dermatology. 2013;227(3):278–84.
66. Drosdzol A, Skrzypulec V, Plinta R. Quality of life, mental health and self-esteem in hirsute adolescent females. J Psychosom Obstet Gynaecol. 2010;31(3):168–75.
67. Alizadeh N, Ayyoubi S, Naghipour M, Hassanzadeh R, Mohtasham-Amiri Z, Zaresharifi S, Gharaei NK. Can laser treatment improve quality of life of hirsute women? Int J Womens Health. 2017;9:777–80.
68. Roche A, Sedgwick PM, Harland CC. Laser treatment for female facial hirsutism: are quality-of-life benefits sustainable? Clin Exp Dermatol. 2016;41(3):248–52.
69. Conroy FJ, Venus M, Monk B. A qualitative study to assess the effectiveness of laser epilation using a quality-of-life scoring system. Clin Exp Dermatol. 2006;31(6):753–6.

Scalp Pruritus

11

Maria Fernanda Reis Gavazzoni Dias, Yuliya Ovcharenko, and Antonella Tosti

Introduction

Scalp pruritus is a common complaint in dermatotrichological practice and has a significant impact on the patient's quality of life. Though the condition is associated with many underlying conditions, determining the proper cause of the symptom is sometimes a great challenge.

Pruritus is defined as an unpleasant tingling or sensation that causes a targeted scratch reflex. Unlike pain, which can be felt throughout the body, itching is only felt on the skin. The mechanism of pruritus is still unknown and has been a long-standing challenge in pathophysiology. The study of pruritus mechanisms can be divided into three directions: stimulus, receptor, and peripheral nerve.

The causes of scalp pruritus are unique and cover the widest range of disorders of dermatological and non-dermatological origin. The relationships between the psyche and pruritus in complexity and interaction have been extensively researched. The "itch—scratch" vicious cycle is often associated with psychiatric comorbidity, including depression and anxiety.

The augmentation of itching owing to the interplay of psychogenic and emotional factors has been well studied. The interdependence between pruritus and psyche can be divided into three groups: pruritic diseases with psychosocial sequelae, pruritic diseases aggravated by psychosocial factors, and psychiatric disorders causing pruritus.

M. F. R. Gavazzoni Dias (✉)
Department of Dermatology, Fluminense Federal University, Rio de Janeiro, Brazil

Y. Ovcharenko
V. N. Karazin Kharkiv National University, University Clinic "Trichology Institute", Kharkiv, Ukraine

A. Tosti
Dr. Phillip Frost Department of Dermatology and Cutaneous Surgery, University of Miami Miller School of Medicine, Miami, FL, USA

Y. Ovcharenko et al. (eds.), *Psychotrichology*,
https://doi.org/10.1007/978-3-031-64083-4_11

To consider all the multifaceted aspects of pruritus, the collective efforts and integration of the dermatotrichologist, the psychiatrist, and the psychologist are needed.

Epidemiology

The specific epidemiology of scalp pruritus is still controversial, given the paucity of data on its prevalence. The incidence ranges from 13 to 45% depending on the population studied [1–3]. Dermatological patients complain mainly of pruritus in psoriasis—80% of cases (moderate), atopic dermatitis—100% (painful, with excoriations) [4], and urticaria—100% [5].

Pruritus Pathophysiology

Although the symptom is frequent, pruritus pathophysiology remains debatable. It has been suggested that pruritus is "pain in miniature," but with a gradual decrease in pain stimulus, the sensation of pain weakens and then completely disappears, leaving no itching. Despite their antagonism under normal conditions, the peripheral and central mechanisms of pruritus and pain share some similarities. It is thought that, in some cases, the intensity of pruritus may exceed that of pain. Destructive itching may be a confirmation of this observation, when the pain from rough traumatization of the skin during scratching temporarily reduces the sensation of intolerable itching in patients.

Understanding the physiological processes of sensitivity is essential for understanding the development of skin sensory syndromes. Afferent nociceptors are classified into two types: A_{β}-fibers and C-fibers. A_{β}-fibers transmit signals of acute and well-localized severe pain or temperature exposure. C-fibers transmit signals implying slow, diffuse aching pain, temperature, pressure, and itching. These fibers stimulate nociceptors in the skin, which in turn stimulate transient receptor potential and purinergic receptors, which transport Na and Ca2 ions across free nerve ending membranes.

Substance P and calcitonin-gene-related peptide are released upon nociceptor activation in the peripheral nervous system, sending a signal from the primary afferent nerve fibers to the anterolateral system. Different stimuli stimulate various C-fibers differently. For example, the stimuli provoked by the administration or application of histamine and cowhage spicules differ.

The sensory innervation of the scalp skin is provided by branches of the trigeminal nerve. The itch receptors are located only in skin and mucous membranes, and C-fibers transmitting the itch signal extend to the dermo-epidermal junction. They account for only 10% of all nerve endings in the skin. Pruritus points are skin areas that have an increased number of thin free endings in the subepidermal layer and epidermis.

Histamine, serotonin, prostaglandin, acetylcholine, cytokines, opioids, bradykinin, and neuropeptides are among the endogenous mediators involved in the mechanism of pruritus. Free nerve endings in the skin release neuropeptides that serve as pruritus mediators in response to nonspecific trigger factors such as scratching, as well as histamine, proteases, cytokines, opioid peptides, eicosanoids, interferon-γ, and neurotropin. Both basophils and eosinophils participate in the histaminergic itch pathway.

Histamine's discovery suggested that its release is the primary cause of pruritus. However, a nonhistaminergic itch pathway exists, in which itch is elicited by nerves expressing a variety of receptors and are activated by pruritogens other than histamine. Proteinases released by bacterial and fungal flora were found to be more active and concentrated in pruritic skin.

In addition to direct itch stimulation by mediators such as histamine and proteinases, two main mechanisms of peripheral and central sensitization have been described that provoke pruritus in various pathophysiological conditions. Itch sensitizers include prostaglandins, interleukins, neurotrophins, and nerve growth factor. The following interleukins have a pruritogenic effect: IL-2, IL-4, IL-13, IL-31. It has been experimentally shown that IL-2 causes pruritus by activating histamine-, bradykinin-, and capsacin-sensitive skin C-fiber populations. Itch mediated by IL-2 does not respond to therapy with antihistamines and nonsteroidal anti-inflammatory drugs. It has been demonstrated that *Staphylococcus aureus*, a known trigger of atopic dermatitis, causes the release of the secretion of IL-31 from Th-2 cells and the microbial peptide cathelicidin-37 from mast cells. According to Gibbs, IL-31 promotes basophil IL-4 and IL-13 secretion and is involved in the differentiation and production of filaggrin. While IL-4 and IL-13 are the leading causes of chronic pruritus, IL-31 contributes to acute itch [6].

It should be noted that in addition to the pathogenic etiologies listed above, leading to scalp pruritus, this area of the body is characterized by the unique neuroanatomy and vasculature, presence of specific neurotransmitters and corresponding receptors, as well as sebum and microflora, which may explain the complaints of itch in patients.

The hair follicle is a recognized neuroendocrine organ. Its innervation is performed by many structures, such as the spear-shaped free nerve endings, Merkel nerve endings, and the pilo-Ruffini complex. Human hair follicle (HF) interacts with the hypothalamic-pituitary-adrenal (HPA) axis, the activation of which represents a systematic biological response to stress. In addition, studies have shown that HF also has a unique ability to synthesize its stress hormones through the equivalent of the HPA axis with established regulatory feedback loops. During periods of stress, systemic corticotropin-releasing hormone (CRH) binds to follicular receptors and stimulates the follicle's intrinsic hormonal axis to locally produce adrenocorticotropic hormone, cortisol, and CRH, leading to further degranulation of mast cells. The degree of hair fiber innervation, neuropeptide expression, and interaction with mast cells depend on the hair growth cycle (see Chap. 1).

In addition, the skin innervation is also affected by neuropeptides in inflammatory skin diseases. In many types of alopecia, scarring or non-scarring, mast cell activation represents one of the pathogenetic links. In alopecia areata (AA), there is an increased number of mast cells among the peribulbar lymphocytic infiltrate. Mast cells tryptase mediates some cellular effects by activating a proteinase-activated receptor-2 (PAR-2). Histopathological studies of atopic dermatitis (AD) also demonstrate an increased number of mast cells. PAR-2 may be a receptor on sensory nerve fibers involved in pruritus induction in both skin conditions.

The scalp is known to have the highest mitotic activity of epidermal cells, which, along with a high density of follicles and sebaceous glands, explains why itchy dermatoses like psoriasis and seborrheic dermatitis (SD) preferentially affect the scalp. Patients frequently refer to new inflamed, scaly lesions as "new pruritic areas," which could indicate disease activity.

Any disruption in the scalp barrier function and changes in the synthesis of epidermal lipids can lead to the development of pruritus. A defect in skin sebum's qualitative and quantitative composition characterizes conditions such as AD, psoriasis, and SD. A pruritic multidirectional communication between the nervous and immune systems within the skin emerges, which may be directed against microbiota components [6]. The presence of a high number of Malassezia species on the scalp skin has been shown to aggravate scalp itch in patients with SD and AD by increasing IL-8 levels. Lipase in these microorganisms hydrolyzes human sebum triglycerides into free fatty acids with irritant and pro-inflammatory properties.

This complex and diverse mechanism of itch development complicates the search for real symptom inhibitors. It has yet to be established whether pruritus is activated directly by receptors or is realized indirectly through mast and endothelial cells. It is believed that the biological purpose of pruritus is to eliminate the action of pruritogens by scratching. One of the scalp's cutaneous sensory abnormalities has been identified as a trichodynia.

Trichodynia

Trichodynia (scalp dysesthesia) is a painful sensation at the skin of the scalp in the absence of any underlying skin condition and abnormal laboratory results. Sultzberg et al. reported it in women with diffuse hair loss in 1960.

According to the literature, 34% of patients with hair loss, including those with chronic telogen effluvium (TE), androgenetic alopecia (AGA), and chemotherapy-induced anagen effluvium (AE), experience scalp pain without any visible pathological somatic manifestations. Symptoms may worsen when combing or brushing one's hair. Women are most frequently affected. The intensity varies from mild to severe.

The majority (76%) of patients with trichodynia suffer from mental disorders, primarily somatoform, obsessive-compulsive and anxiety disorders, and depression. A depressive episode can exacerbate painful dysesthesia. In most patients, the discrepancy between the degree of pain and the clinical picture confirms the existence of somatoform pain disorder.

Recent data demonstrating the localization of the neuropeptide substance P in a patient's scalp suggest a causal relationship with this neuropeptide, which is known to be involved in vascular tone, neurogenic inflammation, and nociception. The role of substance P and other neuropeptides in trichodynia's pathogenesis, especially its relation to the nervous system and emotional stress, needs further elucidation. It is critical to understand that the clinical diagnosis of trichodynia or scalp dysesthesia is not definitive but a starting point for a thorough evaluation and comprehensive symptom interpretation.

Ongoing research into chronic pain syndromes indicates that some may represent a neurological disorder, in some cases associated with a secondary psychiatric component. A physician consulting a patient with complaints of localized pain should consider the possible presence of any underlying psychiatric condition, systemic organ disease, or localized somatic disease. Temporal arteritis, tension headache, migraine, and other diseases are among those linked to symptoms of scalp pain.

Classification of Pruritus

As already noted, scalp pruritus can be caused by various disorders of various etiologies. It can be acute or chronic (over 6 months), localized or generalized.

There is currently no comprehensive classification of pruritus that would account for all clinical presentations and pathophysiology processes of the condition. In 2005, the International Forum for the Study of Itch was held; the same year, the first treatment guidelines were made, and in 2007, the first international classification of pruritus was approved. According to the expert consensus, etiological causes of pruritus, in addition to dermatological origin, can be systemic diseases, neurological disorders, psychogenic causes, mixed cases, and unspecified causes.

From a neuropathophysiology standpoint, a classification considering plausible mechanisms for pruritus development was proposed (Table 11.1).

Clinical classification is based on the disease's clinical picture, anamnesis, and the presence of other chronic conditions (Table 11.2).

Vazquez-Herrera et al. in [7] proposed to classify scalp pruritus into types: with and without dermatological lesions, and with or without hair loss.

Table 11.1 Mechanisms for pruritus

Pruritus	Pruritoceptive	Itch develops in the skin
	Neuropatic	Itch results from change in peripheral nerves
	Neurogenic	Mediators induce itch in the central nervous system without nerve damage
	Psychogenic	Itch caused by psychological factors

Table 11.2 Clinical classification of pruritus

Pruritus	Pruritus of primary inflamed skin
	Pruritus of primary non-inflamed skin
	Pruritus with chronic secondary excoriations

Table 11.3 Hair and scalp diseases associated with pruritus

Alopecia areata
Androgenetic alopecia
Telogen effluvium (including post-COVID)
Lichen planopilaris
Frontal fibrosing alopecia
Fibrosing alopecia in a pattern distribution
Central centrifugal cicatricial alopecia
Discoid lupus erythematosus
Folliculitis decalvans
Dermatomyositis
Cutaneous T-cell lymphoma
Lichen simplex chronicus
Pityriasis amiantacea
Psoriasis
Seborrheic dermatitis
Red scalp syndrome
Involutional xerosis
Atopic dermatitis
Urticaria
Allergic contact dermatitis
Bullous diseases
Infectious diseases (bacterial, viral, fungal, Covid-19)
Parasitic infestations (scabies, pediculosis)

Possible causes of scalp pruritus associated with interfollicular and perifollicular scaling and/or erythema include seborrheic dermatitis (SD), scalp psoriasis, contact dermatitis, early lichen planus follicularis and its related conditions, red scalp disease, tinea capitis, dermatomyositis, and xerosis associated with atopic dermatitis (AD) or skin aging; other less common causes of scalp conditions that can present as pruritus and hyperkeratosis are pityriasis amiantacea, discoid lupus erythematosus; in addition, non-scarring forms of hair loss such as AA, AGA, and TE are associated with pruritus. Pruritus usually accompanies bullous and infectious diseases [8, 9] (Table 11.3).

A thorough clinical examination, including trichoscopy and biopsy in unclear cases, is required for the evaluation of itching scalp. When an infectious agent is suspected, bacterial or fungal culture may be indicated based on clinical suspicion.

Vázquez-Herrera et al. [7] proposed the acronym SCALLP to easily remember some of the most seen causes of scalp itch: Seborrheic dermatitis, Contact dermatitis, Anxiety, Lichen planopilaris, Lice, Psoriasis.

Seborrheic keratosis, keloids, burns, eosinophilic polymorphic, and pruritic eruption associated with radiation (EPPER), and cutaneous cancers are only a few of the additional disorders that might be connected to scalp itch. About 86% of patients with keloids reported having itching, which typically develops at the edge of the scar. Seventy-six percent of burn patients report having pruritus, which is typically categorized as neuropathic pruritus in these cases.

Systemic Diseases Associated with Scalp Pruritus

Although systemic diseases are predominantly accompanied by generalized pruritus in patients without an obvious dermatological explanation, excluding systemic causes of isolated scalp pruritus is important. The systematic approach to chronic scalp pruritus includes various groups of pathologies (Table 11.4).

Some clinical and trichoscopic signs may indicate possible systemic pathology.

Autoimmune diseases associated with scalp pruritus include dermatomyositis, systemic lupus erythematosus (SLE), scleroderma, and Sjögren's syndrome. Pruritus may occur in isolation, or it may be associated with skin lesions. Enlarged interfollicular vessels and erythema are diagnostic trichoscopic signs.

Itching may be a symptom of scalp sarcoidosis. Sarcoidosis can present clinically with a range of symptoms, including diffuse erythema, follicular papules, and erythematous plaques, which are occasionally mistaken for SD. Depending on the clinical presentation, trichoscopy results can vary; however, the presence of yellow-orange patches aids in diagnosis [10, 11].

Table 11.4 Systemic diseases accompanied with pruritus, including on the scalp

Metabolic and endocrine disorders	Chronic renal failure Type 2 diabetes mellitus Hyper/hypothyroidism Carcinoid syndrome Parathyroid gland dysfunction
Hepatobiliary system disorders	Biliary cirrhosis Chronic pancreatitis Drug-induced cholestasis Hepatitis Sclerosing cholangitis Cholestasis of pregnancy Hepatic amyloidosis
Paraneoplastic	Hodgkin's lymphoma Mycosis fungoides Chronic leukemia, myelomatosis, lymphosarcoma Solid tumors of: lungs, colon, brain, breast, stomach, pancreas, prostate, or larynx
Hematological	Iron deficiency anemia Polycythemia vera Hemochromatosis Mastocytosis
Infections	HIV infection Hepatitis C Parasitic infestations
Pharmacological	Drug intoxication Side effects of medications Chemotherapy
Physiological	Pregnancy

Diffuse hair thinning and increased hair shedding are common in systemic connective tissue diseases such as SLE, dermatomyositis, and systemic sclerosis. DLE may cause localized alopecia in SLE.

Pruritus in various solid or hematological malignancies is of particular interest. Severe therapy-resistant itch is one of the first symptoms of Hodgkin's disease, cutaneous T-cell lymphoma, central nervous system (CNS) tumor, occult carcinomas, and other neoplasias. Trichoscopy may be a useful diagnostic tool. Rakowska et al. [12] published the results of diagnostic trichoscopy assessment in 76 patients with erythrodermic cutaneous T-cell lymphoma, which revealed characteristic trichoscopic findings: numerous pili torti, eight-shaped hairs, thick white interfollicular bands, color heterogeneity of the background, and perifollicular arrangement of vessels.

Follicular mucinosis and lymphoproliferative diseases may present with scalp pruritus and diffuse or localized hair loss. The initial sign of multiple myeloma and the disease's progression or relapse may be hyperkeratotic or filiform follicular spicules.

To rule out systemic diseases that cause pruritus, laboratory and instrumental studies and interdisciplinary consultations may be necessary.

Neuropathic Pruritus

If a patient has sensory symptoms like paresthesia, hypoesthesia, and hyperalgesia in the same area and there is no dermatological or systemic cause, neurological causes of pruritus should be suspected. Neuropathic itch is caused by an abnormality in the nervous system's afferent pathway, which can be central or peripheral. Postherpetic itch is an example of peripheral neuropathic pruritus. According to Oaklander et al. [13, 14], this type of itch, which affects at least one-third of herpes zoster patients, is frequently misdiagnosed as postherpetic neuralgia. The study also discovered a link between the severity of pruritus and the severity of neuralgia.

Diabetic patients frequently experience peripheral neuropathic itch, which can affect various body sites as well as the scalp. According to Scribner, controlling the glucose level alleviates scalp itch.

Keloids and burn scars are two more pathologies associated with peripheral neuropathy, both of which present with distinctive skin lesions.

Central causes of neuropathic itch are less frequent than peripheral ones. These include brain tumors, abscesses, strokes, and spinal cord tumors.

A complete neurological exam is required in patients with neuropathic pruritus to evaluate cranial nerve functions and temperature, touch, and pain sensations. A neurologist's consultation, EMG, and nerve conduction study may be required. If a brain tumor is suspected, an MRI may be required.

Psychogenic Pruritus

In the absence of a dermatological, systemic, or neurological cause of scalp pruritus, the symptom may have a psychogenic origin. Managing patients with such complaints is a challenge for a trichologist. A detailed history should be obtained, with questions about the patient's occupation, stressors, and significant life events.

Anamnesis should also include a personal or family history of psychiatric complaints or illnesses, sleep disorders, and drug use. The severity of the itch in these cases may be influenced by a variety of factors, including stress, compulsive behavior, or the use of psychotropic drugs.

According to observations by Yo et al. [15], psychogenic itch is more prevalent in women, particularly between the ages of 35 and 45. The patient with psychogenic pruritus typically presents with a healthy scalp or secondary lesions, such as scratch marks and excoriations, without a primary lesion.

It is important to note that psychogenic causes may exist alongside dermatological or systemic disorders that cause pruritus, which can aggravate the itch. Furthermore, chronic pruritus that does not respond to treatment can lead to depression and have a negative impact on the patient's quality of life. Thus, the interdependence of pruritus and psyche can be classified into three categories: pruritic diseases with psychosocial sequelae, pruritic diseases exacerbated by psychosocial factors, and psychiatric disorders causing pruritus.

Scalp itch can be caused by stress, and it is common to see people scratching their scalps when they are in a stressful situation. Examined the relationship between stressful life events and skin symptoms in 316 patients. Pruritus was discovered to be the most commonly reported symptom (69.3%), with the scalp being the most affected area (59.5%).

Scalp pruritus is frequently observed in patients with mental disorders such as anxiety, depression, obsessive-compulsive disorder, schizophrenia, delusion of parasitosis, tactile hallucinations, and somatoform disorders. Itch was found to affect 42% of psychiatric patients and was more common in those who had an anger trait and had difficulty managing their anger. According to a retrospective study of patients with chronic pruritus, itching of the patient's face and scalp occurs more frequently in psychiatric patients than non-psychiatric patients. The frequency of scalp and face itching was reported to be 16.7% and 10.1% in the first and second groups, respectively [16].

The relationships between the psyche and pruritus in complexity and interaction have been extensively researched. From a neurobiological standpoint, itch develops with the participation of many specific mediators, neural pathways, and signals with central itch processing.

The augmentation of itching owing to the interplay of psychogenic and emotional factors has been well studied. Various mediators involved in the onset and exacerbation of itch (e.g., prostaglandins, histamines, proteases, neuropeptides, cytokines, bile salts, etc.) have been identified. For example, endogenous opioids (e.g., endorphins) expressed throughout the peripheral and central nervous system increase itch. Prostaglandin E2 (PGE2) lowers itch threshold and enhances the subjective perception of itch with histamine provocation.

The psychological aspects of pruritus can be better understood by the famous itch-and-scratch cycle. Focusing on itch leads to an increased perception of itching and suffering. Scratching provides intermediate relief of discomfort and can reduce inner tension, and this negative reinforcement leads to conditioned scratching. A vicious cycle of itch-and-scratch eventually results, often accompanied by a sense of loss of control, despondency, and guilt.

Subjective perception of pruritus is also associated with psychological conditions such as stress and depression. These altered mental states can lower the pruritus threshold through hemodynamic changes, such as blood flow and body temperature disturbances, which increase the peripheral release of histamine, neuropeptides, and inflammatory mediators. In particular, studies have found the effect of depression on the central pathways of increasing opiate activity levels, which enhances the subjective perception of itch.

The French Psychodermatology Group (FPDG) invented the term "functional itch disorder" to describe psychogenic pruritus, defining it as "an itch disorder where itch is at the center of the symptomatology and where psychological factors play an evident role in the triggering, intensity, aggravation, or persistence of the pruritus." Table 11.5 shows the diagnostic criteria proposed by the FPDG.

Neurological causes not accompanied by skin lesions should be ruled out when evaluating psychogenic pruritus. However, in some cases, psychogenic and neurogenic pruritus may coexist. Neurogenic pruritus is usually chronic, more severe, and intense, may manifest unilaterally, and may be associated with sensory changes such as allodynia, dysesthesia, and hyperpathy. It may also be accompanied by persistent paroxysmal pain in specific areas and sleep disturbance.

Unlike neurogenic, psychogenic pruritus is characterized by a chronological relationship with psychiatric symptoms and exhibits a paroxysmal nature with increasing severity, sudden onset/resolution, or intervening asymptomatic periods. A psychiatric consultation is recommended to confirm the diagnosis of psychogenic pruritus.

Treatment for pruritus with concomitant psychosomatic symptoms should target the underlying cause and involve a comprehensive approach that addresses not only the dermatological and somatosensory aspects of the condition but also the cognitive, emotional, and psychosocial aspects. The combined efforts and collaboration of the dermatotrichologist, the psychiatrist, and the psychologist must account for all the complex facets of pruritus.

Table 11.5 Diagnostic criteria for psychogenic pruritus (French Psychodermatology Group 2007)

Diagnostic criteria for psychogenic pruritus		
3 Compulsory criteria	3 out of 7 optional criteria	
1. Pruritus (without primary skin lesion)	1. A chronological relationship of pruritus with one or several life events	5. Predominance during rest or inaction
2. Chronic pruritus (>6 weeks)	2. Psychological repercussions	6. Associated psychological disorder
3. No somatic cause	3. Variations in intensity associated with stress	7. Pruritus that could be improved by psychotropic drugs
	4. Nocturnal variation	8. Pruritus that could be improved by psychotherapies

Diagnostic Algorithm for Scalp Pruritus

The trichologist should use an algorithmic approach to investigate scalp pruritus. It is critical to first investigate the most common causes before ruling out less common etiologies.

Shapiro and Otberg [17] recommended five steps to assess scalp pruritus: history, physical examination, palpation, magnification (trichoscopy), and direct sampling.

The initial task is to establish the cause of the symptom. A physician obtaining history should take into account suspected aggravating factors (shampoos used, exposure to heat) and comorbidities (malignant neoplasms, thyroiditis).

A practical approach to classifying scalp pruritus is based on two conditions: whether or not the symptom of pruritus is accompanied by dermatological lesions, either primary or secondary. Differential diagnosis in patients with dermatological lesions is carried out depending on their type, using a clinical approach and trichoscopy results. It is important to remember that secondary lesions caused by scratching, such as scales and lichen simplex chronicus, can occur even in non-dermatological cases. When making the diagnosis, it is also recommended to consider the presence or absence of hair loss. In some dermatological cases, scalp biopsies may be required. The presence of multiple concurrent causes of scalp itch should also be considered. If a systemic, neurological, or psychogenic cause of pruritus is suspected, a multidisciplinary approach may be necessary, including evaluation by a dermatologist, physician, psychiatrist, and psychologist. Table 11.6 outlines a methodical approach to investigating the most common causes of scalp dysesthesia.

Hair and Scalp Pathologies Associated with Scalp Pruritus

Seborrheic Dermatitis

One of the most common causes of scalp itch is seborrheic dermatitis, which has a prevalence of 16–50% in the adult population. Patients frequently reported sensations of prickling, tightness, pain, and burning. Skin lesions in SD can be so visible that they cause self-esteem loss and have a negative social impact. Pruritus in seborrheic dermatitis typically disappears or decreases in severity after shampooing containing antimycotic agents.

Insights into the etiopathogenesis of SD include the possible role of triggers, among which of great importance is the complex of hormonal, neurogenic, immune, genetic, and metabolic pathomechanisms. Abnormal function of sebaceous glands (change in quantitative and/or qualitative composition of skin sebum) is considered to play a pathogenetic role in the development of SD. This provokes changes in the skin microbiome, which in turn causes a reaction of the macroorganism immune system directed to restoring the balance of microflora.

An increase in lipids on the skin's surface, as well as a change in acidity with a shift to alkalosis, causes desquamation to be disrupted, as well as the displacement

Table 11.6 Clinical and diagnostic algorithm of the most common causes of scalp dysesthesia

Pruritus in primary hair and scalp diseases
Erythema and scaling
Seborrheic dermatitis: trichoscopy
Psoriasis: trichoscopy
Atopic dermatitis: look for other dermatologic signs
Contact dermatitis: patch test required
Primary cicatricial alopecia: trichoscopy/biopsy
Dermatomyositis: trichoscopy/biopsy
Brazilian keratin treatment: clinical history /trichoscopy
Infections and infestations
Tinea capitis: trichoscopy /microscopy /mycological examination
Pediculosis: clinical examination /trichoscopy
No erythema and scaling
Telogen effluvium: clinical history /trichoscopy /phototrichogram
Androgenetic alopecia: trichoscopy /phototrichogram
Alopecia areata: trichoscopy
Involutional alopecia: trichoscopy
Trichodynia
• **Androgenetic alopecia:** trichoscopy
• **Telogen effluvium:** clinical history/trichoscopy/phototrichogram
• **Alopecia areata:** trichoscopy
• **Chemotherapy:** clinical history
• **Involutional alopecia:** trichoscopy
• **Red scalp syndrome**: trichoscopy
• **Coronavirus infection:** clinical history/COVID-19 PCR/COVID-19 antibodies test
Pruritus without hair and scalp diseases
Systemic disease: itch is more often generalized—laboratory tests/consultation
Neurologic disease: peripheral neuropathy or central neuropathy—laboratory tests/consultation
Psychiatric disease: scratching-induced secondary skin lesions
• Psychogenic pruritus: history/trichoscopy/consultation
• Trichoteiromania: history/trichoscopy/consultation
• Neurotic excoriations: history/trichoscopy/consultation
• Delusions of parasitosis: history/trichoscopy/consultation

of acid-resistant flora, which contributes to the reproduction of opportunistic microflora, particularly colonization by Malassezia species. Scalp histamine levels in people with SD are twice as high as those in healthy people.

SD is typically diagnosed based on clinical findings of scaling on seborrhea-affected areas such as the mid-face, upper chest, and back, as well as itch. Adults with SD have classic reddish plaques covered by waxy or moist yellowish scales that easily flake off. The most problematic cases in differential diagnosis of SD and psoriasis are patients with psoriasis onset at puberty and localization exclusively on the scalp. Psoriasis is characterized by more elevated plaques with more significant erythema, more defined borders, white-silver colored scale, and tighter adhesion of scales to the skin.

SD trichoscopic features are interfollicular yellowish scales (Fig. 11.1), and branching vessels, which differ from the typical picture of psoriasis: red dots at low magnification and twisted capillary loops at high magnification.

Treatment. Adults with SD have a chronic course, and spontaneous remissions are uncommon; therefore, ongoing treatment is justified. Identification of

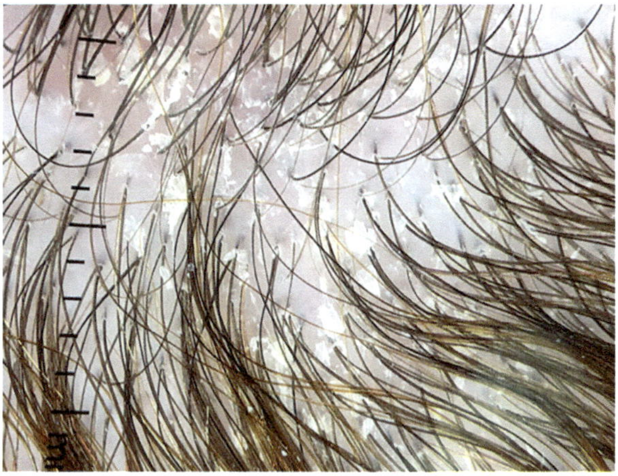

Fig. 11.1 The trichoscopic picture of seborrheic dermatitis shows interfollicular yellowish scales (×20)

contributing factors, such as hyperandrogenism, metabolic disorders, drug exposure, and so on, and, if possible, correction, are critical. The goal of SD therapy should be to normalize the skin microbiome and eliminate scaling and inflammation.

In SD, the first-line treatment option is a combination of antifungal shampoos and topical corticosteroids with low-mild potencies, particularly when pruritus is present. Among commonly used antifungi ingredients such as zinc pyrithione, ketoconazole, miconazole, and ciclopirox, selenium disulfide is recognized as the reference dermatological ingredient with antifungal activity. Due to its potential to cause pruritus, coal tar is not the first treatment option when itching is present, even though it may be effective for SD lesions due to its keratoplastic effect.

Among highly effective dermatocosmetic products for patients with SD are shampoos that combine ingredients of desquamative, anti-inflammatory, antifungal, and conditioning action (sach as VICHY DERCOS DS). The shampoos can be recommended for a long-term use as monotherapy 2–3 times a week, after clearing the signs and symptoms to avoid the excess of corticosteroids use. Shampoos without conditioning additives are poorly accepted by patients, and switching to non-medicated shampoos usually leads to a disease relapse.

Psoriasis of the Scalp

Psoriasis is a recurrent disease of a multifactorial nature with a dominant role in the etiology of genetic factors, characterized by the development of comorbid conditions and a significant negative impact on the quality of life.

The scalp is one of the most common sites of psoriasis, seen in 80% of cases. Clinically, the condition is characterized by well-defined erythematous plaques covered by abundant white-silver lamellar scales.

Psoriatic plaques are characterized by pronounced dryness due to increased transdermal water loss, as well as a deficit in the natural moisturizing factor of the skin. In addition to whitish scales, trichoscopy of psoriatic lesions at low magnification reveals red dots (Fig. 11.2), which are loops of vessels of the papillary dermis,

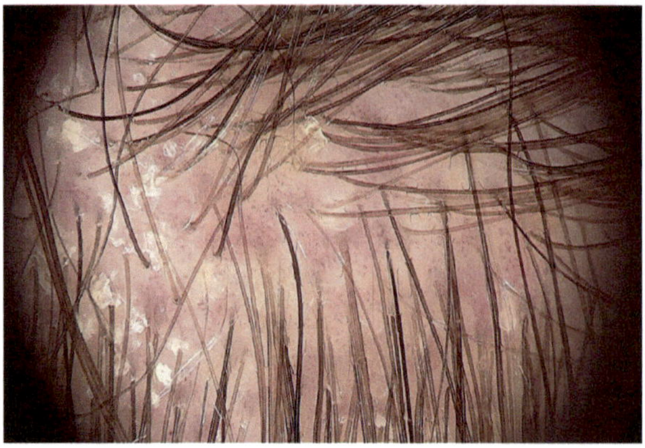

Fig. 11.2 Trichoscopic features of scalp psoriasis: thick lamellar scaling and pinpoint vessels are seen (×20)

elongated and expanded against the background of acanthosis and chronic inflammation. At higher magnification, twisted red loops are often seen; globules and glomerular vessels may be present.

Psoriasis is classified as a dermatological itch with primary skin lesions by the International Forum for the Study of Itch.

According to the literature, pruritus is reported by 67–97% of psoriasis patients, and there is a correlation between the severity of lesions in scalp psoriasis and the severity of itch.

The precise pathogenesis of itch in scalp psoriasis is unknown. Hyperinnervation, neurogenic inflammation, neuropeptide misbalance, abnormal peripheral opioid system function, cytokine release, and vascular abnormalities are all possible mechanisms. It was proposed that retrograde sensory nerve activation and the release of pro-inflammatory and pruritogenic mediators are capable of stimulating angiogenesis and keratinocyte hyperproliferation, chemotaxis, and mast cell degradation. Histamine is not involved in psoriasis-related pruritus, and the role of mast cells in the genesis of pruritus is debatable. In conclusion, the pathogenesis of itch in psoriasis is likely to involve a complex interaction between the nervous, neuroendocrine, immune, and vascular systems, and much remains to be discovered.

Psoriatic pruritus on the scalp can be exacerbated by subsequent Koebnerization with the formation of a vicious cycle leading to the development of new pruritic plaques.

In terms of quality of life, patients recognize pruritus as the most significant factor that hinders productivity, with a negative impact on concentration in 52.5% of cases, according to. The characteristics of pruritus in scalp psoriasis vary; the majority of patients refer to intermittent pruritus, and stress and temperature are the main aggravating factors. According to Ograczyk, psoriatic patients with itch showed worse physical functioning, more stigmatization, depressive symptoms, and sleeping issues.

Treatment of psoriasis should include both inflammation management and lifestyle modification to avoid exposure to trigger factors and prevent possible exacerbations in the future. All therapeutic measures can be divided into the following groups: specialized skin care, topical therapy (topical corticosteroids, topical vitamin D3 analogs), phototherapy, and systemic therapy.

Ineffectiveness of local treatment and phototherapy, as well as psoriasis with damage to the nails or joints, are indications for systemic therapy. Nevertheless, given the special "social significance" of the scalp and the substantial impact of lesions in this area on the quality of life, scalp psoriasis is regarded as a "difficult site" that may necessitate a more aggressive treatment approach. Additional factors to consider systemic treatment for scalp psoriasis are the presence of hair, which complicates topical therapy and limits the effectiveness of phototherapy. In cases of torpid psoriasis, it is advisable to consider systemic therapy and discuss the expected effects and possible risks with the patient.

The most common systemic medications used to treat moderate-to-severe psoriasis are retinoids (acitretin), methotrexate, cyclosporine, apremilast, and biologics (TNF alpha inhibitors, IL 12/23p40 inhibitors, IL17 inhibitors, IL23p19 inhibitors).

In psoriasis treatment, skin care remains the basic therapy and is aimed at normalizing the epidermis condition, moisturizing and softening the skin, as well as eliminating hyperkeratosis and excessive flaking. The antipruritic effect is one of the main targets of such strategies. There are a large number of moisturizers that can also be used on the scalp; however, the use of oily creams is not always convenient for this localization. Therefore, it is preferable to use shampoos with moisturizing components in combination with keratolytics (VICHY DERCOS PSOlution).

Urea (10–30%), salicylic acid (2–5%), lactic, glycolic, and other organic acids are the main agents used for scalp care in psoriasis and SD. The approach of using moisturizing masks after shampooing justifies itself.

Atopic Dermatitis

The scalp is affected in 50% of the patients with atopic dermatitis [18]. Atopic dermatitis may present clinically with erythema and xerosis complicated by lichenification (Fig. 11.3), and scalp itching is one of the secondary diagnostic criteria

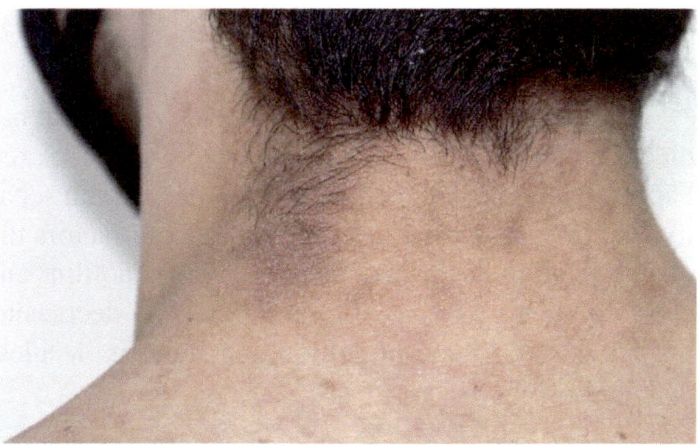

Fig. 11.3 Atopic dermatitis with xerosis, erythema, scaling, and lichenified plaques due to chronic pruritus

according to Hanifin and Rajka. In some cases, histopathology may be required to confirm the diagnosis.

Itch is present in 67% of patients with scalp sensitivity. According to hair loss is also associated with this sensitivity. Genetically determined dry skin plays a significant role in the development of persistent or paroxysmal itch in AD. Recent studies have revealed that dry skin in AD is associated with mutation of filaggrin playing a significant role in the formation of protein-lipid structure of the stratum corneum.

This layer replaces the differentiated keratinocyte plasma membrane, forming a barrier that retains water and can minimize allergen and microorganism exposure. Filaggrin degrades on the skin surface, releasing its components—amino acids. A mixture of hygroscopic amino acids forms the so-called natural moisturizing factor contributing to epidermis hydration and its barrier function. The stratum corneum acids have a pronounced antimicrobial effect. Filaggrin degradation products at its physiological concentration have an inhibitory effect on *Staphylococcus aureus* growth. *S. aureus* induces the secretion of IL-31 from Th-2 cells, and microbial peptide cathelicidin-37 induces its release from mast cells. IL-31 on basophils provokes the release of IL-4 and IL-13. IL-31 plays a role in differentiation and expression of filaggrin. It is reported that the levels of *Malassezia*-specific IgE are elevated in patients with AD.

Treatment. Understanding the mechanism of itch in AD defined the treatment strategy, with external softening and moisturizing of skin playing a leading role. Initial therapeutic recommendations in modern protocols for the prevention and treatment of AD include the use of emollients. Finally, the elimination of skin inflammation caused by histamine release is critical and requires the use of modern antihistamines and anti-inflammatory agents. Systemic immunomodulatory agents used to treat atopic dermatitis include cyclosporine, methotrexate, azathioprine, mycophenolate, and dupilumab, with abrocitinib, baricitinib, tralokinumab, and upadacitinib recently approved in various jurisdictions [19].

Involutional Xerosis

The effects of aging on hair-bearing skin are relatively unnoticeable. The skin covered by hair appears pale and dry. In balding areas of the scalp, photoaging, uneven pigmentation, telangiectasias, and precancerous/cancerous neoplasms are more common.

The main explanation for the pathophysiological mechanism of scalp pruritus in older people has been associated with involutional xerosis. The disruption of skin barrier functions, fluctuations in pH, a decrease in sebaceous and sweat gland activity, and transepidermal moisture loss are all factors that contribute to the development of xerosis. With age, the water-lipid nanofilms and germ layer thin, increasing evaporation from the interstitial dermis and decreasing the amount of acid mucopolysaccharides that normally retain water molecules, leading to process of skin dehydration.

Another cause of itch is photoaging, which is more common in hairless scalps. Dermal elastosis and the deposition of abnormal collagen and elastin fibers are classic histological features of sun-exposed skin. UV-exposed scalp also exhibits a significant change in epidermal thickness and density, uneven melanocyte distribution, and an increase in the number of inflammatory cells. The inflammatory response appears to play a role in photoaging. UV light activates the nuclear transcription factor NF-B, which produces pro-inflammatory cytokines such as interleukin-1 and 6, vascular endothelial growth factor, tumor necrosis factor-alpha (TNF-α), and adhesion molecules. These cytokines provide positive feedback, creating a vicious cycle that amplifies the effects of UV radiation.

Furthermore, impaired skin barrier function may increase susceptibility to irritation caused by external allergens and environmental factors. Fragrances and preservatives in moisturizers and shampoos have been linked to allergic contact dermatitis. Although mild surfactants are thought to cause less irritation, sulfate-free shampoos containing cocamidopropyl betaine (CAPB) may also irritate the scalp. It is recommended that older adults develop a habit of using emollients on a regular basis. Topical steroids can be used for a short period.

Red Scalp Syndrome

The condition is characterized by scalp erythema associated with papules, pustules, and telangiectasias (Fig. 11.4). Patients complain of itching, stinging, burning, and diffuse hair loss. The disorder is considered a variant of rosacea localized to the scalp and may be associated with AGA [20].

Patients frequently express that their symptoms worsen after exposure to the sun, particularly when they experience repeated episodes of scalp sunburn. This suggests chronic UV exposure may be pathogenetic in red scalp syndrome. Trichoscopy in patients with red scalp syndrome reveals dilated and arborizing vessels, which are indicators of photodamaged skin.

The most frequently suggested pathogenesis mechanism in the absence of any dermatological disease is the perifollicular inflammation and increased expression of substance P in the immediate vicinity of the affected HF. In a case series study published by [21] in patients with trichodynia complaining of hair loss, the

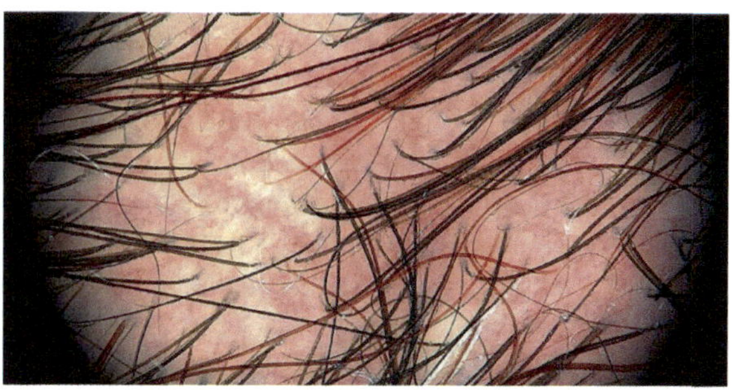

Fig. 11.4 Trichoscopic picture of a red scalp syndrome. Pronounced telangiectasias associated with the symptom of trichodynia are evident

dermatoscopic finding of scalp telangiectasia was found to strongly correlate with the presence of trichodynia.

These findings imply a link between sensory irritation and cutaneous vascular reactivity. The role of perifollicular infiltrate and neuroendocrine factors in the development of somatoform pain and trichodynia has been discussed. Furthermore, it was stated that depressive episodes can exacerbate dysesthesia.

Management of red scalp syndrome is often frustrating for both patients and clinicians. Clinical observations show that the condition is characteristically resistant to treatment with topical steroids and responds to oral tetracyclines. A limited number of publications report varying efficacy in the symptomatic treatment of trichodynia. Among the therapeutic options, of topical treatments have been used with satisfactory results: capsaicin in concentrations 0.075%, tacrolimus 0.1%, lidocaine and compounds including lidocaine, such as TALK (topical amitriptyline 5%, lidocaine 5%, and ketamine 10%), topical gabapentin 10% three times daily [22–24]. In addition, injections of botulinum toxin have been reported to effectively reduce itch [25]. Systemic symptomatic treatments of trichodynia include sedative antihistamines (hydroxyzine hydrochloride 25–50 mg daily) as supportive treatment; anticonvulsants and antidepressants—low doses of oral pregabalin (up to 300 mg/day), gabapentin (up to 3000 mg/day), doxepin (up to 280 mg/day) and naltrexone (3–5 mg/day) are all possible options, but adverse effects may limit their use [26, 27].

Contact Dermatitis of the Scalp

Hair cosmetics such as shampoos, hair dyes, and hair straightening products may lead to contact dermatitis of the scalp (CDS). Pruritus and hair loss are the most commonly reported signs and symptoms of CDS. A late diagnosis may result in chronic scalp eczema with intense lichenification due to long-standing pruritus.

Methyl isothiazolinone and cocamidopropyl betaine are two of the most common ingredients in shampoos that cause allergic contact dermatitis. Rinse substances have brief contact with the skin and have a low sensitizing ability. Sensitization may occur earlier with other products containing the same allergens. Contact dermatitis from rinse hair products can affect the scalp, face, neck, and ears. Lazzarini et al. [28] reported patch test results in 20 CDS patients, and the most common positive allergens were kathon CG, formaldehyde, cocamidopropyl betaine, captan, lauryl polyglucoside, decyl glucoside, methyldibromo glutaronitrile, diazolinidyl urea, balsam of Peru, FM1 (geraniol, cinnamaldehyde, hydroxycitronellal, cinnamyl alcohol, amylcinnamaldehyde, isoeugenol, eugenolo, oak moss), and FM2 (coumarin, lyral, citronellol, farnesol, citralhexyl cinnamic aldehyde).

Hair dyes are another common source of allergen exposure. PPD, or p-phenylenediamine, is regarded as a strong sensitizer capable of causing immediate hypersensitivity reactions and hair loss. PPD toxicity was reported, as well as links to cancer and mutagenicity.

Other potent hair dye contact allergens are resorcinol, m-aminophenol, p-aminophenol, phenylenediamine, amino hydroxytoluene, methylresorcinol, and toluene-2,5-diamine. The branding of the hair dyes products are often marketed to consumers as "natural," "herbal," "antioxidant," which give them the impression of safety.

In addition, hair dye products known as "PPD-free" are available to persons allergic to PPD. They contain PPD substitutes like hydroxyethyl-p-phenylenediamine sulfate (HPPS) or 2-methoxymethyl-p-phenylenediamine. However, allergic contact dermatitis to these substances has also been reported. Herbal hair dye derivates, such as henna, have a low allergy potential and may be an option for those more sensitive. Even so, allergic dermatitis to henna is well described.

The majority of shampoos contain Cocamidopropyl Betaine (CABP), a "sulfate-free" amphoteric surfactant. CAPB is regarded as a sensitizer despite being milder than the traditional anionic sulfate surfactant, lauryl sulfate. Numerous contact allergies in children with atopic dermatitis, including CAPB allergy, are common. It is disputed whether these substances are irritants or allergens in these cases.

The use of formaldehyde and formaldehyde releasers (methylene glycol and glyoxylic acid) in hair-straightening formulations may be a cause of erythema, scaling, and scalp itching. The procedure is called BKT or Brazilian Keratin Treatment. The work of Gavazzoni Dias et al. [29–33] analyzed scalp biopsies of seven patients who developed scalp scurf and erythema shortly after BKT. Only one patient reported pruritus. Clinical lesions were psoriasiform scalp scaling, erythema, lamellar scurf, and skin lesions with erythema, mild desquamation, and sterile pustules.

Erythema, perifollicular, and interfollicular scaling were among the dermoscopic findings. The peripillar desquamation looked like the outer skin layer of the onion bulb (Fig. 11.5).

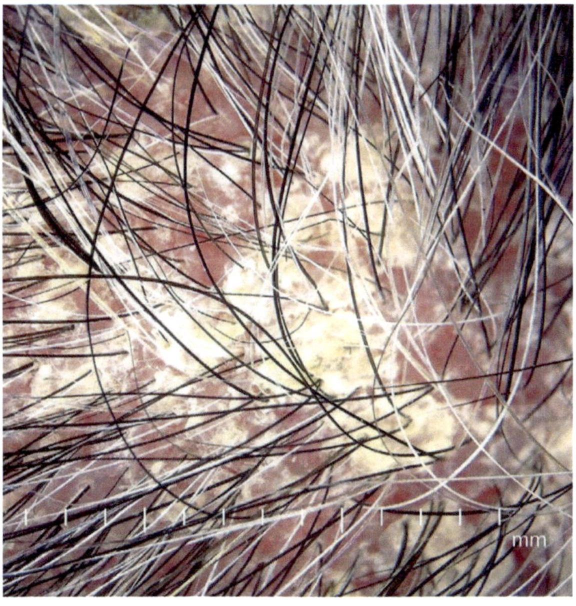

Fig. 11.5 Psoriasiform skin reaction following "Brazilian Keratin Treatment" hair straightening procedure

Psoriasiform and spongiotic psoriasiform patterns were found on histopathology. The features of the first pattern were similar to those described in anti-TNF-psoriasiform reactions. The authors proposed that formaldehyde can cause drug reactions as well as irritant or allergic dermatitis.

It is critical to collect information about the type of hair brush used by patients with suspected contact dermatitis, because contact dermatitis can be caused by nickel, rubber, or plastic.

The most common side effect of topical minoxidil is itchiness. This extremely distressing symptom may be accompanied by scaling (Fig. 11.6). Mild itch may be caused by minoxidil's vasodilator effect. However, irritant or allergic contact dermatitis is more likely to develop as a result of the enhancer, propylene glycol, or, less frequently, as a result of allergy to the minoxidil molecule itself. However, even infrequent, allergic reactions to topical minoxidil were reported with the foam vehicle, which does not contain propilen glycol, and cases of angioedema were reported.

Dermatomyositis

The majority of patients with dermatomyositis complained of burning and itchiness on their scalps. Dermatomyositis that affects the scalp typically results in non-cicatricial alopecia; however, cicatricial lesions are possible to occur (Fig. 11.7a). Scaling, skin atrophy, and diffuse erythema are additional scalp symptoms. Acute

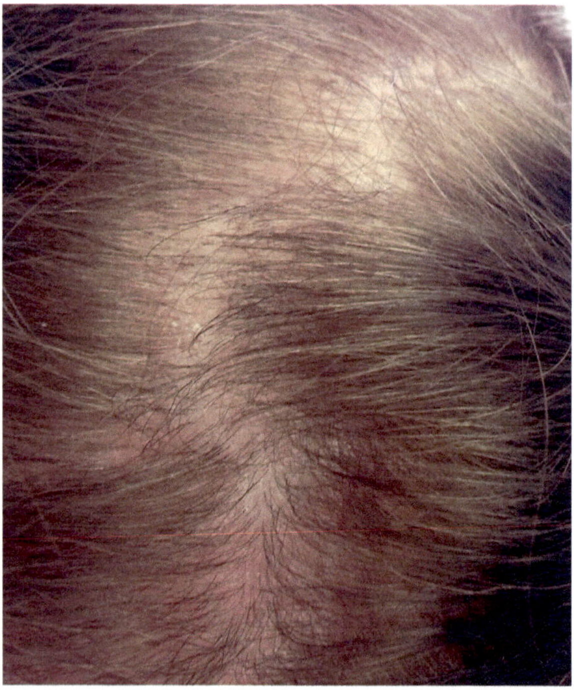

Fig. 11.6 Thin scaling and erythema of the scalp as a result of topical minoxidil use

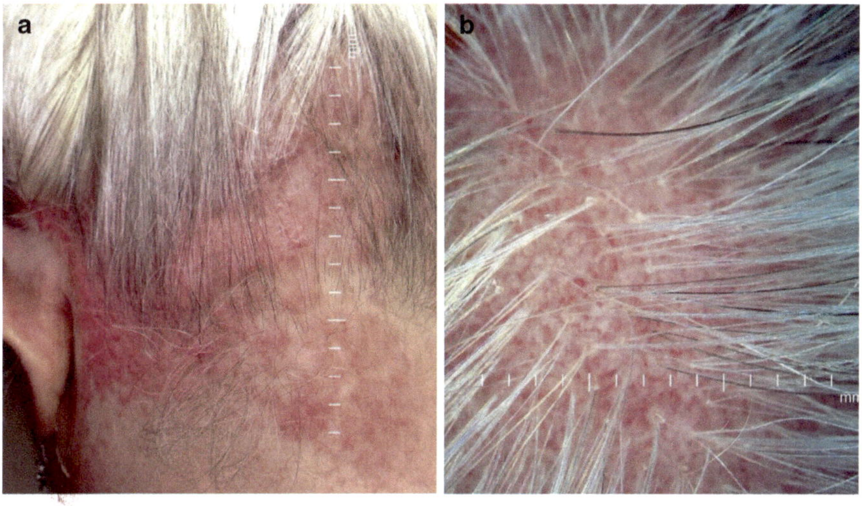

Fig. 11.7 A female patient with dermatomyositis involving the scalp, resulting in cicatricial alopecia: (**a**) severe scalp erythema, scaling, and telangiectasias; (**b**) an increased vascular network, telangiectasias, and polytrichia (more than six hair shafts)

telogen effluvium may also occur. A case of an 80-year-old female dermatomyositis that manifested as progressive hair loss, scalp itching, and histopathological findings of scarring alopecia with interface dermatitis was published by Franciosi et al. [34]. Trichoscopic examination shows enlarged polymorphous interfollicular vessels that are very suggestive of the diagnosis (Fig. 11.7b). Other clinical features, such as proximal muscle weakness, heliotrope rash, Gottron papules and Gottron sign, V-neck sign, shawl sign, periungual changes, mechanic hands, and photosensitivity may be observed on physical examination (Muro et al.). In a patient with dermatomyositis, Hurliman et al. [35] found a significant reduction in the density of epidermal nerve fibers using confocal microscopy, indicating that small fiber neuropathy may be the cause of scalp pruritus in this condition.

Tinea Capitis

Clinically, tinea capitis is characterized by erythema, desquamation, patches of hair loss, and can cause intense scalp itching. The zoophilic *Microsporum canis* and the anthropophilic *Trichophyton tonsurans* are among the dermatophyte species that cause Tinea capitis most frequently, but other dermatophyte species can also infect the scalp. Migrations within a population have an impact on the incidence of various pathogens, which varies by geographic region. In Israel, an increase in Tinea capitis cases among children has been linked to *Trichophyton violaceum* and *Microsporum audouinii*, with children of African immigrants accounting for the majority of these cases. Medium chain length fatty acids in sebum are inhibitory to dermatophyte growth, providing a high resistance to infection in the postpubertal period, which explains the high prevalence in children.

The degree of itch depends on the type of hair invasion, the level of host resistance, and the degree of inflammatory host response. eosinophils are frequently found in inflammatory infiltrates and undoubtedly contribute to the development of pruritus. histamine stimulates the H4 receptor on eosinophils. eosinophils release neurotoxic granule proteins such as eosinophil cationic protein, neurotrophins, and neuropeptides. furthermore, eosinophils can secrete stem cell factor and regulate mast cell function in a paracrine manner

Some researchers distinguish between noninflammatory and inflammatory Tinea capitis. Noninflammatory (epidemic) Tinea capitis is caused primarily by anthropophilic fungi and primarily affects children. Clinical features include foci of short broken hairs at different lengths and black dots (Fig. 11.8)

Mild scaling is occasionally visible. Mild erythema may be present in the noninflammatory tinea capitis caused by *Microsporum canis.* Fungi that are either zoophilic or geophilic typically cause the inflammatory type of tinea capitis. Favus and

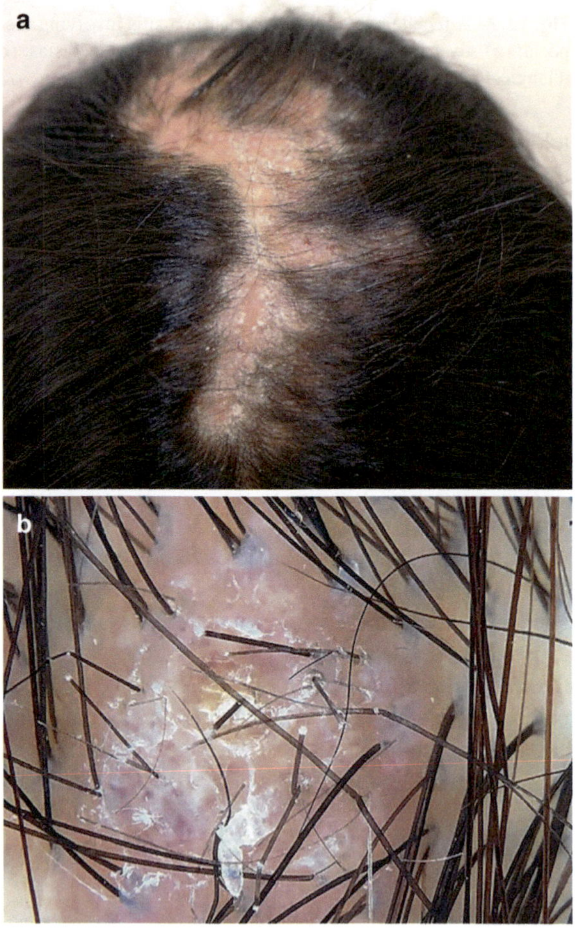

Fig. 11.8 Tinea capitis caused by Microsporum: (**a**) large single erythematous scaly bald patch, (**b**) trichoscopy shows broken hairs, Morse code-like hairs

kerion are two categories for inflammatory lesions. Tinea capitis favosa, also known as favus, is characterized by crusts and amorphous material that contains keratin fragments, dermatophyte hyphae, and hair fragments.

Long-standing infection may result in extensive patchy atrophic cicatricial alopecia.

Folliculitis and perifolliculitis are the initial symptoms of deep trichophytosis of the scalp, which then develops into a painful, constrictive, tumor-like, acute-inflammatory hemispheric infiltrate that is eventually covered in purulent-hemorrhagic crusts. The removal of the crusts reveals follicular openings that resemble honeycombs (kerion). Another diagnostic sign is the presence of lymphadenopathy.

Diagnostics. Mycological examination (microscopic and culture), Wood's lamp examination (for *Microsporum canis*) and modern methods of molecular biological diagnostics are among recognized diagnostic standards. On dermoscopy, the combination of broken hairs, black dots, comma-shaped hairs, and short corkscrew hairs are suggestive of tinea capitis [36] (Table 11.7). Ultraviolet-enhanced trichoscopy may facilitate the detection of fluorescent greenish-bluish hairs infected with *Microsporum canis*.

Treatment. Oral treatment is the gold standard for tinea capitis. Depending on the species of the fungus, medications such as terbinafine, griseofulvin, and azoles, itraconazole, and fluconazole are used. As an adjuvant therapy, topical antifungal treatment can reduce spore transmission. To avoid the development of cicatricial alopecia in kerion lesions, a course of oral corticosteroids in addition to antifungal treatment, as well as systemic antibiotics for secondary bacterial infection, is recommended.

Infestations

Some patients with scalp itch may present with infestations, with the most common being pediculosis and scabies. Scabies usually spares the scalp area in adult cases, but it can affect scalp in children and patients with compromised immune systems.

Pediculosis of the scalp is the most common parasitic infection in children, its causative agent is *Pediculus humanus capitis*. Patients usually report intense

Table 11.7 Trichoscopic features of tinea capitis

Pathogen: Microsporum	Pathogen: Trichophyton
• Morse code-like hairs • Zigzag hairs • Comma hairs • Corkscrew hairs • Block hairs • i-hairs • Diffuse scaling	• Comma hairs • Corkscrew hairs (more common than in Microsporum tinea capitis) • Block hairs • i-hairs

pruritus of the scalp due to an allergic reaction to the saliva that the parasite produces. Scalp itch takes around 4–6 weeks to manifest if it is the first infestation. In subsequent infections, pruritus may take 24–48 h to develop. Other features of pediculosis and scalp pruritus may include hyperkeratosis, secondary bacterial infection, and cervical lymphadenopathy.

Nits are located mainly in the occipital and retroauricular areas of the scalp (Fig. 11.9a). Nits are easily differentiated from hair casts (pseudonits) because they adhere tightly to the hair, while hair casts are easily movable along the hair shaft. Nits can be confused with hair spray residue or scalp scaling. The use of trichoscopy of the material aids in differential diagnosis by displaying a transparent flask-shaped nit that is firmly attached to only one side of the hair shaft and forms a 45° angle with the hair fiber (Fig. 11.9b).

White Piedra can also mimic nits, but the structure of the fungus involves the entire circumference of the hair shaft, as a ring encircling the hair. For a trained clinician pediculosis is not a problematic diagnosis, although trichoscopy will improve visualization of the nits (eggs) and will be helpful in the follow-up. In addition to topical treatments, oral ivermectin (400 g/kg) is a treatment option for children weighing more than 15 kg. It can be taken as a single dose and then repeated 7 days later.

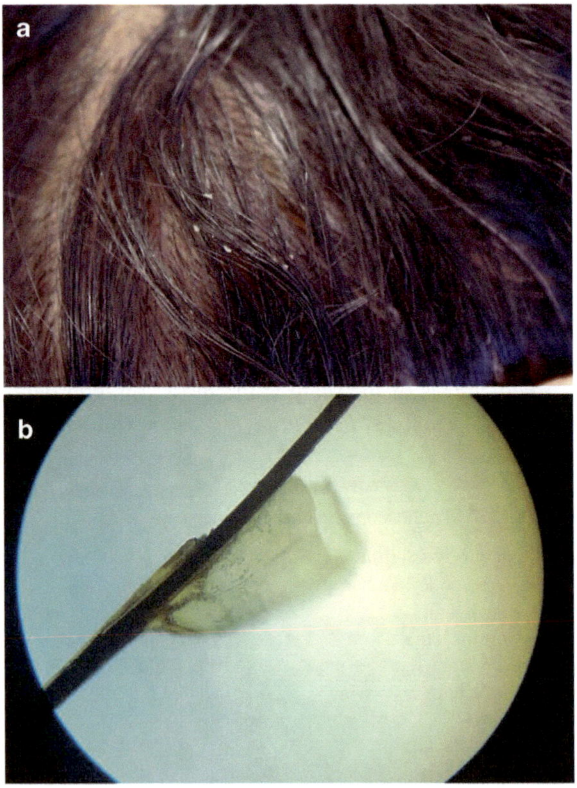

Fig. 11.9 Head lice with nits attached to the hair shafts (**a**). An empty nit (**b**)

Non-scarring Alopecia Associated with Pruritus

Non-scarring alopecia, accompanied by scalp pruritus, includes **androgenetic alopecia**, **telogen effluvium** and, in some cases, active **alopecia areata** and chemotherapy-induced **anagen effluvium**.

Patients with active **AA** often complain of mild itch or burning, which often precedes new lesions. In the work of Yamakoshi et al. Yamakoshi et al. [37], an increased number of mast cells were present in perifollicular lesions of affected hair follicles. Transmission electron microscopy demonstrated that nerve profiles in close apposition to mast cells, which showed signs of degranulation, were located in the center of the lesions. According to the scientists, mast cell release of histamine as well as IL-31 release from the lymphocyte infiltrate are possible triggers of the condition.

Patients with AGA frequently experience comorbid SD, which in some cases can contribute to scalp itching. However, in patients with active TE and TE in combination with AGA, trichodynia, which is thought to be a marker of inflammatory activity, is more frequently reported than scalp pruritus. In a study of Baldari et al. involving 24 patients with AGA, 47 patients with TE, 20 patients with both of these conditions, and 18 patients with TE in remission (109 participants in total), it was concluded that trichodynia accompanied active TE in almost all cases. The prevalence of trichodynia in patients with TE and AGA was statistically highly significant (50.7%, $P < 0.001$) than in patients only with AGA without TE or with TE in remission (4.8%).

Telogen effluvium appears to be the most common trichologic disease associated with COVID-19 infection, though it is unclear whether this is a direct result of the infection or a result of the disease's intense inflammatory cascade. Notably, in the study Trüeb et al, trichodynia was reported in only one of the ten patients with post-COVID-19 TE [38]. According to the findings of a multicentric study published by Starace et al. [23] that evaluated 128 patients after COVID-19 infection, telogen effluvium occurred in 66.3% of patients and trichodynia occurred in 58.4%, with TE associated with trichodynia in 42.4%. The symptoms appeared 4–12 weeks after the infection, and the majority of cases resolved completely. The authors hypothesized that trichodynia could be caused by neuropeptide substance P secretion or COVID-19-associated neuroinflammation.

Chemotherapy-induced **anagen effluvium** (Fig. 11.10a, b) is often associated with trichodynia and scalp pruritus. According to Fabbrocini et al. [39], clinical features of skin lesions during chemotherapy are characterized by a marked xerosis, indicating that the main pathogenetic factor is not the cutaneous adnexa but the keratinocyte itself. The development of itchy follicular papules and pustules at the face, scalp, and upper trunk occur during the use of EGFR-inhibitors. Kanti et al. [40, 41] studied 34 female patients with breast cancer undergoing chemotherapy or endocrine therapy with tamoxifen. In the chemotherapy group, 87% of patients presented with both trichodynia and pruritus; 13% had only trichodynia. In the tamoxifen group, 31% reported scalp sensations, 12% had both, trichodynia and pruritus, 7% had only trichodynia. The symptoms corresponded with the onset and duration of hair loss and the authors suggest a possible correlation. For detailed information about non-scarring alopecia see relevant chapters on individual nosologies (Chaps. 6–9).

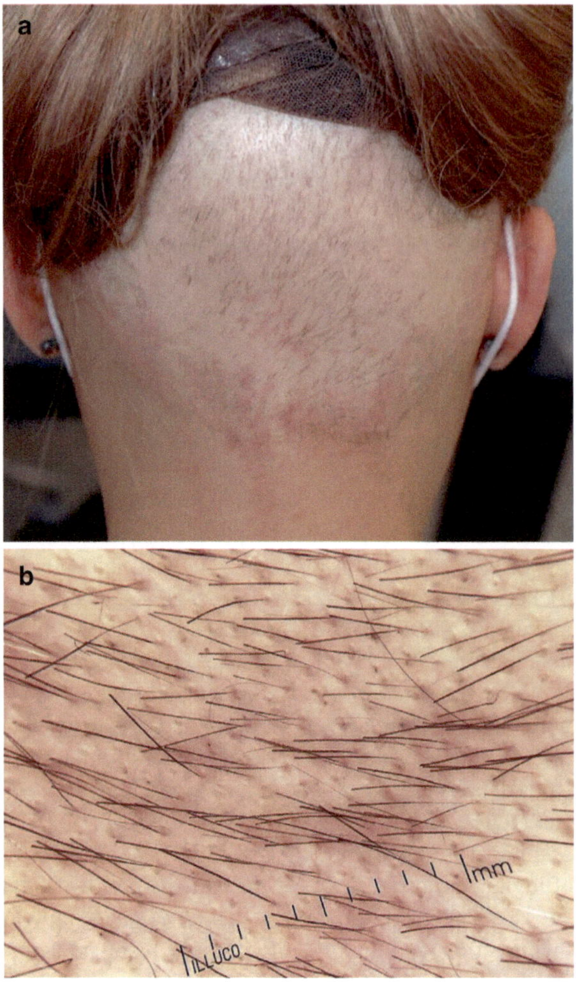

Fig. 11.10 Alopecia after chemotherapy for breast cancer (**a**) clinically, the alopecia with only sparse, thin hair remained; (**b**) the trichoscopy reveals low hair density, short, thin hairs, empty hair follicles, yellow dots, broken hairs, and black dots

Primary Cicatricial Alopecia Associated with Pruritus

Interfollicular and perifollicular scaling and erythema are dermoscopic features found in primary lymphocytic cicatricial alopecias such as **classic lichen planopilaris (LPP)** (Fig. 11.11a, b), **discoid lupus erythematosus (DLE)** (Fig. 11.12a, b), **frontal fibrosing alopecia (FFA)** (Fig. 11.13a, b), **fibrosing alopecia in a pattern distribution (FAPD)** (Figs. 11.14a, b and 11.15a, b), **and central centrifugal cicatricial alopecia (CCCA)** (Fig. 11.16a, b). Early stage of the disease when the inflammation is active is commonly associated with scalp itch or trichodynia.

Reported a case series of 46 LPP patients in which 54.34% of patients reported scalp itching and 6.53% reported scalp burning.

Most patients showed considerable perifollicular erythema. Chieregato et al. [42] reported that 70% of patients with LPP were referred for scalp pruritus. Symptoms were linked to disease activity.

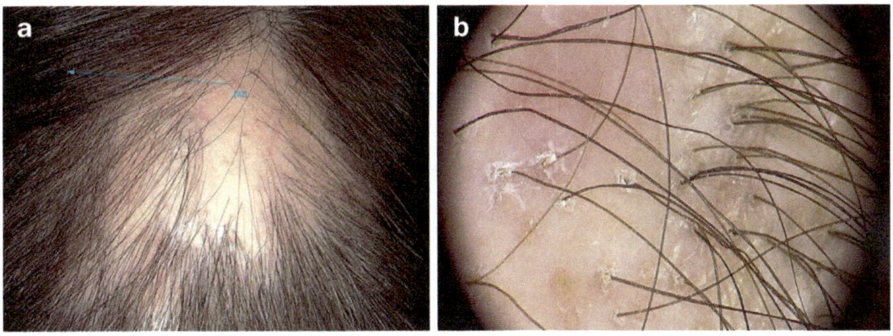

Fig. 11.11 Clinical picture of lichen planopilaris shows alopecia foci with violet areas and perifollicular scaling (**a**); trichoscopic image in the foci of lichen planopilaris visualizes absence of follicular openings, absence of vellus hair, tubular silver-white hair casts, areas of fibrosis, pili torti (×20) (**b**)

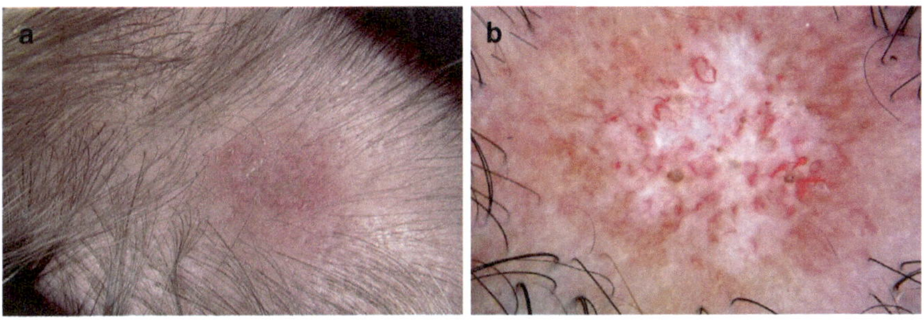

Fig. 11.12 Clinical picture of discoid lupus erythematosus demonstrates alopecia focus with marked erythema, telangiectasias, keratotic plugs, mild interfollicular scaling (**a**); trichoscopic image of discoid lupus erythematosus visualizes loss of follicular openings, large brown-yellow dots, thick arborizing vessels, red dots, and scattered brown discoloration (×20) (**b**)

Tan et al. [43] found scalp pruritus in 65% of DLE patients and 90% of LPP patients in a study of 112 patients with primary cicatricial alopecias.

In the study by Vañó-Galván et al. [44] on 355 patients with FFA, pruritus and trichodynia were observed in 35% and 20% of patients, respectively.

In a retrospective study by Banka et al. [45], 65% of 64 FFA patients had symptoms of scalp itching, pain, or burning. Samrao et al. [46] discovered that 67% of the 36 patients with FFA in their clinical review had scalp pruritus.

In the first description of FAPD by Zinkernagel and Trüeb [47], the authors reported that 37% of the patients complained of scalp pruritus or pain.

Reported itch in CCCA patients. Pruritic lesions responded successfully to treatment with triamcinolone injections of 10 mg/mL, intramuscular triamcinolone injections of 40–60 mg, or oral steroids.

Bin Saif et al. [2] used thermosensory testing and experimental itch models to analyze the C nerve fiber function relating to itch and pain perception in 16 African American women with CCCA and 15 healthy controls. The authors concluded that CCCA activity was linked to a possible role for the protease-activated receptor (PAR)2 and cowhage-induced scalp itch.

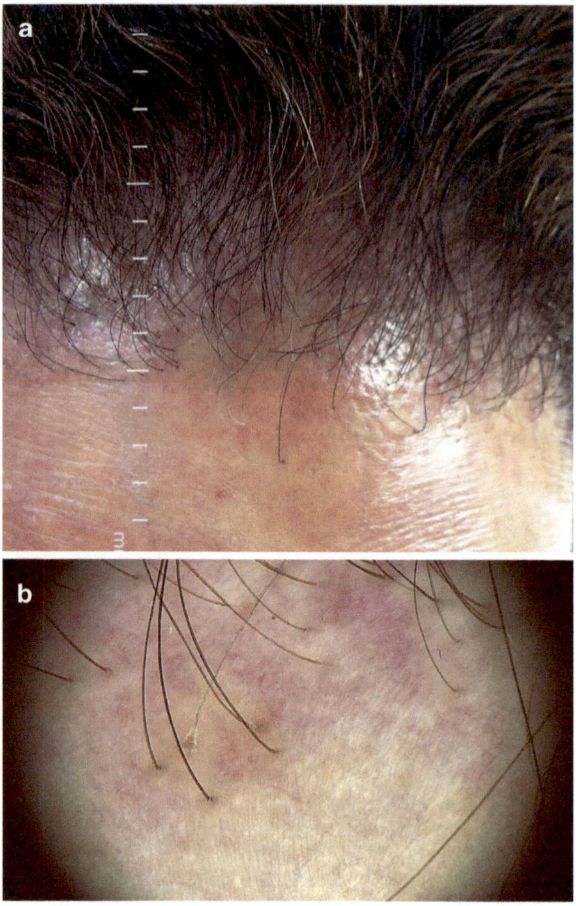

Fig. 11.13 Clinical presentation of frontal fibrosing alopecia (**a**) showing recess of the frontal hair line with marked erythema and scaling. Trichoscopic image of an active severe pruritus lesion in this patient visualizes single hairs, loss of vellus hair, mild scaling, and erythema (×60) (**b**)

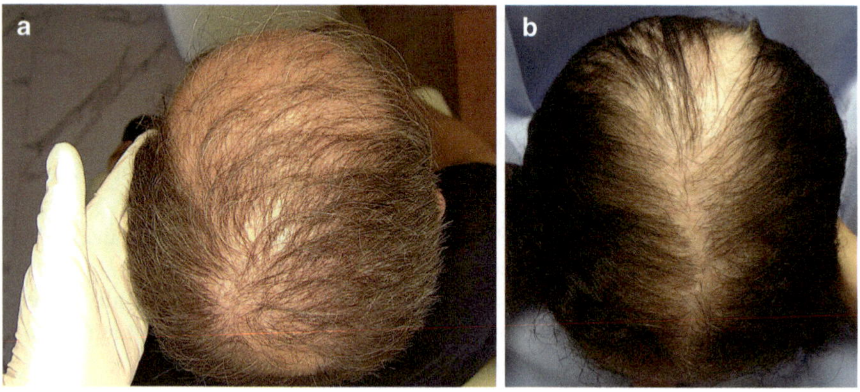

Fig. 11.14 Fibrosing alopecia in a pattern distribution: (**a**) clinical picture resembling male patterns hair loss; (**b**) clinical picture resembling female patterns hair loss

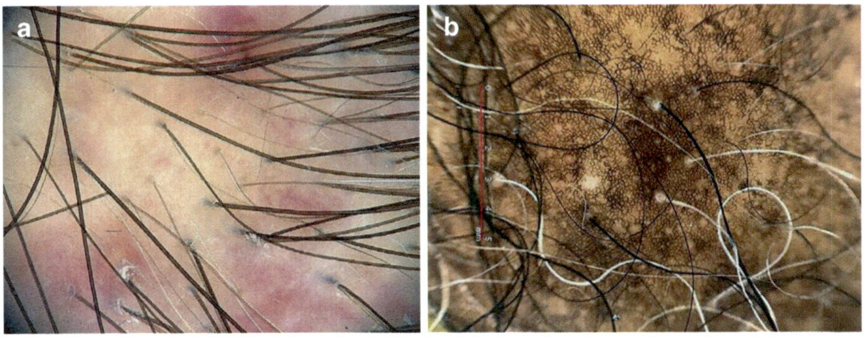

Fig. 11.15 Trichoscopic picture in fibrosing alopecia in a pattern distribution in the affected androgen-dependent zone: (**a**) anisotrichosis and absence of follicular ostia, perifollicular erythema and desquamation are visualized in a patient with a light skin phototype; (**b**) anisotrichosis, absence of follicular ostia, perifollicular white halos (fibrosis) and perifollicular desquamation in the presence of a pigment network are observed in a patient with a dark skin phototype

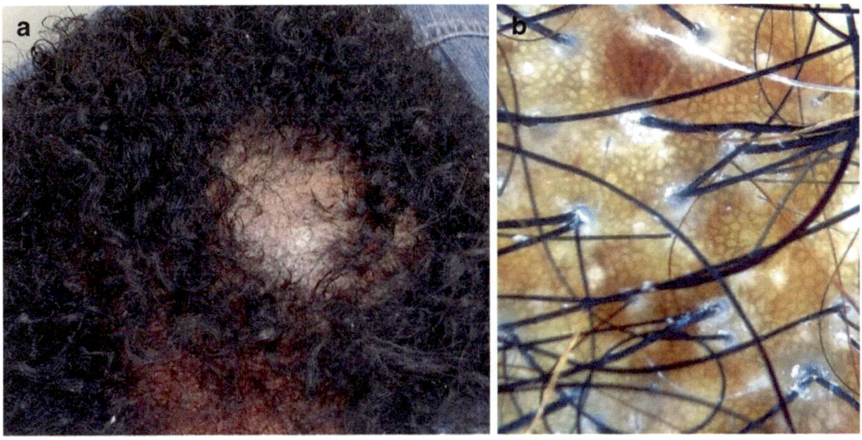

Fig. 11.16 African-descent patient with cicatricial bald patches consistent with central centrifugal cicatricial alopecia (**a**). Trichoscopy of central centrifugal cicatricial alopecia showing single follicular units, anisotrichia, loss of follicular ostia, perifollicular scaling with perifollicular white hallo, and interfollicular dyschromia patches on the contrasting background of the pigment network (×60) (**b**)

The clinical and trichoscopic data, as well as the histological features of the most common scarring alopecia associated with pruritus, are summarized in Table 11.8.

The management of patients with scarring alopecia necessitates a very sensitive approach. Communication about the disease's prognosis and the goal of therapy are critical components of patient consultation. It is necessary to inform the patient that hair regrowth is impossible and that the goal of treatment is to prevent further hair loss. If the lesion is inactive and stable, and there is a suitable donor site, hair transplantation and scalp reduction surgery may be considered. In this case, the patient

Table 11.8 Clinical, trichoscopic, and histological characteristics of the most common scarring alopecias associated with pruritus

Nosology	Clinical signs	Trichoscopy signs	Histological features
Lichen planopilaris	• Whitish areas of atrophy or scarring • Borderline foci scaling • Hair loss (100%) • Pruritus of varying intensity (90%) • Scalp pain (70%) (Kang et al.; [48])	• Lack of follicular openings • Perifollicular scaling • Perifollicular erythema • Broken hairs • Loss of vellus hair (in most cases) [36]	• Lichenoid infiltrate at the dermoepidermal junction surrounding the follicle infundibulum and isthmus • Perivascular infiltrate, may be minimal, superficial, and usually located around the follicle [49]
Frontal fibrosing alopecia	• Progressive frontotemporal hairline recession • Pale and atrophic areas of scarring band-like alopecia • Perifollicular erythema • Glabellar red dots • Perifollicular papules • Loss of eyebrows, eyelashes, facial and body hair • Single hairs • Visible frontal veins • Rosacea-like erythema and telangiectasias on the face • Hyperpigmentation of the upper eyelid • Pruritus of varying intensity (35–67%) • Burning sensation and pain (20%) [29–33, 46, 50, 51]	• Loss of vellus hair • Perifollicular scaling • Perifollicular erythema • Black dots • Men's beard area: Transparency of hair roots • Eyebrow: Hair growing in different directions, pili torti, black dots, broken hairs [36, 44, 52–54]	Histological picture of FFA is similar to LLP, with some differences: • A lesser degree of inflammatory infiltrate and basal layer damage; • A decrease in melanocytes in the follicle's upper part; • The interfollicular epidermis is not damaged [55, 56]

Fibrosing alopecia in a pattern distribution	• Progressive thinning of hair in centroparietal region with a pattern resembling AGA, Ludwig type, or Norwood type • Scalp itch or pain (37%) [47]	• Anisotrichia • Absence of follicular ostia • Hair casts **Additional signs in dark-skinned individuals:** • Perifollicular hyperpigmentation • Peripilar white halos • Interfollicular white areas [57]	• HF miniaturization • Perifollicular lamellar fibrosis associated with lymphocytic infiltration around isthmus and infundibular region of HF • Reduction of sebaceous glands [47]
Central centrifugal cicatricial alopecia	Occurs in dark-skinned individuals: • Noninflammatory scarring alopecia of the central scalp • Centrifugal distribution of alopecia • Patchy alopecia without erythema • Mild itch or soreness at palpation [48]	• Randomly distributed pinpoint white dots • Irregular white areas • Peripilar white-gray halo [36]	**Active disease:** • Perifollicular lymphocytic infiltrate around upper follicle • Concentric lamellar fibroplasia around mid and upper follicles **Advanced disease:** • Perifollicular granulomatous inflammation • Foreign body giant cells in the hair shaft **Late stage:** Follicular fibrosis with erector pili muscle sparing [49]
Discoid lupus erythematosus	• Erythematous foci of alopecia • Follicular hyperkeratosis • Hyperpigmentation or hypopigmentation • Telangiectasias • Pronounced scaling (100%) • Pruritus (65%) • Pain of the scalp (26.2%) [48]	• Lack of follicular openings • Yellow keratotic plugs • Red dots • Enlarged arborizing vessels [36]	• Changes in vacuole edges of follicular epithelium with scattered dyskeratotic keratinocytes, cytoid bodies • Variable density periadnexal and interstitial lymphocytic infiltrate with dermal mucin • Superficial perivascular lymphocytic infiltrate • Atrophy or absence of sebaceous glands [49]

should be informed of the lower graft survival rate compared to AGA and the possibility of recurrence at any time after surgery. Recommendations on various camouflage techniques, such as hair styling, hair replacement systems, chignons, wigs, and coloring, will be beneficial.

Therapeutic Strategies of Scalp Pruritus

When treating a patient complaining of scalp dysesthesia, a physician should consider the possibility of an underlying localized somatic disease, systemic organ disease, or psychiatric disorder. An appropriate therapy approach should be comprehensive and aimed at treating the underlying disease, removing the triggering factors, prescribing targeted topical agents and preventive care, psychocorrection, and improving the patient's quality of life.

Understanding the pathophysiology of pruritus provides physicians with valuable insights for designing a treatment regimen to correct the underlying cause. Concomitant symptoms of anxiety or depression should be treated, regardless of the causal relationship between psychiatric manifestations and skin sensations, because anxious or depressed patients tend to exaggerate all types of complaints.

Therapeutic and preventive care for sensitive skin is the basic therapy and should be aimed at microbiome, mitosis and desquamation normalization, moisturizing, and protecting the skin. Among important targets of such strategies are the prevention of xerosis, antipruritic, anti-inflammatory, and anesthetic effects.

From a dermatotrichology standpoint, care should be exercised in preventing overdose and avoiding alcohol-containing compounds when using various scalp applications. Patch test may be performed to detect any substances causing itch or burning of the scalp. Cosmeceutical products with an optimal pH (4.5–5.5) should be prioritized. The use of "cowashing" or "conditioning washing" proved effective in patients of African descent with sensitive scalp.

Patients who complain of scalp dysesthesia frequently state that their condition got worse after receiving various treatments intended to ease their discomfort. Patients occasionally even experience a negative reaction to a placebo, known as the "nocebo effect." External therapy in these circumstances should be kept to nonirritating cosmetic care.

The elimination of skin inflammation, which is accompanied by histamine release, is critical. This can be accomplished by prescribing modern antihistamines and administering external anti-inflammatory therapy. Topical corticosteroids are the first line of treatment, with foams, lotions, and nongreasy emulsions being the most commonly used steroid formulations on the scalp. Ointment formulations are frequently preferred by patients of African descent.

Traditional systemic therapy for pruritic dermatoses includes antihistamines, systemic corticosteroids, and calcineurin inhibitors. In patients without pronounced changes in mental status, certain psychotropic drugs with nonspecific analgesic and antipruritic effects can be used.

First-generation tricyclic antidepressants, such as doxepin and amitriptyline, are a class of drugs with analgesic effects that have been scientifically proven. This class of medications acts on pruritus by inhibiting serotonin and noradrenaline reuptake. Doxepin has an antihistamine effect and has been shown to be effective in the treatment of urticaria, which is commonly associated with itch. Amitriptyline is well-known for its anesthetic properties and can be used to treat itching that is accompanied by pain.

Mirtazapine is a noradrenergic and selective serotonergic agent with antidepressant, anxiolytic, and antipruritic properties. Because of its sedative properties, the drug is particularly useful for treating nocturnal itch.

Several uncontrolled studies have demonstrated the efficacy of the anticonvulsant agent gabapentin in patients suffering from chronic pain syndromes (postherpetic neuralgia, erythromelalgia, and sympathetic reflex dystrophy) as well as many pruritic conditions such as prurigo nodularis, neuropathic pruritus, uremic pruritus, and lichen simplex chronicus. As a result, this medication, as well as a future generation of specific substance P antagonists being developed for the treatment of depression, may be beneficial in the treatment of scalp dysesthesia.

Anxiolytic benzodiazepines such as alprazolam and clonazepam have been shown to be effective in the treatment of stress-related pruritus. Benzodiazepines have been shown in studies to reduce the frequency and severity of relapses in stress-responsive conditions such as AD and psoriasis. To treat itch, drugs with an antagonistic effect on the neurokinin receptor (NK1) may be prescribed. For example, the efficacy of the NK1 antagonist aprepitant in chronic pruritus unresponsive to conventional therapies was reported, with 80% of subjects experiencing relief.

Thalidomide (TNF-alfa inhibitor) is a sedative immunomodulatory drug. Although it is very effective in treating various causes of pruritus and disrupting the itch-scratch cycle, it is a known teratogenic drug linked to phocomelia, so it should be used with caution and avoided entirely in pregnant women. Neuropathy is another thalidomide side effect that can be irreversible.

It was discovered that the opioid receptor system works by processing itch signals. μ-opioid receptor antagonists naloxone and naltrexone have been shown in studies to be effective in the treatment of pruritus associated with AD and LPP.

If the physician suspects that the sensations described by the patient are hallucinatory in nature (as in chronic tactile hallucinosis), a trial of pimozide may be justified. Antipsychotics such as pimozide, risperidone, olanzapine, and quetiapine can be used to treat nonhistamine-mediated pruritus associated with delusions and psychosis. Antipsychotics should be used in conjunction with other agents, such as selective serotonin reuptake inhibitors (SSRIs), serotonin and norepinephrine reuptake inhibitors (SSRIs), or antihistamines, in patients with pruritus associated with psychosis and delusions.

Patients with various somatic conditions accompanied by pruritic symptoms may have psychiatric comorbidities, which is not uncommon. This is why psychotherapeutic interventions and psychoeducational methods effectively relieve itch and improve patients' quality of life by breaking the vicious itch-scratch cycle. Table 11.9 lists treatment options and recommendations.

Table 11.9 Treatment principles for scalp pruritus

General recommendations
A comprehensive approach
Appropriate treatment focus on the underlying condition
Removal of the triggering factors and psychocomorbidity correction
Topical treatments
Mild to potent corticosteroids
Recommended forms of topical corticosteroid formulations: lotion, emulsions, foams, alcohol-free gels
African-descent patients may prefer ointment vehicle
Treatment and preventive care
Regular use of emollients
Shampoos containing keratolytics, antimycotics, anti-inflammatory/soothing ingredients for the treatment of seborrheic dermatitis and psoriasis
Avoid irritating surfactants and CABP in sensitive scalp patients
Avoid fragrances and preservatives
Cowashing shampoos may help to preserve skin barrier
The use of hair products with pH 4.5–5.5
Itching caused by topical minoxidil
Minor itching is a normal expected symptom
Topical minoxidil: prefer minoxidil foam formulation without propylene glycol
Oral minoxidil: an option for very sensitive patients
Systemic treatments
Systemic antihistamines: hydroxyzine, cetirizine, loratadine, levocetirizine
Doxepin: antihistamine, anxiolytic, and sedative action
Anticonvulsants and pain modulators: gabapentin and carbamazepine
Tricyclic and tetracyclic antidepressants: amitriptyline and paroxetine
Thalidomide (warning: teratogenic concerns)
Psychoeducational and psychotherapeutic methods

The general prognosis for many chronic pain syndromes is improvement or complete resolution of the condition secondary to treatment with psychotropic drugs. When consulting patients with major depression or somatoform disorder at risk of suicide, it is extremely important to actively involve a psychiatrist as part of an interdisciplinary approach in the clinic.

Summary

- In trichology, pruritus is one of the most common symptoms. There is a wide range of its potential causes, which can be attributed to the skin, neurological, systemic, or mental nature. Weighted evaluation and medical examination of the patient will help to avoid misdiagnosis.
- Understanding the complex sensory and immunological neuro connections involved in developing the itch-scratch cycle is of great importance in managing this common complaint.
- In the case of a combination of pruritus and hair loss complaints, in addition to a proper diagnosis of the underlying condition, special caution should be exercised

when selecting topical hair growth stimulants, and special attention should be paid to therapeutic and prophylactic care planning.

- Pruritus treatment with accompanying psychosomatic components should be directed to the underlying cause and requires a holistic methodology for correcting not only dermatological and somatosensory aspects but also cognitive, emotional, and psychosocial components.
- To consider all the multifaceted aspects of pruritus, the collective efforts and integration of the dermatotrichologist, the psychiatrist, and the psychologist are needed.
- Ultimately, knowledge expansion on itch neurophysiology is of great interest to encourage the development of new therapeutic options.

References

1. Bin Saif GA, Ericson ME, Yosipovitch G. The itchy scalp—scratching for an explanation. Exp Dermatol. 2011;20(12):959–68.
2. Bin Saif GA, McMichael A, Kwatra SG, Chan YH, Yosipovitch G. Central centrifugal cicatricial alopecia severity is associated with cowhage-induced itch. Br J Dermatol. 2013;168(2):253–6.
3. Rattanakaemakorn P, Suchonwanit P. Scalp pruritus: review of the pathogenesis, diagnosis, and management. Biomed Res Int. 2019;2019:1268430.
4. Dawn A, Papoiu ADP, Chan YH, Rapp SR, Rassette N, Yosipovitch G. Itch characteristica in atopic dermatitis: results of a web-based questionnaire. Br J Dermatol. 2009;160:642–4.
5. Yosipovitch G, Ansari N, Goon A, Chan YH, Goh CL. Clinical characteristics of pruritus in chronic idiopathic urticaria. Br J Dermatol. 2002;147:32–6.
6. Cevikbas F, Lerner EA, Park M. Physiology and pathophysiology of itch. Physiol Rev. 2020;100(3):945–82.
7. Vázquez-Herrera NE, Sharma D, Aleid NM, Tosti A. Scalp itch: a systematic review. Skin Appendage Disord. 2018;4(3):187–99.
8. O'Neill JL, Chan YH, Rapp SR, Yosipovitch G. Differences in itch characteristics between psoriasis and atopic dermatitis patients: results of a web-based questionnaire. Acta Derm Venereol. 2011;91(5):537–40.
9. Piérard-Franchimont C, Hermanns JF, Degreef H, Piérard GE. From axioms to new insights into dandruff. Dermatology. 2000;200(2):93–8.
10. Pellicano R, Tiodorovic-Zivkovic D, Gourhant J-Y, Catrical C, Ferrara G, Caldarola G, Argenziano G, Zalaudek I. Dermoscopy of cutaneous sarcoidosis. Dermatology. 2010;221:51–4.
11. Torres F, Tosti A, Misciali C, Lorenzi S. Trichoscopy as a clue to the diagnosis of scalp sarcoidosis. Int J Dermatol. 2011;50:358–61.
12. Rakowska A, Jasińska M, Sikora M, et al. Cutaneous T-cell lymphoma in erythrodermic cases may be suspected on the basis of scalp examination with dermoscopy. Sci Rep. 2021;11(1):282. https://doi.org/10.1038/s41598-020-78233-1.
13. Oaklander AL, Bowsher D, Galer B, Haanp M, Jensen MP. Herpes zoster itch: preliminary epidemiologic data. J Pain. 2003;4:338–43.
14. Oaklander AL, Cohen SP, Raju SVY. Intractable postherpetic itch and cutaneous deafferentation after facial shingles. Pain. 2002;96(1–2):9–12.
15. Yo GI, Sipovitch L, Samuel L. Neuropathic and psychogenic itch. Dermatol Ther. 2008;21:32–41.
16. Ferm I, Sterner M, Wallengren J. Somatic and psychiatric comorbidity in patients with chronic pruritus. Acta Derm Venereol. 2010;90(4):395–400.

17. Shapiro J, Otberg N. Hair loss and restoration. 2nd ed. Boca Raton: CRC Press; 2015.
18. Shi M, Zhang H, Chen X, Guo Y, Tao J, Qi H, Gan J, Jiang A, Yu H, Liang J, Chen J, Yang L, Zhuang Y, Yan M, Gu Y, Yu X, Feng X, Yao Z. Clinical features of atopic dermatitis in a hospital-based setting in China. J Eur Acad Dermatol Venereol. 2011;25:1206–12.
19. Drucker AM, Morra DE, Prieto-Merino D, Ellis AG, Yiu ZZN, Rochwerg B, Di Giorgio S, Arents BWM, Burton T, Spuls PI, Schmitt J, Flohr C. Systemic immunomodulatory treatments for atopic dermatitis: update of a living systematic review and network meta-analysis. JAMA Dermatol. 2022;158(5):523–32. https://doi.org/10.1001/jamadermatol.2022.0455. PMID: 35293977; PMCID: PMC8928094.
20. Oberholzer PA, Nobbe S, Kolm I, Kerl K, Kamarachev J, Trüeb RM. Red scalp disease—a rosacea-like dermatosis of the scalp? Successful therapy with oral tetracycline. Dermatology. 2009;219:179–81.
21. Willimann B, Trüeb R. Hair pain (trichodynia): frequency and relationship to hair loss and patient gender. Dermatology. 2002;205:374–7.
22. Lee HG, Grossman SK, Valdes-Rodriguez R, et al. Topical ketamine-amitriptyline-lidocaine for chronic pruritus: a retrospective study assessing efficacy and tolerability. J Am Acad Dermatol. 2017;76:760–1.
23. Starace M, Iorizzo M, Sechi A, Alessandrini AM, Carpanese M, Bruni F, et al. Trichodynia and telogen effluvium in COVID-19 patients: results of an international expert opinion survey on diagnosis and management. JAAD Int [Internet]. 2021;5:11–18. https://doi.org/10.1016/j.jdin.2021.07.006.
24. Starace M, Iorizzo M, Mandel VD, Bruni F, Misciali C, Apalla Z, Silyuk T, Pellacani G, Patrizi A, Piraccini BM, Alessandrini A. Scalp dysaesthesia and lichen simplex chronicus: diagnostic and therapeutic update with literature review. Clin Exp Dermatol. 2022;47(1):3–8. https://doi.org/10.1111/ced.14808. Epub 2021 Aug 30. PMID: 34137059; PMCID: PMC9290567.
25. Lewandowski M, Świerczewska Z, Barańska-Rybak W. Off-label use of botulinum toxin in dermatology—current state of the art. Molecules. 2022;27(10):3143. https://doi.org/10.3390/molecules27103143.
26. Chan S, Reddy V, Myers B, et al. High-dose doxepin for the treatment of chronic, intractable scalp pruritus. JAAD Case Rep. 2020;8:71–3.
27. Sarifakioglu E, Onur O. Women with scalp dysesthesia treated with pregabalin. Int J Dermatol. 2013;52:1398–61.
28. Lazzarini R, Costa LL, Suzuki NM, de Figueiredo Silva Hafner M. Allergic contact dermatitis by shampoo components: a descriptive analysis of 20 cases. An Bras Dermatol. 2020;95(5):658–60.
29. Gavazzoni Dias MFR, De Almeida AM, Cecato PMR, Adriano AR, Pichler J. The shampoo pH can affect the hair: myth or reality? Int J Trichology. 2014;6(3):95.
30. Gavazzoni Dias MRF, Dutra H, Lofeu A, Trüeb RM. Hyperpigmented upper eyelid: a clue to the diagnosis of facial lichen planus pigmentosus in a patient with frontal fibrosing alopecia. Skin Appendage Disord. 2018;121:1–4.
31. Gavazzoni Dias MFR, Dutra Rezende H, Furtado Cardoso de Moraes JR, Dlova N, Ekelem CN, Vilar EAG, et al. New insights into lichen planus pigmentosus associated with cicatricial alopecia. J Eur Acad Dermatol Venereol. 2021;35(3):e200–3.
32. Gavazzoni Dias MFR, Pirmez R, Dutra H. How to select a good shampoo and conditioner. In: Hair and scalp treatments. 2020.
33. Gavazzoni Dias MFR, Rochael M, Vilar E, Tanus A, Tosti A. Eczema-like Psoriasiform skin reaction due to Brazilian keratin treatment. Ski Appendage Disord. 2015;1(3):156.
34. Franciosi E, Blankenship K, Houk L, Rashighi M. Ovoid palatal patch: a clue to anti-TIF1γdermatomyositis. BMJ Case Rep. 2020;13(4):2019–21.
35. Hurliman E, Groth D, Wendelschafer-Crabb G, Kennedy W, Kavand S, Ericson M, et al. Small-fibre neuropathy in a patient with dermatomyositis and severe scalp pruritus. Br J Dermatol. 2017;176(1):209–11.
36. Tosti A. Dermoscopy of the hair and nails. 2nd ed. Boca Raton: CRC Press; 2015.

37. Yamakoshi T, Andoh T, Makino T, Kuraishi Y, Shimizu T. Clinical and histopathological features of itch in patients with alopecia Areata. Acta Derm Venereol. 2013;93(5):575–6.
38. Trüeb RM, Dutra RH, Gavazzoni Dias MFR. What can the hair tell us about COVID-19? Exp Dermatol. 2021;30:288.
39. Fabbrocini G, Cameli N, Romano MC, Mariano M, Panariello L, Bianca D, et al. Chemotherapy and skin reactions. J Exp Clin Cancer Res [Internet]. 2012;31(1):1.
40. Kanti V, Nuwayhid R, Lindner J, Hillmann K, Bangemann N, Kleine-Tebbe A, et al. Evaluation of trichodynia (hair pain) during chemotherapy or tamoxifen treatment in breast cancer patients. J Eur Acad Dermatol Venereol. 2016;30(1):112–8.
41. Kanti V, Röwert-Huber J, Vogt A, Blume-Peytavi U. Cicatricial alopecia. J Dtsch Dermatol Ges. 2018;16(4):435–61.
42. Chieregato C, Zini A, Barba A, Magnanini M, Rosina P. Lichen planopilaris: report of 30 cases and review of the literature. Int J Dermatol. 2003;42(5):342–5.
43. Tan E, Martinka M, Ball N, Shapiro J. Primary cicatricial alopecias: clinicopathology of 112 cases. J Am Acad Dermatol. 2004;50(1):25–32.
44. Vañó-Galván S, Molina-Ruiz AM, Serrano-Falcón C, Arias-Santiago S, Rodrigues-Barata AR, Garnacho-Saucedo G, et al. Frontal fibrosing alopecia: a multicenter review of 355 patients. J Am Acad Dermatol. 2014;70(4):670–8.
45. Banka N, Mubki T, Bunagan MJK, Mcelwee K, Shapiro J. Frontal fibrosing alopecia: a retrospective clinical review of 62 patients with treatment outcome and long-term follow-up. Int J Dermatol. 2014;53(11):1324–30.
46. Samrao A, Chew AL, Price V. Frontal fibrosing alopecia: a clinical review of 36 patients. Br J Dermatol. 2010;163(6):1296–300.
47. Zinkernagel M, Trüeb R. Fibrosing alopecia in a pattern distribution: patterned lichen planopilaris or androgenetic alopecia with a lichenoid tissue reaction pattern? Arch Dermatol. 2000;136:205–11.
48. Ross EK, Tan E, Shapiro J. Update on primary cicatricial alopecias. J Am Acad Dermatol. 2005;53:1–37; quiz 38–40.
49. Whiting DA. Cicatricial alopecia: clinico-pathological findings and treatment. Clin Dermatol. 2001;19(2):211–25.
50. Olsen EA, Bergfeld WF, Cotsarelis G, Price VH, Shapiro J, Sinclair R, et al. Summary of Nort American Hair Research Society (NAHRS)—sponsored workshop on cicatricial alopecia, Duke University Medical Center, February 10 and 11, 2001. J Am Acad Dermatol. 2003;48(1):103–10.
51. Olsen EA, Harries M, Tosti A, Bergfeld W, Blume-Peytavi U, Callender V, Chasapi V, Correia O, Cotsarelis G, Dhurat R, Dlova N, Doche I, Enechukwu N, Grimalt R, Itami S, Hordinsky M, Khobzei K, Lee WS, Malakar S, Messenger A, McMichael A, Mirmirani P, Ovcharenko Y, Papanikou S, Pinto GM, Piraccini BM, Pirmez R, Reygagne P, Roberts J, Rudnicka L, Saceda-Corralo D, Shapiro J, Silyuk T, Sinclair R, Soares RO, Souissi A, Vogt A, Washenik K, Zlotogorski A, Canfield D, Vano-Galvan S. Guidelines for clinical trials of frontal fibrosing alopecia: consensus recommendations from the International FFA Cooperative Group (IFFACG). Br J Dermatol. 2021;185:1221. https://doi.org/10.1111/bjd.20567. Epub ahead of print. PMID: 34105768.
52. Vañõ-Galván S, Molina-Ruiz AM, Fernández-Crehuet P, Rodrigues-Barata AR, Arias-Santiago S, Serrano-Falcõn C, et al. Folliculitis decalvans: a multicentre review of 82 patients. J Eur Acad Dermatol Venereol. 2015;29(9):1750–7.
53. Vañó-Galván S, Saceda-Corralo D, Blume-Peytavi U, Cucchía J, Dlova NC, Gavazzoni Dias MFR, et al. Frequency of the types of alopecia at twenty-two specialist hair clinics: a multicenter study. Skin Appendage Disord. 2019;5(5):309.
54. Cervantes J, Miteva M. Distinct trichoscopic features of the sideburns in frontal fibrosing alopecia compared to the frontotemporal scalp. Skin Appendage Disord. 2018;4(1):50–4. https://doi.org/10.1159/000479116. Epub 2017 Aug 5. PMID: 29457017; PMCID: PMC5806192.

55. Poblet E, Jiménez F, Pascual A, Piqué E. Frontal fibrosing alopecia versus lichen planopilaris: a clinicopathological study. Int J Dermatol. 2006;45(4):375–80. https://doi.org/10.1111/j.1365-4632.2006.02507.x. PMID: 16650161.
56. Gálvez-Canseco A, Sperling L. Lichen planopilaris and frontal fibrosing alopecia cannot be differentiated by histopathology. J Cutan Pathol. 2018;45(5):313–7. https://doi.org/10.1111/cup.13112. Epub 2018 Feb 23. PMID: 29369400.
57. Griggs J, Trüeb RM, Gavazzoni Dias MFR, Hordinsky M, Tosti A. Fibrosing alopecia in a pattern distribution. J Am Acad Dermatol. 2021;85(6):1557–64. https://doi.org/10.1016/j.jaad.2019.12.056. Epub 2020 Jan 8. PMID: 31926219.

Psychopharmacological Treatment of Hair Disorders

12

Mohammad Jafferany

Introduction

A comprehensive understanding of individual psychotrichological disorders is an important basis for potential clinical applications; however still further research is required to identify novel molecules and specific mediators in the pathogenesis of conditions resulting in hair disease.

During the consultation, the trichologist needs to pay attention to the psychological aspect of the disease, inform the patient about the relationship between skin, hair and psyche, identify psychosocial factors and concomitant psychiatric comorbidity.

The choice of psychotropic medications is based upon the nature of underlying psychopathology. The most common psychopathologies in hair disorders are depression, anxiety, psychosis, and obsessive behaviors. These conditions could be treated by anxiolytics, antidepressants, antipsychotics, or mood stabilizers in individual situations [1]. It should also be acknowledged that a dermatologist's prescription of psychotropic medication is more likely to be accepted by patients than a psychiatrist's prescription, owing to the social stigma associated with mental illness and visiting the psychiatrist.

Antidepressant Use in Hair Disorders

There are four types of antidepressants used in psychotrichological disorders, which include selective serotonin reuptake inhibitors (SSRIs), serotonin-norepinephrine reuptake inhibitors (SNRIs), atypical antidepressants, and tricyclic antidepressants (TCAs) (Table 12.1). Antidepressants work on serotonin and norepinephrine

M. Jafferany (✉)
Department of Psychiatry and Behavioral Sciences, Central Michigan University, College of Medicine, Saginaw, MI, USA
e-mail: jaffe1m@cmich.edu

Y. Ovcharenko et al. (eds.), *Psychotrichology*,
https://doi.org/10.1007/978-3-031-64083-4_12

Table 12.1 Antidepressants

Active ingredient	Trade name	Daily dose (mg/day)	Side effects
Selective serotonin reuptake inhibitors (SSRIs)			
Fluoxetine	Prozac®, Daforin®	10–80	Nausea, insomnia, anorexia, anxiety, drug interactions
Sertraline	Zoloft®, Tolrest®, Assert®	25–200	Dry mouth, nausea, diarrhea, insomnia, sexual dysfunction, hyperhidrosis
Paroxetine	Paxil®, Pondera®, Aropax®	20–60	Drowsiness, weakness, dizziness, hyperhidrosis, anxiety, insomnia, dry mouth, headache, vision changes
Fluvoxamine	Luvox®	50–300	Dry mouth, headache, nausea, insomnia, anxiety, drug interaction, diarrhea, sexual problems, muscle pain
Citalopram	Celexa®	20–60	Dry mouth, hyperhidrosis, nausea, somnolence, insomnia, headache, drowsiness, tachycardia
Escitalopram	Lexapro®, Reconter®	5–20	Drowsiness, insomnia, dry mouth, hyperhidrosis, loss of appetite, nausea, yawning, weight changes
Serotonin-norepinephrine reuptake inhibitors (SNRIs)			
Desvenlafaxine	Pristiq®, Khedezla®	50–400	Nausea, dizziness, insomnia, decreased appetite, hyperhidrosis, xerostomia
Duloxetine	Cymbalta®, Drizalma®, Sprinkle®	40–60	Nausea, dizziness, headache, insomnia, constipation
Levomilnacipran	Fetzima®	40–120	Nausea, dizziness, dry mouth, headache, increased blood pressure/pulse, insomnia
Milnacipran	Savella®	50–100	Nausea, dizziness, dry mouth, headache, increased blood pressure, insomnia, constipation, hyperhidrosis
Venlafaxine	Effexor®	75–375	Nausea, constipation, hyperhidrosis, headache, increased blood pressure, anxiety, and insomnia
Atypical antidepressants			
Vilazodone	Viibryd®	10–40	Nausea, dizziness, dry mouth, diarrhea, vomiting, insomnia
Nafazodone	Serzone®	100–250	Drowsiness, headache, nausea, dizziness, dry mouth, diarrhea, vomiting, insomnia, vision problems, increased appetite
Vortioxetine	Trintellix®, Brintellix®	5–20	Nausea, headache, dry mouth, diarrhea,vomiting, insomnia, dizziness, itchy skin
Duloxetine	Velija®, Cymbalta®	40–60	Nausea, dizziness, loss of appetite, dry mouth, sleepiness, fatigue, eye pain, hyperhidrosis, constipation
Bupropion	Welburtrin®, Zetron®	250–450	Jitteriness, flushing, seizures, anorexia, tachycardia, psychosis
Venlafaxine	Effexor®, Zyvifax®, Zaredrop®	75–300	Nausea, headache, dry mouth, increased blood pressure, diarrhea, vomiting, insomnia, dizziness, itchy skin, sexual dysfunction

(continued)

Table 12.1 (continued)

Active ingredient	Trade name	Daily dose (mg/day)	Side effects
Trazodone	Donaren®, Desyrel®, Oleptrol®	150–600	Drowsiness, blurred vision, confusion, dizziness, sedation, dry mouth, ventricular irritability, anorexia, tachycardia, psychosis
Mirtazapine	Remeron®, Zispin®, Norest®	10–45	Somnolence, drowsiness, dry mouth, increased appetite, constipation, weight gain, neutropenia, muscle pain, tremor
Tricyclic antidepressants			
Nortriptyline	Pamelor®, AventlyHCI®	10–150	Nausea, vomiting, loss of appetite, insomnia, dry mouth, vision changes, sexual dysfunction
Amitriptyline	Amytril®, Tryptanol®, Elavil®	10–150	Nausea, constipation, headache, diarrhea, vomiting, insomnia, dizziness, rash, breast swelling, sexual dysfunction
Clomipramine	Anafranil®	10–250	Nausea, drowsiness, constipation, dry mouth, diarrhea, vomiting, insomnia, dizziness, sexual dysfunction, flushing
Doxepin	Silenor®, Sinequan®	100–300	Drowsiness, blurred vision, dry mouth, constipation, urinary retention, weight gain/loss, rash, low blood pressure, hepatitis
Protriptyline	Vivactil®	15–60	Nausea, anxiety, dry mouth, diarrhea, vomiting, insomnia, sexual dysfunction, constipation, blurred vision
Imipramine	Tofranil®	150–300	Nausea, headache, loss of appetite, dry mouth, dizziness, vomiting, weigh gain/loss, weakness, diarrhea, vomiting, sexual dysfunction, constipation, blurred vision

receptors mainly to help with anxiety, depression, and obsessive symptoms associated with various hair disorders and improve functioning and quality of life in these patients [2].

The side effect profile of antidepressants is determined by their major action on an individual neurotransmitter. Serotonin is the main neurotransmitter, but several antidepressants also act upon norepinephrine, histamine, and dopamine neurotransmitter, which lead to side effects especially attributed to those neurotransmitters. Common side effects attributed to antidepressants are: nausea, vomiting, diarrhea, dizziness, tiredness, headache, weight gain, insomnia, lack of appetite or increased appetite. Sexual side effects are a major concern for noncompliance in the treatment. Some of the antidepressants, for instance, paroxetine is pregnancy category D antidepressant and should not be used in pregnant patients.

SSRI withdrawal syndrome or discontinuation syndrome should be kept in mind when a person suddenly stops taking antidepressants:

- Flu-like symptoms
- Insomnia
- Nausea

- Imbalance
- Sensory disturbances
- Hyperarousal

Excessive use of SSRI antidepressants such as in situations like intentional overdoses or taking too many pills accidentally poses a risk of serotonin syndrome, characterized by the following triad: altered mental status, neuromuscular abnormalities, and autonomic hyperactivity symptoms. Clinical picture depending on the severity may differ:

- Mild symptoms include: mild hypertension, tachycardia, mydriasis, diaphoresis, shivering, tremors, myoclonus, and hyperreflexia
- Moderate symptoms include: fever, flatulence, ocular clonus, agitation, hypervigilance, and pressured speech
- Severe symptoms include: extremely high fever, high blood pressure, delirium, and muscle rigidity. Severe cases are often complicated by seizures, rhabdomyolysis, myoglobinuria, metabolic acidosis, renal failure, acute respiratory distress syndrome, respiratory failure, coma, and death

Mood Stabilizers in Hair Disorders

The use of mood stabilizers in psychotrichology focuses on problems with poor impulse control and obsessive-compulsive spectrum-related disorders such as trichotillomania and its variants. Mood stabilizers basically affect glutamatergic neurotransmission. Glutamate, which is an excitatory neurotransmitter is a key regulator of synaptic strength and plasticity and plays a major role in the neurobiology of learning, memory, and general cognition.

The psychotrichologist should be familiar with common side effects associated with mood stabilizers such as sedation, tremors, dizziness, cognitive difficulties, aplastic anemia, and syndrome of inappropriate diuretic hormone. Valproic acid and carbamazepine are pregnancy category D medication and thus should be avoided in pregnant patients. Lamotrigine is linked to high risk of rash, which could lead to Stevens Johnson Syndrome.

Lithium is well-known for causing more dermatological side effects than any other mood stabilizer, including acneiform rash, geographical tongue, and psoriasiform rash. Monitoring of lithium levels is required until the patient is on lithium therapy.

Lithium levels in the blood must first be checked 2 months after the start of treatment and then every 6 months after that. Since lithium has a very small therapeutic window, any change in the level should prompt an urgent patient referral to the emergency room. Common mood stabilizers, their doses, and side effects are shown in Table 12.2.

Table 12.2 Mood stabilizers

Active ingredient	Trade name	Daily dose (mg/day)	Side effects
Lithium carbonate	Lithobid®, Eskalith®, Litium®	150–1800	Hand tremors, mild thirst, increased urination, diarrhea, vomiting, drowsiness, weakness, blurred vision, dermatological side effects
Sodium valproate	Depakote®, Depakene®	125–2000	Bleeding gums, bloating, confusion, cough, diarrhea, dysphoria, fever, headache, nausea, liver dysfunction
Lamotrigine	Lamictlal®, Lamitor®	25–400	Ataxia, skin rash, headache, insomnia, nausea, dyspepsia, infection, drowsiness, constipation
Carbamazepine	Tegretol®, Tegrex®, Carbatrol®, Equetro®, Epitol®	200–1600	Ataxia, dizziness, pruritus, amblyopia, xerostomia, nausea, vomiting, drowsiness, blurred vision
Topiramate	Topamax®, Trokendi®, Qudexy XR®	50–400	Anxiety, ataxia, confusion, diarrhea, diplopia, fatigue, headache, insomnia, nausea, dyspepsia, dizziness, anorexia, drowsiness, weight loss
Pregabalin	Lyrica®	25–600	Infections, ataxia, headache, dyspepsia, infection, blurred vision, drowsiness, dizziness
Gabapentin	Neurontin®, Gralise®	100–3600	Ataxia, fatigue, fever, sedated state, insomnia, nausea, dyspepsia, infection, tremor, drowsiness

Antipsychotics in Hair Disorders

Antipsychotic drugs in hair disorders are used for either augmenting SSRIs and mood stabilizers to treat depression and anxiety or for psychotic symptoms. Some hair disorders need long-term steroid treatment and those patients are more prone to develop steroid psychosis, which could be prevented by antipsychotics. Antipsychotics are dopamine receptor antagonist acting mainly on dopamine D2 receptors.

Antipsychotics may be divided into two broad groups: typical and atypical or first-generation and second-generation drugs. Several of the newer antipsychotics approved in the last few years have relatively less side effects. The difference between typical and atypical antipsychotics is binding to and affinity for D2 receptors. The typical antipsychotics bind more tightly, thus, are more notorious for extrapyramidal side effects. Antipsychotics that have been developed recently, as well as atypical or second-generation antipsychotics, have a lower affinity for the D2 receptor and thus cause fewer side effects, including a lower incidence of extrapyramidal side effects.

Antipsychotic side effects include postural hypotension caused by alpha-1 receptor blockade, weight gain, and sedation caused by histamine H1 blockade, and constipation, urinary retention, dry mouth, pupil dilatation, and tachycardia caused by anticholinergic effects. The high potency agents are characterized by extrapyramidal symptoms such as dystonia, akathisia, Parkinsonism, and tardive dyskinesia.

In rare cases, neuroleptic malignant syndrome, a severe and potentially fatal reaction characterized by tachycardia, increased blood pressure, fever, rigidity, and Parkinsonism, may develop. Common laboratory abnormalities in this syndrome include leukocytosis, elevated creatine phosphokinase, elevated liver function tests, and myoglobinuria. Antipsychotics can also cause weight gain, amenorrhea, galactorrhea, blood dyscrasias, photosensitivity, and cholestatic jaundice as side effects. Tables 12.3 and 12.4 provide comprehensive details on atypical and novel antipsychotic medications.

Table 12.3 Atypical antipsychotics

Active ingredient	Trade name	Daily dose (mg/day)	Side effects
Clozapine	Clozaril®	100–900	Constipation, drooling, weight gain, dry mouth, blurred vision, drowsiness, dizziness, headache, tremors, confusion, fainting, fever, hyperhidrosis
Risperidone	Risperdal®	2–8	Extrapyramidal effects, dizziness, sedation, dry mouth, headache, nausea, vomiting, cough, insomnia, cough, skin rash, muscle spasms, galactorrhea
Olanzapine	Zyprexa®	5–20	Loss off balance control, muscle trembling, blurred vision, weight gain, dizziness, dry mouth
Quetiapine	Seroquel®	75–800	Chills, confusion, cold sweats, dizziness, drowsiness, nausea, vomiting, stomach pain, weight gain, mood changes, nightmares
Ziprasidone	Geodon®	40–160	Cough, sedation, fever, loss of balance control, drooling, restlessness, sneezing
Aripiprazole	Abilify®	5–30	Weight gain, blurred vision, nausea, vomiting, headache, anxiety, insomnia, dizziness, drowsiness, anxiety
Asenapine	Saphris®	2.5–20	Restlessness, uncontrolled movements, sticking out of tongue, constipation, dry mouth, insomnia, drowsiness, dizziness, upset stomach and weight gain, suicidal ideation
Lurasidone	Latuda®	20–160	Loss of balance control, muscle trembling, restlessness, slow reflexes, nausea, dizziness, drowsiness, shaking, diarrhea
Iloperidone	Fanapt®	1–24	Blurred vision, cough, drooling, fever, headache, loss of voice, restlessness, runny nose, hyperhidrosis, drowsiness, dizziness
Paliperidone	Invega®	6–12	Drooling, loss of balance control, muscle trembling, shuffling walk, uncontrolled movements, drowsiness, dizziness, nausea, cough, dry mouth, blurred vision

Table 12.4 Novel antipsychotics

Active ingredient	Trade name	Daily dose (mg/day)	Side effects
Lumateperone	Caplyta®	42	Neuroleptic malignant syndrome, tardive dyskinesia, seizures, dizziness, allergic reaction, drowsiness, dry mouth, nausea, fatigue, vomiting, decreased appetite
Brexpiprazole	Rexulti®	1–4	Anxiety, dizziness, drowsiness, fatigue, dyspepsia, nasopharyngitis, increased creatinine phosphokinase in blood specimen, tremor, hypersomnia, weight gain
Cariprazine	Vraylar®	1.5–6	Blurred vision, dizziness, drooling, drowsiness, fever, muscle trembling, tremor, weight gain, nervousness, restlessness
Pimavanserin	Nuplazid®	10–34	Peripheral edema, confusion, nausea, rapid weight gain, bloating, weigh gain/loss, hallucination, walking abnormally

Anxiolytics and Hypnotics in Hair Disorders

The role of anxiolytics in psychotrichology is limited to severe anxiety reactions and sleep difficulties associated with hair disorders. Anxiety medications could be divided into two major groups: benzodiazepines (BDZs) and non-benzodiazepines (NBDZs). BZDs act by potentiating the gamma aminobutyric acid (GABA)-A receptor. GABA is a known inhibitory brain neurotransmitter and has three subtypes: A, B, C.

Side effects of BZDs manifest through the central nervous system by excessive sedation, impairment of motor function, tiredness, and stupor. BZDs with longer half-life tend to accumulate and can lead to memory impairment. They may intensify the effects of anticonvulsants, antipsychotics, and narcotic analgesics. Therefore, patients receiving other agents should be monitored carefully. Chronic use can also lead to tolerance (uncontrollable desire to increase the use of a substance in order to achieve the same effect) and dependence: psychological (cravings and preoccupation with obtaining the substance) and physiological (manifests as physical withdrawal symptoms).

NBDZs are also used to treat anxiety and sleep difficulties in these patients. Compared to BDZs, NBDZs have different mechanisms of action. While zaleplon has less cognitive side effects, Rozerem works on the melatonin receptors, zolpidem acts as a partial benzodiazepine but has no anticonvulsant properties. Eszopiclone is well-known for its long-term use in treating insomnia [3]. The summaries of hypnotic and anxiolytic drugs are found in Tables 12.5 and 12.6.

Table 12.5 Benzodiazepines

Active ingredient	Trade name	Daily dose (mg/day)	Side effects
Long acting			
Chlordiazepoxide	Librium®	5–75	Dizziness, drowsiness, tiredness, nausea, vomiting, headache, skin rash, swelling, blurred vision, constipation, hallucinations, hyperactivity, trouble walking
Diazepam	Valium®	2–40	Hypotonia, shakiness and unsteady walk, loss of balance control, trembling, tiredness, blurred vision, drowsiness, dizziness
Flurazepam	Dalmane®	15–30	Confusion, headache, dizziness, vertigo, insomnia, irritability, weakness, heartburn, blurred vision, loss of coordination
Intermediate-acting drugs			
Alprazolam	Xanax®	0.25–4	Ataxia, cognitive dysfunction, constipation, drowsiness, dysarthria, fatigue, anxiety, blurred vision, skin rash, insomnia, sexual dysfunction
Lorazepam	Ativan®	0.5–10	Sedation, dizziness, drowsiness, sleepiness
Clonazepam	Klonopin®	0.25–4	Muscle weakness, drowsiness, dizziness, confusion, cough, abnormal thinking
Temazepam	Restoril®	7.5–30	Dizziness, insomnia, lethargy, irritability, muscle weakness, headache, blurred vision
Oxazepam	Serax®	15	Drowsiness, dizziness, insomnia, vertigo, irritability, confusion, insomnia, headache, blurred vision, amnesia, swelling
Triazolam	Halcion®	0.25–0.5	Dizziness, insomnia, irritability, tiredness, depression, headache, blurred vision
Midazolam	Versed®	Intravenous only	Dizziness, tiredness, insomnia, irritability, loss of coordination, headache, itching, blurred vision

Table 12.6 Sedative-hypnotics

Active ingredient	Trade name	Daily dose (mg/day)	Side effects
Short acting			
Triazolam	Halcion®	0.125–0.25	Dizziness, insomnia, tiredness, irritability, headache, blurred vision, loss of coordination, agitation
Intermediate-acting drugs			
Estazolam	Prosom®	0.5–2	Hypokinesia, clumsiness or unsteadiness, dizziness, and sleepiness
Temazepam	Restoril®	7.5–45	Dizziness, insomnia, lethargy, irritability, amnesia, headache, depression, blurred vision
Long acting			
Flurazepam	Dalmane®	15–45	Dizziness, irritability, weakness, headache, loss of coordination, stomach ache, blurred vision
Quazepam	Doral®	7.5–15	Drowsiness, dizziness, vertigo, insomnia, confusion, headache

(continued)

Table 12.6 (continued)

Active ingredient	Trade name	Daily dose (mg/day)	Side effects
Nonbenzodiazepines			
Zolpidem	Ambien®	5–20	Dizziness, hallucination, dry mouth, nausea, constipation, weakness, headache, diarrhea
Zaleplon	Sonata®	5–20	Dizziness, drowsiness, amnesia, nausea, headache, anxiety, depression, constipation, dry mouth, back pain
Eszopiclone	Lunesta®	2–3	Infection, drowsiness, unpleasant taste in mouth, nausea, dizziness, xerostomia
Melatonin receptor agonists			
Ramelteon	Rozerem®	8	Dizziness, drowsiness, fatigue, sleepiness, nausea, tiredness
Barbiturate-like drugs			
Chloral hydrate	Notec®	500–1500	Drowsiness, diarrhea, vomiting, nausea, headache, stomach pain
Natural agents			
	Melatonin	0.3–2	Dizziness, insomnia, depression, headache, stomach cramps
	Valerian root	400–900	Headache, excitability, uneasiness, insomnia, mental dullness

Summary

- To manage psychotrichological patients, the clinical dermatologist and trichologist should become acquainted with the therapeutic options available, both nonpharmacological and psychopharmacological, and determine the limits of what can be accomplished in the psychotrichology practice setting.
- If the trichologist is serious about treating these patients with psychopharmacological agents, their decision should be based on the underlying psychopathology.
- To provide effective and safe treatment, the trichologist must have a basic understanding of psychopharmacology.

References

1. Jafferany M, Ferreira BR, Abdelmaksoud A, Mkhoyan R. Management of psychocutaneous disorders: a practical approach for dermatologists. Dermatol Ther. 2020a;33:e13969. https://doi.org/10.1111/dth.13969. Epub ahead of print. PMID: 32621633.
2. Jafferany M, Stamu-O'Brien C, Mkhoyan R, Patel A. Psychotropic drugs in dermatology: a dermatologist's approach and choice of medications. Dermatol Ther. 2020b;33:e13385. https://doi.org/10.1111/dth.13385. Epub 2020 Apr 20. PMID: 32268440.
3. Torales J, Melgarejo O, González I, García O, Barrios I, Jafferany M. Psychopharmacology in dermatology: treatment of primary psychiatric conditions in dermatology. Dermatol Ther. 2020;33:e13557. https://doi.org/10.1111/dth.13557. Epub ahead of print. PMID: 32396243.

Psychotherapy in Hair Pathology 13

Ruta Barkauskaite

"Sorrow has no hierarchy. Suffering is not a sport.

There is no final ranking". (From character's speech, "The New Pope" series, episode 9, by P. Sorentino.)

Introduction

It is known that a large number of hair problems can have mental and psychosomatic causes. In this case, a purely biomedical principle of therapy does not justify itself and is a partial solution to a complex issue. An approach, which is based on the biopsychosocial paradigm of understanding these diseases with the integration of interdisciplinary methods of diagnostics and therapy, is needed.

The social significance of hair is an important clue in understanding the condition of a patient visiting both a trichologist and a psychotherapist. The psychological and social effects of hair loss can be devastating. Suffering of these patients is not related with the life-threatening or loss of health potential nature, but a loss of social potential, which determines the direction, opportunities, and quality of life.

Medical professionals caring for patients with hair diseases should focus on forming a therapeutic relationship based on partnership and trust, which will be used as the resource for joint work.

Another important message of this chapter, addressed not only to psychologists and psychotherapists, is the desire to inspire hope that psychological help is a real way out of the crisis for both patients and their relatives.

R. Barkauskaite (✉)
Faculty of Human and Social Studies, Institute of Psychology, Mykolas Romeris University, Vilnius, Lithuania

Y. Ovcharenko et al. (eds.), *Psychotrichology*,
https://doi.org/10.1007/978-3-031-64083-4_13

Psychology in Psychotrichology

It should be noted that it is the psychology of health that finds application in the field of health and disease, and that it has "absorbed" the most important achievements of psychosomatic medicine, behavioral medicine, and medical psychology, and that it studies the psychological aspects of diseases, among other things.

Since the 1970s, when Robert Ader pioneered psychoneuroimmunology, Western medicine has accepted that the mind and body are related and that this relationship causes them to be constantly interconnected via chemical substances and cellular receptors.

Since those observations, new data has been added every day, and science has provided new insight into what was previously a true dogma in allopathic medicine, which held that the cause of diseases is solely physical matter and could only be altered through material means. Energy, mind, and emotions were not taken into account in the onset or progression of disease, and even less so in healing and health.

A great deal of research and evidence that the mind and body are inseparable has led to a growing interest in new knowledge among doctors, broadening their vision and the resources they use in what is known as mind-body medicine, integrative medicine, or biopsychosocial medicine.

This concept takes into account the reality that most diseases are multifactorial, being formed by previous situations whose effects are accumulating in the body. The whole life history of the person gives indications of circumstances in which each one is exerting a certain role to culminate in some clinical picture.

Thus, gestational and birth conditions, previous illnesses, parents' lifestyle, family environment, physical environment in childhood, physical and emotional traumatic experiences in childhood, emotions felt as a result of how one was treated, traumatic experiences in adolescence, the moment of disease onset, worsening conditions in its evolution, the patients' tendency for positive or negative thoughts, family, social, sexual, financial conditions, and belief system are all unique factors for each person. These factors combine to make the disease a one-of-a-kind condition. And thereby, biological, psychological, emotional, social, and spiritual factors all contribute to the onset and progression of disease.

Trichology has recently become involved in this scientific advancement. Psychotrichology is a relatively new field of scientific research that investigates issues related to trichology, psychiatry, and psychology.

There are numerous hair-related disorders that are linked to psychological disorders, with some causing psychological disorders and others being caused by psychological disorders, creating a vicious cycle in which hair disorders worsen psychological disorders and vice versa. It is the subgroup of psychotrichological disorders that confirms the appropriateness of taking psychology into account when considering this issue.

However, paying attention to the psychological aspects of skin and hair care is not a new concept. In his writings, Hippocrates (460–377 BC) mentioned the relationship between stress and its effects on skin, describing people who tore their hair out in response to emotional stress [1]. Further attempts to address the effect of psychological factors on skin and hair diseases can be found in the works of several dermatologists, including Beard, Took, Buckley, and Winkler, around the turn of the nineteenth and twentieth centuries.

Today's research is centered not only on the development of new treatments, but also on the enhancement of functioning and coping with hair diseases. The study of patient quality of life is an important field of research that aims to identify the most problematic aspects of quality of life as well as the impact of individual factors (medical, psychological, demographic, etc.). It is well acknowledged that searching for a single cause of the disease and treating it alone is insufficient in the majority of cases, and that a holistic approach is required to address patient needs and achieve the best care for patients with hair disorders.

Social and cultural significance of hair is quite an interesting topic. Rituals associated with hair could highlight the exclusive position of a person in the social hierarchy, humiliate this person forever or give a spiritual status. The symbolism of hair is inexhaustible, and we will not find a single culture or subculture where hair would not be important for a person's social identity.

Nowadays, the role of hair has not diminished at all. Hair care rituals and meanings are evolving, but they continue to influence a person's social status. In today's world, a full head of hair is an ideal that defines a desirable member of society for both men and women.

Success, high social status, well-being, youth, health, and beauty are sought-after values. Everything that goes beyond the ideals is negatively perceived by the society, is stigmatized, and even may be downgraded to a "marginal" status.

Hair is only one of the body's defining characteristics, but nothing makes a person more vulnerable than changes or damage to the hair. Our "visiting card" is our face and hair. Any hair distortion can result in disfigurement and has social consequences, which can be severe. As a result, apparent or subjectively perceived hair loss is not a loss of a vital organ, but a loss of a part of social identity, which is accompanied by a chronic feeling of "failure to comply" with social appearance requirements, which provokes depressive feelings and changes a person's attitude toward self.

In light of the foregoing, psychotrichology should be regarded as a distinct field of modern medicine as well as a concept that applies to all trichology. When it includes the group of disorders classified as psychotrichological, it is considered a subspecialty. In a broader sense, the psychotrichological approach encompasses all hair diseases, as they can all have reflexes in people's moods and mental and emotional balance [2].

As a result, patient management necessitates a comprehensive psychotrichological approach. The trichologist must be prepared to identify mental and emotional states associated with hair diseases and to provide psychological support, starting with a highly effective physician–patient relationship, stress management, and even primary psychopharmacological and psychological treatments. However, in specific cases the trichologist will need the integration with professionals in psychology and psychiatry.

This collaboration between dermatologist and psychologist is critical when there is a predominant psychological event as the starting point of the hair disease or when a trichological condition has a damaging and unbalancing effect on the psyche. In these situations, a professional psychologist must perform a psychodiagnosis and provide effective treatment. In other situations, such as mental disorders accompanied by trichological symptoms or cases where hair disorders are accompanied by or result from anxiety, depression, hypochondria, delusions, and hallucinations, the trichologist must rely on the psychiatrist to provide the appropriate psychopharmacological management.

As a result, psychotrichology is a field that integrates three specialties without which it would be impossible to provide the patient with the necessary care. It should be added that the participation of psychology and psychiatry will not always result in the elimination of the disease. In many cases the objective is not a complete cure but the attention to the mental and emotional states that are part of the clinical picture. In these circumstances, the patient should be at least given resources to deal with the problem in a balanced and autonomous manner.

Life with Hair Problems: Psychosocial Processes

Individuals with hair diseases perceive their illness as a complex situation associated with many psychosocial problems, and it is this aspect that psychology studies. Chronic trichopathies, due to their progressive and recurrent nature, force patients to constantly adapt to changes in their appearance. So they learn to cope not only with deviations from their usual appearance, but also with a change in their bodily image. In turn, according to numerous scientific reports, the bodily image is closely related to self-esteem, which, as indicated above, is significantly lower in people suffering from psychotrichological diseases.

On the other hand, there is a common misconception that hair diseases do not pose a serious risk, as they are not associated with an immediate life threat and do not affect daily functioning. However, these diseases can cause embarrassment, curiosity, disgust, stigmatization, or even discrimination in those who surround patients with hair disorders. It's important to remember that in the past, any changes in appearance, particularly in the skin, were regarded as punishment for living a sinful life. In the Middle Ages, patients with psoriasis were considered possessed by the devil and were expelled from society or even burned at the stake. Even today, some people believe that scars, particularly those covered in hair, appear as a result of contacts with the devil (Devils or Witch mark) or wild animals.

In this regard, it is reasonable to assume that the negative perception of people suffering from dermatotrichological diseases stems, at least in part, from the belief that these people are directly responsible for their own disease.

It is also important to keep in mind that hair disease patients' psychosocial lives become more complicated, and that some conditions limit patient activity, make daily tasks more difficult, and make symptoms like insomnia, irritability, anxiety, and embarrassment worse.

The impact on social functioning entails, first and foremost, difficulties communicating with others, limitations on various activities (including sexual activity), limitations in visiting public places, and avoiding situations that involve exposing one's scalp.

Problems and difficulties with social functioning described above are caused by fear of becoming the object of close attention of others, embarrassment due to the skin and hair condition, or one's own "corruption". There are also problems with the performance at the workplace.

Chronic recurrent hair disorders contribute to a sense of loss of control and can lead to obsessive attention to hair condition, which can lead to compulsive grooming and cosmetic procedures. Furthermore, people suffering from hair diseases tend to blame themselves for their bad mood and inability to cope with difficulties, comparing their condition to diseases that pose a direct threat to life.

Chronic stress caused by a hair disease can manifest as a variety of mental disorders. Numerous studies show that mental disorders are much more common in dermatosis patients, both adults and children, than in the general population. It has been reported that 30–60% of patients with dermatological diseases exhibit symptoms of depressive and anxiety disorders, as well as delusional disorders or suicidal ideation and tendencies [3–6].

Picardi et al. [6] found a high prevalence of psychiatric disorders in dermatological outpatients: 25% in leukoderma, 26% in psoriasis, 32% in acne, 27% in parasitic infestations, 34% in urticaria group and the highest rate of 35% in patients with hair loss.

Among factors with modulating effect on mental disorders are the disease type, degree and severity of changes, their chronicity and duration, as well as sociodemographic variables.

Identity and Self-Image

Identity is a concept that encompasses both personal and social aspects of human life. Social identity asserts social definitions of individual's self-concept: gender, race, ethnicity, profession, job, marital status, etc. To achieve a certain social definition, such as "beauty," a society presents stereotypes, puts forward a hierarchy of requirements and expectations, creates specific levers of pressure and mechanisms of competition in order to let the "best" win. Individual's social identity is formed under the influence of a plethora of social requirements at any stage of life. The self-concept as an intrapsychic phenomenon in response to the environment is embedded in this picture. Self-awareness is formed in the individual's mental aspect and during the course of the individual's integral development through physical, psychological, and sociocultural factors. This is accompanied by both positive and negative feelings about oneself: awareness of oneself as "valuable" or "non valuable," perception of oneself as "normal" or "defective," and perception of oneself as attractive or repulsive. In general, all these create the "self-image" or "I-concept."

What Is Happening to Self-image, Identity, and Psychosocial Functioning in People with Alopecia?

According to studies, anyone who has experienced hair loss, whether partial or complete, has issues with both social and personal identity. Trichotillomania, alopecia areata, and androgenetic alopecia are among the most researched psychotrichological disorders from a psychological standpoint.

Trichotillomania. Self-destructive forms of hair loss are most commonly reported in children aged 7–13. The etiopathogenesis of trichotillomania is not fully understood, but symptoms frequently appear secondary to events that cause suffering, such as when parents argue or divorce, a change in school, the birth of a new sibling in the family, chronic illness, separation from loved ones or friends, loss of a loved one, friend, or pet, moving to another town or country, or other traumatic experiences. It is commonly reported in the medical literature that childhood emotional, physical, or sexual abuse can result in hair-pulling symptoms. However, in young children, the symptom may have another cause, such as when a child develops a bad habit while playing with hair.

Psychotrauma is widely regarded as one of the most important factors in the development of trichotillomania. Difficult, intense, and overwhelming experiences severely damage the child's ability to cope. These processes result in constant mental tension and anxiety. To escape the "inner hell," the child chooses a self-destructive form of relief: pulling out his or her hair. This behavior becomes more frequent and expansive over time, involving larger areas of the body. Hair-pulling becomes a depressing, compulsive (uncontrollable) action until "problem solving," i.e., avoiding difficult inner experiences, becomes a problem in and of itself. A vicious circle emerges: hair pulling action provides temporary relief, but hair bearing areas exposed by this action become a new source of anxiety, which is suppressed once more by hair pulling. Patients with trichotillomania describe hair pulling as pleasantly painful, especially when the scalp becomes irritated and inflamed as a result of repeated damage. Over time, this behavior develops into an addiction or obsession that is difficult to overcome.

According to psychological research, self-image and psychosocial functioning are affected the most in patients with trichotillomania. Due to hard experience and disfigurement, their self-esteem lowers, they can see themselves as "defective," "abnormal," their self-confidence gets affected.

It is very likely that the child, adolescent, or adult has been suffering from these oppressive feelings long before any symptoms appeared. When the hair-pulling becomes obvious, this obsessive behavior may cause additional aggravation. The suffering patients feel guilty and ashamed about their inability to stop, which worsens their poor self-perception and draws them further into a vicious cycle of misery. A rather typical behavior in trichotillomania is social isolation, which involves avoiding friends and social gatherings. Children and teenagers who have this problem at school may become targets of bullying. This can have an impact on academic learning and lead to apathy toward social interests and pursuits. Unresolved internal conflicts are likely to have an impact on psychological development and even self-identity in adulthood.

Alopecia Areata (AA). This disease is distinguished by its "out of nowhere" onset and the severity of partial or complete hair loss. Extensive hair loss can occur over a few days to several months and can be severe, resulting in extensive or total loss of scalp hair or even all body hair. More often than not, the scalp and body are covered with remaining hair, but when the foci of hair loss can no longer be hidden by the remaining hair, the person's appearance changes in a disfiguring way.

The psychological response is closely related to progressive hair loss. Psychotrauma, loss and despair, and psychological crisis are all documented experiences. Studies on the psychological state of AA patients frequently concentrate on the social component of one's subjective impression of one's appearance and reactions within a close and distant social environment, including cultural stereotypes, attitudes that cause mental frustration, and attitudes that have a negative impact on one's self-esteem. In evaluating this impact, it is important not to lose sight of the most significant psychological aspect in patients with AA.

If a person doubted his or her own attractiveness prior to a drastic change in appearance, doubts can turn into self-denial with baldness. In this case, triggers include not only integrated external attitudes or stereotyped assessments, but also a direct sense of self. And it is perceived as belonging to someone else, as "not me." Self-denial is a self-inflicted trauma, exacerbated in the worst case by the external environment. The severity and complexity of the trauma depends on the extent of the lost self-worth. The trauma of self-denial is the awareness and experience of alienation, strangeness, unfamiliarity of a new appearance for oneself. In other words, the new "package" cannot be identified with the person's inner self. The process of self-identification is disrupted: previous mechanisms are damaged and replaced with something barely acceptable, if not terrible. When AA patients talk about "turning into a beetle" (as in Kafka's "The Metamorphosis"), "becoming a Gollum" (as in J. R. R. Tolkien's works), or "becoming an alien," these are not figures of speech. It is a feeling of doom to live with oneself as with a stranger.

Such a picture does not represent all individual experience, but rather it is extreme manifestation during a crisis and reflects the most difficult period in the life of an AA patient. However, whether with or without professional assistance, an individual's self-perception may change on the path to self-acceptance. And there is a way out of this situation. The fixation of a "distorted" self-image for decades is possible, but there are cases when patients with alopecia completely change their lives, perceiving alopecia as a "school of life."

In patients with AA, psychosocial functioning may even be paralyzed for a time. A person with extensive hair loss has to look for means for masking one's appearance. And this is a separate science and practice, when patients spend years looking for ways to create a satisfactory appearance both for others and for themselves. The close and distant social environments can either complicate or facilitate this stage of identity reconstruction. It is exacerbated by other people's conversations, which are traumatic scenarios for someone with alopecia. There have been published descriptions of paranoid states in which a patient suffering from hair loss becomes almost obsessed with other people discussing his or her appearance. Mockery of appearance and rejection in a close environment constitute the most unfavorable situation.

The sufferer may not overcome the crisis, as a result of which mental disorders may develop.

Obviously, high level of anxiety and stress may lead to a decrease in productivity at work or study, multiplication of everyday problems, and worsening of social isolation. AA affects all areas of human life, sometimes leading to the loss of a job or close relationships. Like those suffering from trichotillomania, patients with AA may avoid public places and refuse social benefits.

Gender-Specific Aspects. Published data are limited in their ability to distinguish gender-specific aspects. The research suggests that men and women of young age perceive complete hair loss of AA differently. For women, hair with its social and personal values is woven into their understanding not only of their femininity, which is mostly identified with beauty, naturalness, but also into their self-perception as a human in general. In other words, baldness affects not only identity, but also self-perception. The words "monster," "egg," and "alien" are frequently used by women when discussing their experiences with alopecia. They either place the blame on themselves, feeling that it was somehow deserved for some of their behaviors or "wrong" actions, or they think that their body failed them as a result of being under a lot of stress. Men experience alopecia as something that "just happened" whereas women actively "got involved" in what had occurred.

The identity crisis in women is complicated by the absence of a generally accepted positive social image of "normality" associated with head and face hair loss. This can cause feelings of hopelessness and desperation; these negative feelings intensified by women's perception of reaction to their new look from others, especially in the closest environment. These women need support like air. However, things do not always turn out well. The path of overcoming the identity loss and accepting a new look can be hindered by the distress of loved ones. But this factor is not determinative.

Under these circumstances, women can still believe that their new look is "viable," that they are not "defective" in a truly human sense, and that they remain women even when they lose the societally recognized attributes of beauty. They may rediscover these values for themselves, or they may be trapped in their grief for the rest of their lives.

The works of prof. Thomas Cash are dedicated to men with alopecia. He emphasized that even male pattern baldness, common to everybody, does not go unnoticed for the men themselves. Postmodern society has given rise to a new attitude of men toward themselves. They care more about their look, which has become an important criterion for their social status and personal success. Both for women and men, appearance has become more valuable, and therefore, in the event of hair loss, men also lose "beauty," "attractiveness," and "health." Hair loss affects their social status and social power. In author's own study on the AA impact on the psycho-emotional sphere, male patients, regardless of social status, reported that they became more vulnerable in the eyes of their employers, subordinates, or business partners. They felt they were perceived as members of the fringe of punks or skinheads, or as people suffering from a serious illness.

Age-specific aspects. The experience of alopecia is perceived differently at different ages. Children present population the least studied from their own perspective due to natural limitations—lack of self-reflection and self-awareness. Children may feel rejected by others because of their appearance, but they do not perceive themselves as "ugly" or "alien," this assessment children get from others. Thus, child's self-image and self-assessment are completely dependent on the outside world: child's self-perception will be identical to the image perceived by family members, at kindergarten, school, by doctor, etc.

Teenagers have quite different experience of alopecia. At this stage of life, a person is already self-aware and capable to actively form self-image. Years of neurological, hormonal, somatic, and psychological development precede the completion of the stabilization process. Alopecia usually appears as a natural disaster during this period, which is full of changes for the teenagers themselves, and might lead to a psychological crisis. Self-rejection by a teenager, as well as rejection by peers or people in their close circle, increases the likelihood of psychotrauma.

Adolescents' major tasks, such as gaining recognition and approval from at least one peer; their first romantic relationships and awareness of self-attractiveness; academic success as proof of ability, talent, and social success, may become more complicated in this situation. In the worst-case scenario, a teenager with alopecia may become an outcast, a loner, abandon favorite activities, stop studying and going to school, and begin thinking about suicide.

Alopecia in adulthood has not been thoroughly studied; however, general trends indicate that the ability to tolerate hair loss increases with age, as life experience, the stability of social, professional, sexual, family, and other identities, as well as the stability of the created lifestyle, become resources for overcoming various crises, including alopecia. Despite this, baldness is a painful experience at any age.

The Impact of Hair Disease on Family Members

Hair diseases can disrupt the lives of entire families due to both treatment and medical condition limitations. This can result in disagreements, misunderstandings, and feelings of guilt. According to reports, some people with AA do not want to have children because they are afraid of hereditary transmission of the disease.

If the patient is a child, the medical condition has the greatest negative impact on family members. A parent of a child with severe alopecia may experience "parental grief," denial of the disease, shame and guilt, overprotection, focusing on the needs of the sick child while ignoring other children, or, in some cases, rejection and ignoring the sick child, depression, and fatigue.

For parents, their child's medical condition can be perceived as a loss of the so-called "normalcy," resulting in a shift in their own perception and concept of the family, with subsequent adjustments to roles, plans, and dreams, as well as the use of entirely new coping mechanisms.

Adaptation to Hair Disease

The fight against hair disease is largely dependent on cooperation with a physician and adherence to a medical treatment regimen. In this case, of major importance are psychological factors. Adaptation to alopecia, among other things, depends on its course, and this aspect, along with adaptation to the disease in general, is the study subject of health psychology. The disease may have progressive, episodic, or acute course. Progressive diseases develop in a predictable way (androgenetic alopecia). Patients know what to expect and they are ready for it. On the other hand, any deviation from the usual course of events can provoke great anxiety (available information about the disease is usually very superficial).

Chronic remitting diseases are distinguished by periods of worsening and improvement in health status. This creates uncertainty and requires the patient to adapt to changes in appearance.

The psychological and physiological adaptation to a disease is also affected by whether it is congenital or acquired. Patients with episodic acquired conditions must exert less adaptive effort. Long-term symptoms, on the other hand, necessitate a longer adaptation.

In the case of congenital alopecia or alopecia manifesting in early childhood, parents will have to deal with more significant problems with adaptation: The way they cope and their attitude toward the child can affect the success of the child's and their own adjustment. The reaction of parents determines the child's attitude to hair changes. When observing anxiety or helplessness in parents, the child, will more likely react in the same way. Parents who view their child's illness as a complex situation, a crisis from which there is no way out and which requires many sacrifices, transmit this perception of the physical condition to the child. In the future, this can lead to a refusal to fight the disease, a loss of faith in remission, and a decrease in motivation for hair care.

Reactions to torpid hair loss may include anger, feeling of helplessness, and blaming parents or other family members having same symptoms. Patients may perceive their state of health as a burden of fate through an unfortunate set of events. In this situation, the patient does not feel personal responsibility and blames no one. This attitude makes it easier to adapt to certain limitations, which are habitual inconveniences for the family.

In the case of acquired diseases, a person is forced to adjust to his or her "new" appearance, the reactions of others, and, in many cases, lifestyle changes. Patients with an unknown etiology may form their own assumptions about the disease's cause and progression, and develop a behavior pattern that gives them confidence that they can control their condition. Contrary to popular belief, people suffering from life-threatening diseases frequently prioritize their appearance, as in the case of temporary chemotherapy-induced hair loss in cancer patients.

A patient with a hair disease has to go through a period of psychological adaptation, allowing coming to terms with changes in patient's body. With massive hair loss and the onset of adulthood, the patient would be left in a state of mourning after losing their "normal" appearance. The patient's initial reaction is one of grief over the loss. Periods of shock, denial, anger, and sadness precede acceptance of one's illness.

Maintaining eye contact with the person commenting on the patient's appearance, quickly responding to a snarky remark, or redirecting the attacker's attention by shifting the conversation to another topic are all task-oriented ways of dealing with hair and skin disease. Emotional coping strategies encompass changing the way you think and perceive the situation that causes anxiety. Their effectiveness is context-dependent: when the patient is in control, task-oriented strategies will be more effective; in the absence of control, it is rational to choose emotional strategies.

According to Picardi et al. [7], people frequently attribute worsening health to stress, even when stress is not present in their lives. Problem exaggeration serves as the basis for justifying one's disease.

People with personality disorders, particularly those on the hysterical and narcissistic spectrums, have significant difficulties adapting to changes in body image because of their excessive focus on visual appeal, need for approval, and increased sensitivity to the opinions of others. Individuals suffering from borderline disorders see their dermatological condition as a major threat to their body image and independence [8].

Patient–Physician Relationships

Studies of patient–physician relationships show a general trend of fragmentation between evidence-based physician decisions and patient expectations. This fragmentation can lead to treatment discontinuation, so it is necessary to achieve compliance with therapy in accordance with patient's desires and needs. The patient is the active party of the treatment. No doubt, patients would have increased motivation to follow the treatment plan if they took part in its creation and understood the proposed alternatives and possible prognosis.

A recent study in AA patients on expectations from medical care showed that patients do not feel that doctors hear them, understand their condition, and take it seriously [9]. In the course of the author's study of the psychological state of patients caused by the psychosocial consequences of alopecia, respondents met with "insensitivity," "neglect," and lack of support. Patients claimed that doctors frequently trivialize the condition by saying things like, "It's just hair, you're healthy, rejoice," and "other health conditions might be worse, you're doing well."

The latest research confirms that physicians do not have necessary psychological knowledge to work with psychotrichological patients. Lack of competences and skills to determine patient's psychological state leads to sustaining the false hope, which forms nonadaptive strategies for overcoming the crisis. Patients might receive care for many years. The desire to grow hair again is natural in and of itself, but treatment objectives must be established along with an explanation of anticipated outcomes. Acceptance of oneself, with or without hair, encourages self-realization. When self-acceptance is not achieved, it is possible to fixate on the traumatic experience of “deformed, spoiled oneself,” with attempting to achieve hair regrowth being the way to “correct” oneself. Many patients have spent decades attempting to correct this “deformity” through medical means, despite the fact that only psychological assistance is required.

Information, Education, Referral

The information obtained from the doctor is crucial for the patient. The expectations of patients are centered on the body. It is important that they understand what happened to their bodies and what they can do about it. Keeping medical history records alone is insufficient; patients require detailed explanations and answers to their questions. They are hoping for reassurance and that the doctor has a solution. Situations in which doctors do not express their views on contentious or uncertain issues cause patients anxiety. Discussing the real situation, no matter how unpleasant, is preferable to “competent silence.”

According to research, physician–patient communication is closely related to the physician’s perception of the patient's emotional state. Because the doctor does not always have appropriate competency, patients frequently leave the doctor's office without advice on how to deal with their emotions. Professional assistance is required to improve a patient’s psychological state. This component is critical because trichological treatment will be ineffective in a patient experiencing a severe psychological crisis.

AA is not a widely discussed condition. A patient with this experience may not be aware that there are AA support groups. In some countries, there are reimbursement programs covering two wigs a year that can be advantageous for the patients. A physician has to convey this information to the patient. A patient who does not receive answers to questions cannot feel he or she is a part of the treatment process. Perhaps patient’s education, detailed explanation of the diagnosis, coordination of a treatment plan, and referral to related specialists take more time than a doctor can spare due to the limitations of actual medical setting. Being aware of this fact, it is necessary to find forms of communications through referral to related specialists who are ready to consult the patient.

Patient Management by Other Specialists: Pediatrician, Family Doctor, Hair Transplant Surgeon

A pediatrician seeing parents with a child with hair problems is required to determine who actually the patient in the office is. A child with AA, as a rule, does not suffer from alopecia the same way as his/her parents. A family psychotherapist is required to explain to parents the potential hazardous effects of their attitude toward their child’s problem and encourage them to change their emotional response if needed.

Physicians’ attitudes in relation to AA treatment in a child are very important. They can be “comforting” for parents, but do more harm than good specifically for the child.

Family doctor often acts as manager of such cases. Family doctor has all the means to inform the patient about related medical professionals involved in solving problems associated with alopecia. Since the family doctor may be the first person addressed, they are responsible for further referral. Before making a decision, for example, about a hair transplant, it is worth discussing a patient's visit to a trichologist. It is also worth seeking psychological help or attending a support group for people with alopecia. Psychologists successfully practicing in the field of psychotrichology are in great demand. Special training programs in psychotrichology for trichologists and psychologists have just begun to develop. Despite these limitations, decisions must be made here and now, which means using the available options.

Trichologists may recommend surgical hair transplantation in some cases. Certainly, there is a high level of ethical responsibility in this situation because it is related to the patient's financial means, but more importantly, with the hope of regaining lost appearance. The most important aspects of patient management are informing the patient about all options, risks, and prognosis. The surgeon should pay special attention to the patient's psychological state, which requires at least a basic understanding of psychotrichology. Intervention during a patient's acute mental state has been shown to be ineffective. As a result, consultations with a psychologist should be included in treatment planning.

Psychological Help for People with Hair Pathology

Psychopharmacological treatment is required in the management of severe mental disorders (for example, major depression, anxiety disorders, and so on) that develop in individuals suffering from torpid extensive or uncontrolled hair loss. Of course, psychiatry also deals with primary mental disorders associated with trichodermatological symptoms (e.g., trichotillomania, delusional dermatoses).

Psychotherapy in combination with psychotropic drugs also requires taking into account the typological characteristics of mental disorders.

Psychological care for people with hair pathology includes a variety of psychotherapeutic approaches, ranging from psychoanalysis to hypnosis, cognitive and behavioral therapy with educational methods, indirect suggestion elements, and relaxation techniques. Dealing with patients suffering from progressive hair loss and alopecia entails taking steps to assist them in coping with and adapting to their condition's difficulties and limitations. It's been shown that psychotherapeutic interventions have a beneficial effect on the disease course and promote remission.

However, existing data on the efficacy of psychotherapeutic approaches in this population of patients are based on case reports or small-scale uncontrolled studies.

Along with the technique's theoretical efficacy, it's crucial that the therapist is comfortable using the technique and is convinced of its effectiveness, and that patients have faith in their ability to heal. The effectiveness of contact and the therapeutic relationship between patient and physician are the most crucial factors for a successful healing process, according to scientific research.

The ability to connect with patients and create therapeutic relationships is something that can be learned over time with practice. More experience than theoretical knowledge is involved here. And these competencies are necessary for any specialist who wants to advance in their field of expertise.

Psychoanalysis leads to the release of repressed feelings, the understanding and awareness of real needs and desires, and a clear awareness of the differences between the real and imaginary worlds, among other things. One more task of psychoanalysis is to overcome a person's reluctance to describe their current state of health. Existing problems become less severe or disappear when they are verbally expressed. Spontaneous associations, clarification and confrontation, interpretation and processing are some of the therapeutic techniques used [10].

In some cases, such as chronic idiopathic telogen effluvium, hair disease can be an expression of emotional difficulties. The therapy aims to resolve developmental and psychological conflicts and shortcomings by focusing on the phenomena of transference and countertransference. Analysis, interpretation, and confrontation are the most commonly used methods. This type of therapy is especially beneficial when the disease is accompanied by personal issues caused by the patient's previous traumatic experience.

Empathy and understanding, as well as patience and long-term problem analysis, are extremely important for therapists. In this regard, psychoanalysis focuses on assessing the patient's current mental state and its underlying causes, as well as developing appropriate strategies to effectively promote positive change.

The psychodynamic approach is used in the treatment of anxiety, depression, and low self-esteem, which frequently accompany dermatological and hair-related medical conditions [11].

There are published reports on the use of hypnosis in the complex treatment of AA patients. Willemsen et al. (2008) reported data on 28 patients with extensive AA who were refractory to previous conventional treatment and were treated with a hypnotherapeutic approach that combined symptom-oriented suggestions to improve self-esteem. The authors reported that all patients experienced a significant reduction in anxiety and depression, and 12 patients experienced significant hair growth. This suggests that hypnosis can boost a person's immunity while also improving their psychological well-being.

The cognitive and behavioral approaches are increasingly used in individuals with compulsive disorders, and they teach coping with specific medical problems (e.g., pruritus) and restrictions through the introduction of principles of self-monitoring, reducing harmful habits, distracting attention from medical problems, changing convictions about the medical condition and one's own functioning, and teaching the healthy and functional ways of express emotions. All of this may help improve patients' quality of life ([12]; Fortune 2004*). The techniques proposed include questioning mistakes in thinking, "the worst-case scenario technique," monitoring thoughts, keeping a diary, stopping thoughts, distracting attention, relaxation, and memorizing the positive aspects of one's appearance

The goals of cognitive-behavioral intervention are as follows:

- The affected individual becoming aware and understanding their psychophysical condition;
- Identifying and naming the symptoms and difficulties experienced
- Acquiring knowledge of treatment options
- Facilitating decisions concerning the affected individual undergoing treatment
- Discussing difficulties in contacts with other people
- Analysis of difficulties related to the medical condition itself, and separation of those factors and behaviors that strengthen them
- Improvement in one's body image and self-esteem
- Becoming aware of erroneous beliefs about the medical condition and reformulating them
- Identifying and improving the effectiveness of previously used coping methods
- Identifying existing, but not yet utilized, resources that are to improve coping with the medical condition
- Becoming aware of practical ways of coping with difficult situations (e.g., being persistently stared at by other people) and applying them
- Becoming aware of psychological issues that are not directly related to the medical condition

The primary goal of this therapy is to educate the patient about the pattern of occurrence of disorders in hair diseases, in which visible changes and their consequences result in the development of maladaptive reactions.

Individuals suffering from dermatotrichological conditions may not realize they require psychotherapy at first. Their main problem is the condition of their hair, which they strive to improve. Most of the time, they only see a psychotherapist after pharmacological treatment has failed to produce the desired results and the somatic condition and/or emotional problems make daily functioning difficult. Given the complexity of issues related to medical conditions, comprehensive interdisciplinary care that includes treatment from a psychologist, psychiatrist, dermatologist, and nurse is required. Taking into consideration the complexity of problems associated with medical conditions, comprehensive interdisciplinary care is needed (by a psychologist, psychiatrist, dermatologist, and a nurse), along with the provision of information about the biological aspects of a particular disease and methods of its treatment, training in hair care, providing explanations about the role of stress, offering cognitive behavioral therapy, as well as training in relaxation techniques, identifying cognitive mistakes and improving adaptability, self-confidence, etc.

The significance of support groups for people with hair and skin diseases, participation in which can aid in overcoming the experience of social rejection, has been established. These groups allow people to share their experiences and meet other people who are affected. The purpose of support groups is to educate people about the medical condition and how to cope with it.

General Aspects of Alopecia Areata Psychotherapy

There is still much to learn about the etiopathogenesis of AA. A disease's pathogenesis is currently thought to involve a unique interaction of genetic, endogenous (mental and physical), and possibly exogenous factors. Even though some researchers classify AA as a psychosomatic disorder and a number of hypotheses regarding the emergence of mental disorders in pre-morbidity have been put forth, this does not explain the occurrence of the universal form of AA in a 9-month-old infant.

Some researchers proposed psychogenic causes of AA when the disease occurs after a traumatic experience such as the death of a loved one, divorce (of the patient or parents), and so on. However, it was demonstrated that such an experience cannot be attributed to all AA patients. As a result, when advancing theories about baldness as a possible complication of psychotrauma or mental processes, it is important to avoid taking a preconceived position and instead study the patient's actual experience. Life with alopecia undoubtedly causes an acute psychological reaction, and all psychotherapeutic steps should be based on dealing with the psychosocial consequences of AA.

Characteristics of the Alopecia Areata Psychological Crisis

A patient who experiences sudden, unexplained hair loss may "paralyze" and enter a psychological crisis. Crisis psychology techniques are helpful in this situation. A patient must simultaneously deal with numerous health-related issues, learn how to handle reactions from others, deal with their own distress, and deal with the practical aspects of regaining their appearance. Great anxiety results from losing control over situation. It is essential that the patients gain control as soon as possible and to the best of their ability.

Patient's expectations may be unrealistic until the patient is armed with sufficient knowledge of the condition. For example, it is important for the patient to understand that hair loss may be irreversible, that attempts at treatment are worthwhile, but do not give guarantees for hair regrowth, that relapse is possible.

A sudden change in a patient's appearance elicits an **emotional response** from the surrounding environment that can range from extreme care and empathy to rejection and neglect of the suffering patient. In some cases, patients hide their alopecia from loved ones, who are unaware that a "secret" exists. Others' imagined or real reactions, in one way or another, contribute to the present crisis. The way others perceive the patient, what feelings and reactions are elicited, can be a source of strength or a drama that aggravates the process of mourning and self-acceptance.

A **sense of self or identity** disorder manifests itself in the following questions: "who am I now?", "what kind of creature is this?", "how can this creature live on?", "what will happen to my future?", "I can't show this version of myself to anyone," "this is a terrible monster, scarecrow," "my life is over," and so on. In cases of severe abrupt hair loss, experiencing loss of self is a long process, but it is critical that therapists accept that when the patient speaks this way of themselves, it is not just an exacerbated interpretation. To those who have never experienced this condition, it may appear that a person exaggerates the significance of losing an organ so insignificant to survival.

However, it is the encounter with such an experience that reveals to a person the invisible and intangible structure of merciless social reality. The patient requires acceptance and understanding of their grief. An untimely confrontation of ideas can transform a sudden sense of doom into severe loneliness: "no one will understand me."

Another layer of crisis experiences associated with everyday functioning lies in matters of physical appearance. The bald or apparently bald person is totally confused as to how to "get oneself in order." Experience has shown that answers to these practical questions can be found in public organizations, support groups for people who have lived with similar conditions for years, have tried a lot of methods, and can give practical advice on how not to get lost in the ocean of services and goods offered on the market. It is worth referring the patient to these organizations.

Main Topics in Managing Patients with Hair Problems

The topic of **social identity** affects patients with both extensive and small-scale, but already noticeable to others, hair loss. In case of solving problems with appearance, it makes no difference which way the hair loss occurred. Studying patient's life circumstances will reveal not only the significance of hair loss, but also how much hair loss affects patient's life: whether there are problems in social and intimate relationships, and which ones specifically, whether baldness has an impact on professional activity.

Self-image and a more comprehensive sense of self are another aspect of identity. Feelings toward oneself and one's vision of oneself must be worked through. Although generalizations are not appropriate for various types of alopecia, the disfiguring effect of hair loss may be a common denominator. Patients may express a need to regain "normality" of appearance and again be "like everyone else" or not be dismissed as "not normal." The resolution of this internal conflict as a whole can determine the patient's quality of life in both slowly progressive hair loss such as androgenetic alopecia and acute hair loss such as AA and chemotherapy-induced alopecia.

It is not rare that the patient gets stuck in perceiving and feeling oneself as "defective," "in need of correction" or "faulty." This condition is classified as a **body dysmorphic disorder** secondary to hair disease. The main diagnostic criterion for this condition is the presence of significant loss of scalp or facial hair, resulting in a visible disfigurement that elicits a genuine reaction from others. This differs from primary body dysmorphic disorder in that the patient has a primary mental disorder, whereas body dysmorphia develops as a result of an emphasis on minor signs of appearance with an exaggerated system of fantasies regarding the patient's perception. A thorough psychotherapeutic diagnosis and deconstruction of the patient's experience are required to understand the origins of body dysmorphic disorder in a specific patient. Sudden changes in a person's appearance, such as those seen in the universal form of AA, can be extremely traumatic. In this case, self-denial is a violent but natural reaction to oneself, often fueled by real rejection rather than fantasies about how others perceive you. Thus, differential diagnosis is critical for comprehending psychological processes and devising a therapeutic strategy.

Images of people with alopecia, with whom they are sometimes jokingly identified, are of particular interest. The evolutionary idea that "everyone will eventually go bald" and that they are "a new race" becomes popular among AA patients. Because alien beings are generally thought to be more advanced, the image of "alien" includes both "alienness" on the one hand and "unusualness," "peculiarity" on the other. These images are thought to be reflections of the same social pursuit of ideals as in the presence of hair. These images are comforting and create a sense of exclusivity, but becoming engrossed in them is dangerous because they focus on appearance. In any case, this critical aspect is vulnerable. To what extent does this attitude toward oneself as an "alien" describe the person realistically for themselves or others, reducing everything to mere appearance? What happened to the rest? According to the author's experience and the experiences of several "alopecia survivors," it is necessary to find, acquire, and develop human qualities: talents and abilities, in order to develop a new, positive self-identity. In this case, the emphasis shifts from physical appearance, which, without a doubt, must be corrected in accordance with one's ideals, to other factors such as family, work, profession, achievements, and simply living.

There are certainly occupations and lifestyles where physical attractiveness is simply required. Work with the external image should be permanent in this situation. An illustration would be a woman with alopecia who, while working as a character guide, switches out five wigs and headpieces in a week. She realizes she doesn't need a single, constant self-perception because she is "anyone," "one of many," and "different," and she does this by switching between various images.

The most difficult process is resolving the patient's conflict with oneself, because mental self-perception is inextricably linked with perception of the surrounding world. If relatives, for example, find it difficult to accept changes, they may feel ashamed or "make amends" by engaging in different behaviors. This "resistance and rejection" on their part can cost the person experiencing hair loss dearly. External acceptance, support, and reinforcement encourages the patient's self-acceptance.

The therapist must maintain a neutral attitude toward the patient's appearance. In cases of AA, the dynamics of the hair disease itself, with regrowth and relapses, can make it a permanent event in the patient's life. The "fight of faith" for hair growth does not have the same therapeutic effect as avoiding emphasis on appearance and accepting oneself and one's life in disease dynamics.

Examples of positive images are important when working with patients who have a negative self-image. The search is complicated by the fact that baldness is stigmatized in social life, and a positive image is not offered. There are two options. One option is to openly live with partial or complete baldness and become a positive social model, filling the positive image niche. Acceptance of change, as well as sufficient resistance to social pressure associated with physical appearance, are required elements. As history has shown, this position elicits a positive social reaction.

But if a person is not planning to live in solitude or rebel against the rules and stereotypes of society, he or she will be forced to adapt and resort to disguise. These choices are individual: a solution for one person may be a problem for another. The task of therapy is to help the patient make the choice and comprehend it.

Hypnotherapy, group therapy, as well as support groups, helping others suffering from hair loss are already proven their efficacy for the patient. The group can become a safe haven for finding new values, information, and acceptance.

Self-Identity Using the Camouflage

Today, there are different services and products available for people with hair problems. Only 20 years ago, a woman with hair loss had difficulty finding a wig, and now she is lost in the plethora of procedures to simulate scalp hair, as well as hair prostheses.

It is well-known that men have more difficulty camouflaging than women due to cultural norms. Men who have lost some or all of their hair are much less likely to choose cosmetic brow and eyelash shaping (trichopigmentation). The usual headgear, glasses, a hood, or cap is more popular. As a result, when confronted with social pressure, men must navigate the "open battlefield" of self-identity. In contrast to male pattern baldness, the "impersonality" of the face without brows and eyelashes is not regarded as a social norm.

As a rule, for women who have lost their hair, beauty care is often forced and expensive. And this is another possible obstacle in the process of forming a stable self-identity. An unnatural looking wig can make things worse: an attempt to mask the absence of hair with a low-quality product only makes it more evident—unravels the most terrible "secret." The risk of exposing this secret can cause constant anxiety and fear in social communications. The more natural looking and higher the quality of the product that creates a new image, the more protection it gives a woman. But does it bring closer to solving the problem?

Hair systems that are securely attached to the head and provide complete freedom of movement, a sense of social security, and natural beauty have the potential to put an end to this epic of suffering. But we have our doubts when we see the emotional pain in the eyes of a young girl who should be happy with a hair system on her head. Unfortunately, even the best prosthesis will not heal mental wounds. A genuine restoration of a positive self-image is impossible without accepting the loss of one's former self and gaining a new, changed self. Of course, a well-designed appearance can provide the necessary support in daily life, while psychological trauma can be treated.

Gender identity in hair diseases is another facet of the general identity problem, with its own gender specificity.

Research confirms that alopecia has a crushing effect for the female femininity. Social stereotypes of beauty, health, attractiveness, sexuality, and naturalness get destroyed. In this case, the rehabilitation of all areas of functioning is the task of the psychotherapist. Of importance is a realistic confrontation of ideas associated with rigid stereotyped concepts, and the search for others with a sensitive attitude to painful feelings. As mentioned above, there is a risk of trivialization of experiences, for example, "sexuality is not inherent in hair at all," "let's take a bunch of examples from life." And yet it is amazing how great is the significance of this part of the human body, which does not affect the vital functions. However, a woman is experiencing a real loss of this significance, and it is very important to wait until she is ready to accept the relative damage of alopecia in the physical sense or to see the beauty of her head without hair, dare, with the help of a therapist, to accept her unusual, exotic appearance, but most importantly—vitality. The topic of physical attractiveness and sexuality is very interesting, and the therapist should be prepared to deal with these issues, keeping in mind the gender difference/match between the therapist and the patient. What is the essence of attractiveness and sexuality is a universal question that must be answered individually. It is critical to help the patient understand that the hair is only a part of the entire picture.

The condition of men with androgenetic alopecia (AGA) is better researched than any other. Although male baldness is a common occurrence, for the man himself, this issue may not be so simple. The problem will be deemed serious if a patient seeks help of a psychotherapist. We can foresee in advance what of personal experience lies behind such a seemingly "insignificant" detail of appearance. Studies report AGA-associated suicidal ideation in men. It is known that in alopecia gender identity is affected in women as well as in men. Psychological problems are more characteristic for young men, since hair loss is perceived as a marker of "aging," which for a man means loss of strength, youth, and associated opportunities. Just like in women, it is related to issues of attractiveness and sexuality. Therefore, the goal of therapy is to explore patient's real resources, expand their understanding of these resources, and shift the emphasis from appearance to more durable and long-term aspects. Nevertheless, appearance itself remains an important issue, the solution of which requires the search for aesthetic means congruent with the image of oneself.

A Message for Patients and Their Relatives

The first thing that should be said: alopecia is not a sentence. Indeed, it turns life upside down, and a person facing with alopecia will never be the same again. But where the past life ends, a new one begins. It is still unknown, but it is worth taking a step—and it becomes clear.

"Alopecia survivor" is the name for those who went through this experience and regained what was lost: beauty, health, femininity, masculinity, attractiveness, sexuality. It is amazing for how many people this experience became the revelation. They were "stripped naked," stripped of social simulacra, and put face to face with exposed reality. This meeting will not be forgotten even after the hair grows back.

Alopecia is a spiritual school. You learn to walk again, breathe again, your molecules are rearranged, and you go through nine circles of transformation. You can't buy anything like this anywhere, this cannot be learned from the most advanced spiritual master. Harsh, but cool and useful.

It is critical to allow yourself time for each stage: to suffer, to allow the pain to subside, to not close in on yourself, but to go through the pain. With or without assistance, but preferably with assistance. Find books, movies, people, or any images you can hold onto. The most difficult to bear is pain that turns into anger. Accepting this blow humbly is extremely difficult... You do not want to be treated in this manner. You want things to be the same as they were before. But reality is cruel. And it is preferable to engage in constructive dialogue rather than engage in a fight.

It is worthwhile to reclaim oneself as a person with whom one desires to live, rather than to escape and hate. Happiness isn't as important as inner peace and harmony. This is frequently perceived as a defeat: if I accept myself as I am, I will bury my belief that I can return to the past; I cannot give up. For a while, hiding your head in the sand works. Humbleness does not eliminate the possibility of hair growth. On the contrary, inner peace and harmony relieve anxiety, tension, feelings of guilt and shame, and the pain of loss. This is the best "soil" for hair follicle restoration.

Furthermore, the family is in distress. The same shock, confusion, impotence to do anything, to prevent, to help. Often the first healthy reaction of a family is to see a doctor. This is a mandatory step, because a timely diagnosis can define the course of the disease. If the disease in a child is difficult to treat, progresses to a state of complete hair loss, it is important to change your attitude. Attitude of the whole family.

The hardest thing is when the child says to parents: "I will take money from you if you want me to visit another doctor" (a real story), still the parents keep tirelessly looking for a specialist for years. Seeking help is normal, but then again, why is this being done after many fruitless atempts? Are parents ashamed of their child, do they need to "fix" their child? If a neighbor drop by, will they be hiding their child under a scarf or a wig or in another room? It's scary for the future of a child without hair, especially a girl, so it's better to let her stay in her parents' house for life? Is the parents' guilt so limitless that they are willing to sacrifice child's life's goals for the sake of hair? Chasing for the child's "happiness" might leave the child alone in own darkness. In cases of bullying child might get traumatised therefore it is crucialy important that parents and/or relatives do their best and talk to their child, talk themselves out in the therapy or parent's support group. Also, focusing on child's life, development, goals is far more productive direction rather then giving the child a constant idea that he or she must be treated at all cost. It takes time and effort to heal from the grief: open up to the emotional crisis in family members, accepting the reality of hair problem, overcoming the social stereotypes, reframing the concepts of normality, beauty, femininity or masculinity, and much more. Nothing helps a child, teenager, or adult better than accepting alopecia by the closest ones. There is a way out of the crisis.

Summary

- Numerous life aspects of patients suffering from hair diseases have recently become the subject of interest in psychology. This applies both to causes of numerous trichopathies and factors that aggravate their course and affect treatment.
- Moreover, of extreme importance for this group of diseases is the impact on patient's social life.
- Helping psychotrichological patients involves joint efforts of trichologists, psychiatrists, and psychologists.
- The absence of this care for patients reduces the dermatological consultations to attempts to repair the effects without seeking causes, making patients captive attendants of the services without offering a perspective of solution.
- In psychological practice, it is recommended to introduce programs aimed at improving the functioning of patients and increasing the efficiency of their adaptation to the existing condition, as well as the creation of support groups.

References

1. Rodriguez-Cerdeira C, Pera-Grasa J, Molares A, Isa-Isa R, Arenas-Guzmin R. Psychodermatology: past, present and future. Open Dermatol J. 2011;5:21–7.
2. Ovcharenko Y. Serbina I. Psychotricological approach in the management of patients with hair disorders. In: Abstract book EHRS 2023, Sheffeld, United Kingdom; p.
3. Gieler U. Psyche and skin: what's new? J Eur Acad Dermatol Venereol. 2003;17:128–30.
4. Gupta MA, Gupta AK. Psychiatric and psychological co-morbidity in patients with dermatologic disorders. Am J Clin Dermatol. 2003;4:833–42.
5. Makowska I, Gmitrowicz A. Psychodermatology—the interface between dermatology, psychiatry and psychology. Psychiatria i Psychologia Kliniczna. 2014;14:100–5.
6. Picardi A, Abeni D, Melchi CF, Puddu P, Pasquini P. Psychiatric morbidity in dermatological outpatients: an issue to be recognized. Br J Dermatol. 2000;143:983–91.
7. Picardi A, Abeni D, Renzi C, Braga M, Melchi CF, Pasquini P. Treatment outcome and incidence of psychiatric disorders in dermatological out-patients. J Eur Acad Dermatol Venereol. 2003;17:155–9.
8. Ginsburg IH. The psychosocial impact of skin disease. An overview. Dermatol Clin. 1996;14:473–83.
9. de Vere HI, McNiven A, McPherson T. A qualitative exploration of the experiences of adolescents with alopecia areata and their messages for healthcare professionals. Br J Dermatol. 2021;184(3):557–9.
10. Januszewski A. Fundamentals and characteristic elements of psychoanalytic therapy for skin diseases. In: Szewczyk L, Kulik A, editors. Selected issues in clinical and personality psychology. Lublin: TN KUL; 2001. p. 97–117.
11. Miniszewska J. Psychodermatology from the perspective of a psychologist. Health Psychol Rep. 2015;3(4):269–80.
12. Fortune D, Richards H, Kirby B, Bowcock S, Main C, Griffits C. A cognitive-behavioral symptom management programme as an adjunct in psoriasis therapy. Br J Dermatol. 2002;146:458–65.

Final Comments

The pathophysiology of hair diseases is extremely complex, including many factors and signaling pathways. Hormones, the "brain-hair follicle" axis and the "environment-hair follicle" axis affect the hair follicle, opposing its regulatory circuits, and in the absence of strategies to counter this attack, they can eventually block the internal mechanisms of follicle control. The result is a harmful self-sustaining inflammatory cascade as the new status quo. Restoring hair follicles to a state of homeostasis requires a different approach to therapy.

The concepts of suppressing and correcting the adverse effects of psycho-emotional stress on hair growth, which are the basis of the chain of molecular pathogenesis, offer useful pharmacotherapeutic support that allows patients with hair loss to break out of the depressive psycho- and socio-dynamic vicious circles of the disease. However, most modern treatment methods are focused on separate goals. A paradigm shift in the treatment of hair diseases from mono-target to multi-target therapeutic approaches is necessary, and the development of an individual route for each patient must take into account the phenotype, pathobiology, clinical phenomenology, somatic comorbidity, and psychostatus.

This strategy suggests the principle of treatment of psychotrichological disorders based on a polyprofessional approach combining trichotropic treatment with psychopharmacotherapy supplemented with psychocorrective effects (cognitive-behavioral psychotherapy with the inclusion of educational methods, elements of indirect suggestion, and relaxation techniques).

Psychotrichology basically follows the principles of psychosomatic medicine in the implementation of a complex biopsychosocial approach to the patient, taking into account the interaction and mutual influence of the psychic and somatic in normal and pathological conditions.

As a scientific and practical direction, psychotrichology is a modern concept of health care that takes into account complex psychosomatic and somatopsychic interactions, as well as the interaction of an individual with social environment during the onset, course and treatment of diseases, and uses the knowledge gained in the prevention and treatment of psychotrichological disorders. This means that psychotrichology is focused on the study of relationships between the personal

Y. Ovcharenko et al. (eds.), *Psychotrichology*, https://doi.org/10.1007/978-3-031-64083-4

psychological characteristics of individuals, present hair pathology, and developed mental disorders.

These circumstances dictate the features of medical management of psychotrichological patients, which involves interdisciplinary interaction of dermatotrichologists, psychiatrists, psychologists, and general practitioners.

Summarizing, psychotrichology may be regarded as a branch of clinical and experimental medicine, within the framework of which coexisting trichopathies and functional mental disorders are considered, in the occurrence and course of which psychosocial factors play a significant role. The data of studies and clinical observations not only convincingly confirm the significant importance in the development and course of hair diseases many of psychosomatic and somatopsychic mutual influence, but also bring us closer to the knowledge of the complex patterns underlying them.

Index

Y. Ovcharenko et al. (eds.), *Psychotrichology*, https://doi.org/10.1007/978-3-031-64083-4

GPSR Compliance

The European Union's (EU) General Product Safety Regulation (GPSR) is a set of rules that requires consumer products to be safe and our obligations to ensure this.

If you have any concerns about our products, you can contact us on ProductSafety@springernature.com

In case Publisher is established outside the EU, the EU authorized representative is:

Springer Nature Customer Service Center GmbH
Europaplatz 3
69115 Heidelberg, Germany

Batch number: 09013545

Printed by Printforce, the Netherlands